Recent Research on Human Papillomavirus (HPV) Infection and Vaccination

Recent Research on Human Papillomavirus (HPV) Infection and Vaccination

Guest Editors

Li Shi
Yufeng Yao

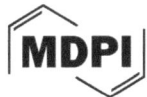

Basel • Beijing • Wuhan • Barcelona • Belgrade • Novi Sad • Cluj • Manchester

Guest Editors

Li Shi
Institute of Medical Biology
Chinese Academy of Medical
Science and Peking Union
Medical College
Kunming
China

Yufeng Yao
Institute of Medical Biology
Chinese Academy of Medical
Sciences and Peking Union
Medical College
Kunming
China

Editorial Office
MDPI AG
Grosspeteranlage 5
4052 Basel, Switzerland

This is a reprint of the Special Issue, published open access by the journal *Vaccines* (ISSN 2076-393X), freely accessible at: https://www.mdpi.com/journal/vaccines/special_issues/4F60P5B77K.

For citation purposes, cite each article independently as indicated on the article page online and as indicated below:

Lastname, A.A.; Lastname, B.B. Article Title. *Journal Name* **Year**, *Volume Number*, Page Range.

ISBN 978-3-7258-3863-9 (Hbk)
ISBN 978-3-7258-3864-6 (PDF)
https://doi.org/10.3390/books978-3-7258-3864-6

© 2025 by the authors. Articles in this book are Open Access and distributed under the Creative Commons Attribution (CC BY) license. The book as a whole is distributed by MDPI under the terms and conditions of the Creative Commons Attribution-NonCommercial-NoDerivs (CC BY-NC-ND) license (https://creativecommons.org/licenses/by-nc-nd/4.0/).

Contents

Danhong Song, Peiyi Liu, Dadong Wu, Fanghui Zhao, Yueyun Wang and Yong Zhang
Knowledge and Attitudes towards Human Papillomavirus Vaccination (HPV) among Healthcare Providers Involved in the Governmental Free HPV Vaccination Program in Shenzhen, Southern China
Reprinted from: *Vaccines* **2023**, *11*, 997, https://doi.org/10.3390/vaccines11050997 1

Dominik Pruski, Sonja Millert-Kalińska, Jan Haraj, Sandra Dachowska, Robert Jach, et al.
Knowledge of HPV and HPV Vaccination among Polish Students from Medical and Non-Medical Universities
Reprinted from: *Vaccines* **2023**, *11*, 1850, https://doi.org/10.3390/vaccines11121850 15

Jihye Choi, Efrat K. Gabay and Paula M. Cuccaro
School Teachers' Perceptions of Adolescent Human Papillomavirus (HPV) Vaccination: A Systematic Review
Reprinted from: *Vaccines* **2024**, *12*, 361, https://doi.org/10.3390/vaccines12040361 25

Julie H. T. Dang, Alexandra Gori, Lucy Rios, Angelica M. Rolon, Jingwen Zhang and Moon S. Chen, Jr.
"You Don't Know If It's the Truth or a Lie": Exploring Human Papillomavirus (HPV) Vaccine Hesitancy among Communities with Low HPV Vaccine Uptake in Northern California
Reprinted from: *Vaccines* **2024**, *12*, 372, https://doi.org/10.3390/vaccines12040372 42

Gbadebo Collins Adeyanju, Tene-Alima Essoh, Annick Raissa Sidibe, Furaha Kyesi and Muyi Aina
Human Papillomavirus Vaccination Acceleration and Introduction in Sub-Saharan Africa: A Multi-Country Cohort Analysis
Reprinted from: *Vaccines* **2024**, *12*, 489, https://doi.org/10.3390/vaccines12050489 57

Lara S. Savas, Ross Shegog, Erica L. Frost, C. Mary Healy, Dale S. Mantey, Sharon P. Coan, et al.
Effect of an HPV Vaccination Multi-Level, Multi-Component Program on HPV Vaccination Initiation and Completion in a Pediatric Clinic Network
Reprinted from: *Vaccines* **2024**, *12*, 510, https://doi.org/10.3390/vaccines12050510 74

Mirjana Štrbac, Milko Joksimović, Vladimir Vuković, Mioljub Ristić, Goranka Lončarević, Milena Kanazir, et al.
Overview of the Implementation of the First Year of Immunization against Human Papillomavirus across Different Administrative Units in Serbia and Montenegro
Reprinted from: *Vaccines* **2024**, *12*, 803, https://doi.org/10.3390/vaccines12070803 91

Jordan Jacobs, Eugene Chon and Karl Kingsley
Longitudinal Screening for Oral High-Risk Non-HPV16 and Non-HPV18 Strains of Human Papillomavirus Reveals Increasing Prevalence among Adult and Pediatric Biorepository Samples: A Pilot Study
Reprinted from: *Vaccines* **2024**, *12*, 895, https://doi.org/10.3390/vaccines12080895 105

Ni Guo, Zhixin Niu, Zhiling Yan, Weipeng Liu, Lei Shi, Chuanyin Li, et al.
Immunoinformatics Design and In Vivo Immunogenicity Evaluation of a Conserved CTL Multi-Epitope Vaccine Targeting HPV16 E5, E6, and E7 Proteins
Reprinted from: *Vaccines* **2024**, *12*, 392, https://doi.org/10.3390/vaccines12040392 119

Molly R. Braun, Anne C. Moore, Jonathan D. Lindbloom, Katherine A. Hodgson, Emery G. Dora and Sean N. Tucker
Elimination of Human Papillomavirus 16-Positive Tumors by a Mucosal rAd5 Therapeutic Vaccination in a Pre-Clinical Murine Study
Reprinted from: *Vaccines* **2024**, *12*, 955, https://doi.org/10.3390/vaccines12090955 . . . . **135**

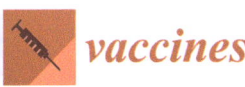

Article

Knowledge and Attitudes towards Human Papillomavirus Vaccination (HPV) among Healthcare Providers Involved in the Governmental Free HPV Vaccination Program in Shenzhen, Southern China

Danhong Song [1], Peiyi Liu [2], Dadong Wu [2], Fanghui Zhao [1], Yueyun Wang [2,*] and Yong Zhang [1,*]

[1] National Cancer Center/National Clinical Research Center for Cancer/Cancer Hospital, Chinese Academy of Medical Sciences, Peking Union Medical College, Beijing 100021, China; songdh@student.pumc.edu.cn (D.S.)
[2] Affiliated Shenzhen Maternity & Child Healthcare Hospital, Southern Medical University, Shenzhen 518000, China
* Correspondence: wangyueyun@126.com (Y.W.); zhangyong@cicams.ac.cn (Y.Z.)

Abstract: No research has been conducted to explore the variables associated with healthcare providers' (HCPs) knowledge and attitudes toward the human papillomavirus vaccine (HPV) since the vaccine was approved for free use in some Chinese cities. In Shenzhen, southern China, a convenience sample strategy was used to distribute questionnaires to HCPs involved in the government's HPV vaccination program from Shenzhen. There were 828 questionnaires collected in total, with 770 used in the analysis. The mean HPV and HPV vaccine knowledge score was 12.0 among HCPs involved in the government HPV vaccination program (with a total score of 15). the average scores for HPV and HPV vaccine knowledge varied among different types of medical institutions. District hospitals had the highest mean score of 12.4, while private hospitals ranked fourth with a mean score of 10.9. Multivariate logistic regression results revealed significant disparities in the type of license and after-tax annual income across HCPs ($p < 0.05$). The future education and training for HCPs should focus on private community health centers (CHCs), HCPs whose license type is other than a doctor, and HCPs with low after-tax annual income.

Keywords: HPV vaccine; healthcare provider; knowledge; recommend; influencing factor

1. Introduction

Cervical cancer is the only cancer with a known cause that is both preventable and treatable, yet it is the world's fourth most common gynecologic cancer, with a significant disease burden in China [1,2]. In 2020, there were 119,300 new cases of cervical cancer and 37,200 deaths, placing the country sixth and seventh in terms of cancer incidence and mortality among Chinese women [2]. In China, the incidence and mortality rates of cervical cancer have increased by varying degrees over the past 20 years [2], and the average age of onset has decreased [3]. Human papillomavirus (HPV) is one of the most common sexually transmitted infections worldwide. High-risk types of HPV are associated with various types of cancer, such as cervical cancer, other anogenital cancers (including penile, vaginal, vulvar, and anal cancers), head and neck cancers (including oral cavity, oropharynx, and larynx cancers), as well as benign warts [4]. The human papillomavirus is responsible for more than 90% of cervical cancer incidences [5]. Clinical studies have demonstrated that HPV vaccines are effective in preventing HPV-related illnesses and reducing the burden of related diseases [6–9]. Since its introduction in 2006, the HPV vaccine has been gradually implemented in numerous countries. In November 2020, the World Health Organization announced a "Global strategy to accelerate the elimination of cervical cancer as a public health problem", which included one of the three mid-term strategic objective values for 2030, which aimed for 90% of girls to complete HPV vaccination by the age

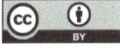

of 15, achieving primary prevention against HPV infection [10]. As of August 2021, 114 (59%) out of the 194 Members States of the World Health Organization have included HPV vaccination in their national immunization plans [11]. In 2016, China licensed the first HPV vaccinations. However, due to the late adoption of HPV vaccination in China, the government has been gradually implementing a trial program that provides free HPV vaccinations to local governments. At present, the vaccine has not yet been included in the National Immunization Program (NIP). Studies have shown that the cumulative estimated HPV vaccination rate in the female population aged 9–45 in China is only 2.24%, which is relatively low [12]. Awareness and attitudes about the HPV vaccine are not encouraging [13–15]. According to a recent school-based nationwide study in China, only 17.1% of adolescents had knowledge of the HPV vaccine [14]. Healthcare provider (HCPs) recommendations are a significant factor that motivates the general population and parents to vaccinate their children against HPV [16–19]. Additionally, knowledge of HPV-related issues is a crucial predictor of HCP confidence and a willingness to recommend HPV vaccines [20–22]. Previous studies have also identified various factors that impact HCPs' knowledge of HPV and HPV vaccines, including their profession, type of license, age, education level, and job title [23,24]. As Shenzhen is one of the pilot cities for free HPV vaccination, it is essential to assess whether the HCPs participating in the program have the necessary knowledge and willingness to recommend HPV vaccines to school girls.

We conducted a survey of HCPs involved in the free HPV vaccination program for schoolgirls in Shenzhen to describe their current state overall, as well as their knowledge and attitudes toward the HPV vaccine. The survey also aimed to assess the factors that may impact their knowledge and recommended behaviors regarding the vaccine.

2. Methods

2.1. Study Design and Participants

A cross-sectional study on HPV vaccine knowledge and attitudes among HCPs in Shenzhen was conducted between June 2022 and November 2022. Convenience sampling was used to cover all districts in Shenzhen. The inclusion criteria for the study population included HCPs involved in the governmental free HPV vaccination program in Shenzhen who voluntarily participated in the survey. The exclusion criterion was a refusal to participate in the questionnaire. The survey for this study was collected by sending electronic questionnaires to HCPs who attended training for the free HPV vaccination program in Shenzhen.

2.2. Data Collection and Questionnaire

The Chinese online survey application "Questionnaire Star" (https://www.wjx.cn/ (accessed on 1 April 2023)) was utilized to collect the data for this study. Respondents were directed to complete the electronic questionnaire by scanning a QR code or clicking on the link generated by the "Questionnaire Star". The questionnaire was devised through a collaborative process involving epidemiologists and (HCPs), utilizing the previous literature and extensive discussions. To ensure its validity and effectiveness, the questionnaire was initially tested on a group of 90 HCPs, and adjustments were made to the content and language based on their feedback. The questionnaire was ultimately divided into three sections to cover different aspects of HPV awareness and knowledge. The questionnaire mainly consisted of the following three parts: (1) Socio-demographic data such as age, gender, degree of education, marital status, and income level. (2) Knowledge of HPV and HPV vaccines, such as HPV transmission channels, HPV transmission targets, HPV infection symptoms, and the best time for HPV vaccination. (3) Behavior for recommending HPV vaccination. To calculate the knowledge score, the questionnaire was assigned one point for each correct answer and no points for each incorrect answer. The questionnaire was administered electronically, and it was sent to project training sessions and working groups related to the free HPV vaccination program for schoolgirls in Shenzhen.

2.3. Statistical Analysis

HCPs involved in the governmental HPV vaccination program were classified into four groups based on their medical institution and type of employment: Level I/Regional community health center (CHC), Level II CHC, Private CHC, and District Hospitals. The HCPs mainly included obstetricians, gynecologists, general practitioners, public health doctors, and nurses. Chi-square tests were used to compare sociodemographic information between the subgroups, while Kruskal–Wallis H tests and Kruskal–Wallis 1-way ANOVA (k samples) were used to compare knowledge levels. To investigate the characteristics associated with levels of HPV vaccine knowledge, dichotomous logistic regression and multi-variable logistic regression were used(including age, gender, education level, marital status, major, type of license, job title, employment type, after-tax annual income, years of work, and medical institution type). The Mann–Whitney U test was used to compare disparities in the HPV and HPV vaccine knowledge scores among healthcare professionals who recommended the HPV vaccine and those who did not make such recommendations. The Odds Ratio (OR), 95% confidence interval (CI), and p-value were determined. Two-tail tests were considered statistically significant if their p-values were less than 0.05. SPSS 26.0 (Armonk, NY, USA) was performed for analysis.

3. Results

3.1. Demographic Characteristics

In total, 828 questionnaires were collected for the study. However, 58 of these questionnaires had missing information or logical errors and were, therefore, excluded from the analysis. The final analysis included 770 records (with a usability rate of 93.0%). Table 1 shows the respondents' socio-demographic characteristics. The majority of respondents in Level I/Regional CHC (42.3%, n = 115), Level II CHC (41.6%, n = 128) and Private CHC (22.0%, n = 20) were between the ages of 31 and 40. The female respondents' population was extremely high (94.1%). HCPs from various healthcare institutions differed significantly in age, gender, education level, Major, type of license, job title, employment type, after-tax annual income, and years of work, indicating significant differences ($p < 0.05$) (Table 1).

3.2. Knowledge of HPV and HPV Vaccine among Different Types of Medical Institutions

This study found that the mean HPV and HPV vaccine knowledge score was 12.0 among HCPs involved in the government HPV vaccination program (with a total of score 15) and a total knowledge score of 15.0. However, there were several knowledge items that had a correct rate of less than 70%, including: "The body naturally creates high quantities of HPV antibodies to prevent re-infection?" and "HPV can be spread by contact with the skin, oral mucosa, and others" "Who is eligible to receive the HPV vaccine?" This study found that the average scores for HPV and HPV vaccine knowledge varied among different types of medical institutions. District hospitals had the highest mean score of 12.4, while private hospitals ranked fourth with a mean score of 10.9. Further analysis revealed significant differences in the knowledge scores between private community health centers (CHCs) and other medical institution types (adjusted $p < 0.001$), while the other three types of medical institutions did not differ significantly from each other (adjusted $p = 1.000$) (Table 2).

3.3. Factors Associated with Knowledge of HPV and the HPV Vaccine among All Participants

Multivariate logistic regression was used to analyze influencing factors regarding HPV and HPV vaccine knowledge levels among the 770 HCP who participated in the government HPV vaccination program. The results revealed significant disparities in the type of license and after-tax annual income across HCPs ($p < 0.05$). Nurses (aOR = 0.26, 95% CI: 0.18–0.38) and other HCPs (aOR = 0.25, 95% CI: 0.12–0.51) were lower than physicians. This study found that HCPs with higher after-tax annual incomes had higher HPV and HPV vaccine knowledge scores. Using an after-tax annual income of 100,000 RMB as a reference, HCPs with incomes of 100,000–200,000 RMB (aOR = 1.61, 95% CI: 1.07–2.42),

200,000–300,000 RMB (aOR = 2.16, 95% CI: 1.24–3.76), and >300,000 RMB (aOR = 2.39, 95% CI: 0.89–6.42) had higher adjusted odds ratios for higher knowledge scores (Table 3).

3.4. HPV Vaccination Recommendation Behavior

Out of 770 participants, a total of 729 (94.7%) reported recommending the HPV vaccine to others. This included 259 (94.9%) in Level I/Regional CHCs, 292 (94.8%) in Level II CHCs, 86 (94.5%) in Private CHCs, and 92 (93.9%) in district hospitals. However, some respondents reported a reluctance to recommend the HPV vaccine to others, citing several reasons. The main three reasons for this included: "Vaccine promotion is not my responsibility," "Fear of trouble caused by recommending self-pay vaccines to service recipients" and "Uncertainty of the HPV vaccination process" (Table 4).

In addition, the Mann–Whitney U test was used to analyze the differences in HPV and HPV vaccine knowledge scores between healthcare professionals who recommended the HPV vaccine and those who had not recommended it. The results showed that the distribution of HPV and HPV vaccine knowledge scores between the two groups of healthcare professionals was inconsistent. The average knowledge score of healthcare professionals who recommended the HPV vaccine was 12.09 ± 2.02, while that of healthcare professionals who did not recommend the HPV vaccine was 10.76 ± 2.67. The average rank of knowledge scores for healthcare professionals who had recommended the HPV vaccine was 392.15, while that of healthcare professionals who had not recommended the HPV vaccine was 267.30. The Mann–Whitney U test results indicated that there was a statistically significant difference in HPV and HPV vaccine knowledge scores between healthcare professionals who had recommended the HPV vaccine and those who had not recommended it (U = 10,098.500, $p < 0.001$).

Table 1. Demographic characteristics of HCPs involved in the governmental HPV vaccination program (n = 770).

Variables		Total		Level I/Regional CHC * (%)		Level II CHC * (%)		Private CHC * (%)		District Hospitals (%)		X^2	p
		770		273		308		91		98			
Age [a]	≤30	161	21.00%	61	22.40%	56	18.20%	32	35.20%	12	12.40%	51.542	<0.001
	31–40	299	38.90%	115	42.30%	128	41.60%	20	22.00%	36	37.10%		
	41–50	246	32.00%	83	30.50%	105	34.10%	20	22.00%	38	39.20%		
	>50	62	8.10%	13	4.80%	19	6.20%	19	20.90%	11	11.30%		
Gender	Male	56	7.30%	16	5.90%	23	7.50%	13	14.30%	4	4.10%	8.941	0.03
	Female	714	92.70%	257	94.10%	285	92.50%	78	85.70%	94	95.90%		
Education level	Junior High School/High School/Vocational High School/Junior College	21	2.70%	6	2.20%	5	1.60%	9	9.90%	1	1.00%	31.293	<0.001
	College/University	688	89.40%	250	91.60%	273	88.60%	81	89.00%	84	85.70%		
	Master's degree or above	61	7.90%	17	6.20%	30	9.70%	1	1.10%	13	13.30%		
Marital Status	Unmarried	126	16.40%	52	19.00%	42	13.60%	20	22.00%	12	12.20%	6.801	0.34
	Married	607	78.80%	208	76.20%	252	81.80%	67	73.60%	80	81.60%		
	Divorced/widowed	37	4.80%	13	4.80%	14	4.50%	4	4.40%	6	6.10%		
Major	Clinical Medicine	409	53.10%	153	56.00%	163	52.90%	46	50.50%	47	48.00%	26.661	0.002
	Preventive Medicine	48	6.20%	14	5.10%	17	5.50%	2	2.20%	15	15.30%		
	Nursing	221	28.70%	84	30.80%	80	26.00%	31	34.10%	26	26.50%		
	Other HCP	92	11.90%	22	8.10%	48	15.60%	12	13.20%	10	10.20%		
Type of license	Doctors	511	66.40%	181	66.30%	219	71.10%	49	53.80%	62	63.30%	39.891	<0.001
	Nurse	218	28.30%	83	30.40%	83	26.90%	30	33.00%	22	22.40%		
	Other HCP	41	5.30%	9	3.30%	6	1.90%	12	13.20%	14	14.30%		

Table 1. Cont.

Variables	Total		Level I/Regional CHC * (%)		Level II CHC * (%)		Private CHC * (%)		District Hospitals (%)		X^2	p
Job title												
Lower than primary	27	3.50%	6	2.20%	5	1.60%	9	9.90%	7	7.10%	105.31	<0.001
Primary	204	26.50%	74	27.10%	65	21.10%	47	51.60%	18	18.40%		
Intermediate	437	56.80%	164	60.10%	207	67.20%	26	28.60%	40	40.80%		
Deputy senior/Senior	102	13.20%	29	10.60%	31	10.10%	9	9.90%	33	33.70%		
Employment Type [b]												
temporary employment	247	32.20%	94	34.60%	102	33.20%	20	22.20%	31	32.00%	83.807	<0.001
Contract Employment	325	42.40%	113	41.50%	127	41.40%	62	68.90%	23	23.70%		
Formal staffing	175	22.80%	58	21.30%	75	24.40%	0	0.00%	42	43.30%		
Retirement and re-employment	19	2.50%	7	2.60%	3	1.00%	8	8.90%	1	1.00%		
After-tax annual income												
<100,000 RMB	158	20.50%	54	19.80%	40	13.00%	48	52.70%	16	16.30%	89.923	<0.001
100,000–200,000 RMB	438	56.90%	150	54.90%	201	65.30%	40	44.00%	47	48.00%		
200,000–300,000 RMB	143	18.60%	58	21.20%	57	18.50%	2	2.20%	26	26.50%		
>300,000 RMB	31	4.00%	11	4.00%	10	3.20%	1	1.10%	9	9.20%		
Years of work [c]												
<5 years	151	19.70%	53	19.50%	60	19.50%	26	28.90%	12	12.20%	31.078	0.002
6–10 years	138	18.00%	63	23.20%	47	15.30%	16	17.80%	12	12.20%		
11–15 years	127	16.60%	44	16.20%	56	18.20%	13	14.40%	14	14.30%		
16–20 years	136	17.70%	44	16.20%	66	21.50%	8	8.90%	18	18.40%		
>21 years	215	28.00%	68	25.00%	78	25.40%	27	30.00%	42	42.90%		

* CHC: community health center. [a] Two-missing value in HCPs involved in the governmental HPV vaccination program age. [b] Four missing values in HCPs involved in the governmental HPV vaccination program Employment Type. [c] Three missing value in HCPs involved in the governmental HPV vaccination program in years of work.

Table 2. Knowledge of HPV and HPV vaccines among different medical institution types ($n = 770$).

Question/Correct	Total N	Total %	Level I/Regional CHC N	Level I/Regional CHC %	Level II CHC N	Level II CHC %	Private CHC N	Private CHC %	District Hospitals N	District Hospitals %
HPV-related questions										
The majority of HPV infections in people do not cause any symptoms?	626	81.3%	224	82.1%	256	83.1%	63	69.2%	83	84.7%
Autoimmune therapy can cure the majority of HPV infections?	541	70.3%	192	70.3%	222	72.1%	46	50.5%	81	82.7%
The body naturally creates high quantities of HPV antibodies to prevent re-infection?	402	52.2%	134	49.1%	169	54.9%	57	62.6%	42	42.9%
The patient or the individual who has the virus are not the source of HPV transmission?	559	72.6%	209	76.6%	225	73.1%	59	64.8%	66	67.3%
HPV can be spread through sexual contact?	731	94.9%	263	96.3%	290	94.2%	84	92.3%	94	95.9%
During childbirth, a mother's genital tract HPV infection may pass to the baby?	549	71.3%	189	69.2%	233	75.6%	63	69.2%	64	65.3%
HPV can be spread by contact with the skin, oral mucosa, and others?	483	62.7%	175	64.1%	193	62.7%	42	46.2%	73	74.5%
Only women can contract HPV?	706	91.7%	259	94.9%	277	89.9%	75	82.4%	95	96.9%
Women exclusively contract HPV in their cervix?	672	87.3%	243	89.0%	268	87.0%	71	78.0%	90	91.8%
Regular cervical cancer screening for women is an important measure to prevent the disease?	739	96.0%	260	95.2%	296	96.1%	86	94.5%	97	99.0%
HPV vaccine-related questions										
Who is eligible to receive the HPV vaccine?	500	64.9%	186	68.1%	199	64.6%	47	51.6%	68	69.4%
Who is the front-runner for the human papillomavirus (HPV) vaccine?	580	75.3%	208	76.2%	236	76.6%	59	64.8%	77	78.6%
What time of year is ideal for receiving the human papillomavirus (HPV) vaccine?	713	92.6%	255	93.4%	292	94.8%	75	82.4%	91	92.9%
The human papillomavirus (HPV) vaccine guards against the virus?	708	91.9%	250	91.6%	290	94.2%	75	82.4%	93	94.9%
After receiving an HPV vaccine, routine cervical cancer screenings are no longer necessary?	748	97.1%	267	97.8%	296	96.1%	89	97.8%	96	98.0%
Overall mean score	12.0	80.0%	12.1	80.7%	12.1	80.7%	10.9	72.7%	12.4	82.3%

Kruskal–Wallis H: H = 28.441, $p < 0.001$. Kruskal–Wallis one-way ANOVA (k samples): Private CHC-Level I/Regional CHC (adjsted $p < 0.001$); Private CHC-Level II CHC (adjsted $p < 0.001$); Private CHC-District Hospitals (adjsted $p < 0.001$); Level I/Regional CHC-Level II CHC (adjsted $p = 1.000$); Level I/Regional CHC-District Hospitals (adjsted $p = 1.000$); Level II CHC-District Hospitals (adjsted $p = 1.000$).

Table 3. Factors associated with the knowledge of HPV and the HPV vaccine among all participants ($n = 770$).

Variables	Average Score	Score < 12	Score ≥ 12	Uni-Variate Logistic Regression OR (95% CI)	p	Multi-Variate Logistic Regression AoR (95% CI)	p
Age [a]	12.02 ± 2.08				0.060		0.127
≤30	11.68 ± 2.17	63	98	1.00		1.00	
31–40	12.01 ± 2.11	100	180	1.28 (0.86–1.90)	0.224	-	0.714
41–50	12.33 ± 1.87	66	199	1.75 (1.15–2.68)	0.009	-	0.429
>50	11.85 ± 2.28	23	39	1.09 (0.60–2.00)	0.780	-	0.027
Gender					0.289		
Male	11.84 ± 2.05	22	34	1.00		*	*
Female	12.04 ± 2.09	231	483	1.35 (0.77–2.37)	0.289	*	*
Education level					<0.001		0.230
Junior High School/High School/Vocational High School/Junior College	10.33 ± 2.24	15	6	1.00		1.00	
College/University	12.01 ± 2.09	226	462	5.11 (1.96–13.35)	0.001	-	0.465
Master's degree or above	12.79 ± 1.56	12	49	10.21 (3.27–31.85)	<0.001	-	0.775
Marital Status					0.879		
Unmarried	11.85 ± 2.31	43	83	1.00		*	*
Married	12.04 ± 2.01	199	408	1.06 (0.71–1.60)	0.771	*	*
Divorced/widowed	12.30 ± 2.42	11	26	1.23 (0.55–2.71)	0.618	*	*
Major					<0.001		0.577
Clinical Medicine	12.54 ± 1.76	95	314	1.00		1.00	
Preventive Medicine	12.71 ± 1.58	8	40	1.51 (0.68–3.34)	0.306	-	0.309
Nursing	10.83 ± 2.32	120	101	0.26 (0.18–0.36)	<0.001	-	0.358
Other HcCP	12.22 ± 1.90	30	62	0.63 (0.38–1.02)	0.062	-	0.586
Type of license					<0.001		<0.001
Doctors	12.61 ± 1.72	110	401	1.00		1.00	
Nurse	10.82 ± 2.31	120	98	0.22 (0.16–0.32)	<0.001	0.26 (0.18–0.38)	<0.001
Other HCP	11.12 ± 1.98	23	18	0.22 (0.11–0.41)	<0.001	0.25 (0.12–0.51)	<0.001
Job Title					0.001		0.803
Lower than primary	10.89 ± 2.26	15	12	1.00		1.00	
Primary	11.44 ± 2.21	84	120	1.79 (0.80–4.01)	0.160	-	0.838
Intermediate	12.21 ± 2.00	129	308	2.98 (1.36–6.55)	0.006	-	0.630
Deputy senior/Senior	12.71 ± 1.76	25	77	3.85 (1.59–9.31)	0.003	-	0.521

Table 3. Cont.

Variables	Average Score	Score < 12	Score ≥ 12	Uni-Variate Logistic Regression		Multi-Variate Logistic Regression	
				OR (95% CI)	p	Aor (95% CI)	p
Employment Type [b]					0.007		0.697
Temporary employment	11.90 ± 2.17	85	162	1.00		1.00	
Contract Employment	11.70 ± 2.09	122	203	0.87 (0.62–1.23)	0.441	-	0.937
Formal staffing	12.82 ± 1.66	39	136	1.83 (1.18–2.85)	0.007	-	0.407
Retirement and re-employment	11.74 ± 2.68	6	13	1.14 (0.42–3.10)	0.802	-	0.380
After-tax annual income					<0.001		0.029
<100,000 RMB	10.88 ± 2.28	81	77	1.00		1.00	
100,000–200,000 RMB	12.09 ± 1.99	136	302	2.34 (1.61–3.39)	<0.001	1.61 (1.07–2.42)	0.023
200,000–300,000 RMB	12.80 ± 1.62	30	113	3.96 (2.38–6.59)	<0.001	2.16 (1.24–3.76)	0.007
>300,000 RMB	13.35 ± 1.56	6	25	4.38 (1.71–11.27)	0.002	2.39 (0.89–6.42)	0.083
Years of work [c]					0.557		
<5 years	12.09 ± 2.08	48	103	1.00		*	*
6–10 years	11.75 ± 2.14	53	85	0.75 (0.46–1.21)	0.239	*	*
11–15 years	11.92 ± 1.94	42	85	0.94 (0.57–1.56)	0.820	*	*
16–20 years	12.01 ± 2.36	43	93	1.01 (0.61–1.66)	0.975	*	*
>21 years	12.24 ± 1.94	64	151	1.10 (0.70–1.73)	0.680	*	*
Medical institution Type					0.002		0.187
Level I/Regional CHC	12.14 ± 1.81	83	190	1.00		1.00	
Level II CHC	12.15 ± 2.15	92	216	1.03 (0.72–1.46)	0.889	-	0.667
Private CHC	10.89 ± 2.41	46	45	0.43 (0.26–0.69)	0.001	-	0.038
District Hospitals	12.35 ± 1.94	32	66	0.90 (0.55–1.48)	0.680	-	0.769

[a] Two-missing value in HCPs involved in the governmental HPV vaccination program age. [b] four missing value in HCPs involved in the governmental HPV vaccination program Employment Type. [c] Three missing value in HCPs involved in the governmental HPV vaccination program in years of work * Not included in multifactorial analysis—Variables not included in the equation.

Table 4. HPV Vaccine recommendation behavior (n = 770).

Variables	Total		Level I/Regional CHC		Level II CHC		Private CHC		District Hospitals	
	N	%	N	%	N	%	N	%	N	%
Have you ever advised a client to receive an HPV vaccine?	770		273		308		91		98	
Yes	729	94.70%	259	94.90%	292	94.80%	86	94.50%	92	93.90%
No	41	5.30%	14	5.10%	16	5.20%	5	5.50%	6	6.10%
The reason you did not recommend HPV vaccination to your clients (multiple choice)										
Workplaces are not allowed to recommend self-funded vaccines to clients	5	12.20%	4	28.60%	1	6.30%	5	100.00%	0	0.00%
Uncertain who the HPV vaccine is intended for.	6	14.60%	1	7.10%	4	25.00%	0	0.00%	1	16.70%
Uncertain of the HPV vaccination process	12	29.30%	2	14.30%	7	43.80%	2	40.00%	1	16.70%
Uncertain about safety of HPV vaccine	8	19.50%	3	21.40%	3	18.80%	1	20.00%	1	16.70%
Uncertain effectiveness of HPV vaccine	7	17.10%	2	14.30%	3	18.80%	0	0.00%	2	33.30%
Fear of trouble caused by recommending self-pay vaccines to service recipients	14	34.10%	4	28.60%	7	43.80%	2	40.00%	1	16.70%
Vaccine promotion is not my responsibility	15	36.60%	4	28.60%	8	50.00%	1	20.00%	2	33.30%
Other	6	14.60%	4	28.60%	0	0.00%	1	20.00%	1	16.70%

4. Discussion

In the context of the gradual introduction of the free HPV vaccination program in Chinese cities since 2020, there has been a need for evaluation studies on HCPs associated with this program. This study aimed to assess the level of HPV and HPV vaccine knowledge among HCPs and examine differences between the knowledge levels among HCPs in various types of medical institutions. In addition, we explored the factors that influenced the level of HPV and HPV vaccine knowledge among HCPs and identified the reasons for not recommending the HPV vaccine. The findings of this study provided valuable insights for improving the overall knowledge of HCPs involved in the program and promoting the quality of program implementation in the region.

This study found that HCPs in private CHCs had lower knowledge levels about HPV and the HPV vaccine compared to HCPs in the other three public medical institutions. The difference in knowledge levels between the four medical institutions was significant. However, the recommendation behaviors of HCPs across the four medical institutions were consistent. This study also identified that HCPs' knowledge of the HPV vaccine was influenced by their type of license and after-tax annual income. Additionally, the most common reason given for not recommending the HPV vaccine to their clients was that "vaccine promotion is not my responsibility". These findings highlight the importance of targeted education and training programs for HCPs, particularly those working in private CHCs, to improve their knowledge and recommendation behavior around the HPV vaccine. It also suggests the need for greater emphasis on the importance of HPV vaccination and the role of HCPs in promoting it to their patients. The survey revealed significant differences in the sociological characteristics of HCPs involved in the government HPV vaccination program across the four types of medical institutions, except for marital status. HCPs working in private CHCs had a lower age distribution, a higher percentage of male HCPs, fewer preventive medicine majors, fewer doctors, more nurses, no formal staffing, lower education levels, lower job titles, and a lower after-tax annual income. Additionally, their years of work were primarily distributed between more than 21 and less than 5 years. These findings suggest that private CHCs may face challenges in terms of their talent pool, as their HCPs tend to have lower qualifications and experience when compared to those in other medical institutions. Addressing these disparities may require targeted efforts to improve the recruitment and retention of qualified healthcare professionals, as well as targeted education and training programs to improve their knowledge and skills.

Our findings are consistent with the findings in the Pearl River Delta region [25,26]. Owing to Shenzhen's developed economy and recent emphasis on the construction of primary medical institutions, as well as the good stability and high credibility of public medical institutions, studies have noted a trend in staff from private CHCs migrating to public health institutions after gaining several years of training and experience. This has resulted in lower talent levels in private CHCs compared to public medical institutions. Addressing this issue may require efforts to improve the recruitment and retention of qualified healthcare professionals in private CHCs, as well as targeted education and training programs to improve the knowledge and skills of their HCPs.

This study found that the mean (SD) HPV and HPV vaccine knowledge score among participants in Shenzhen was 12.02 (2.08) out of 15 [27–29]; this suggests that there is room for improvement in HCPs' knowledge and understanding of HPV and the HPV vaccine in Southern China. This could be due to China's late approval of the HPV vaccine and the absence of NIP implementation. More than 96.0% correctly identified "regular cervical cancer screening is required after HPV vaccination" based on the correct rate of each knowledge item. "Regular cervical cancer screening for women is an important preventive measure". This may be because cervical cancer screening has been a national public health program since 2009. However, only 52.2% were aware that "the body's natural infection with HPV has a low level of resistance that is insufficient to fight off another virus attack". Less than 65% were aware that "HPV could be transmitted through contact with the skin, oral mucosa, and other body fluids" and that "HPV vaccination is available for both men and women". This suggests that while most HCPs are familiar with HPV and the HPV vaccine, they lack in-depth knowledge of HPV infection pathways and modes of transmission. Future educational programs or training courses should take care to explain these items of knowledge. Studies in countries with HPV vaccination programs have also revealed that medical personnel's knowledge of HPV and HPV vaccines is frequently incomplete, with the potential to spread misinformation [27,30,31]. Furthermore, studies in countries with established HPV vaccination programs also revealed that medical personnel's knowledge of HPV and HPV vaccines was frequently incomplete, which could lead to the spread of misinformation. Therefore, it is important for educational programs to be based on accurate and up-to-date information and to be regularly updated as new research emerges. In doing so, HCPs can be better equipped to provide accurate information and recommendations to their patients, leading to improved vaccination rates and reduced rates of HPV-related diseases.

A comparison of the four types of medical institutions revealed that there was no difference in the level of knowledge between the three types of public medical institutions but there was a significant difference between private CHC and the other three types of public medical institutions. This disparity could be attributed to the lower overall quality of medical staff in private CHCs compared to public medical institutions. Therefore, it is critical to increase HCPs' knowledge of HPV and HPV vaccines, improve access to HPV and HPV vaccine information in private CHCs, and strengthen HPV education for HCPs in CHCs. These efforts are necessary to ensure that HCPs are equipped with the information and skills required to offer effective HPV prevention and treatment to patients. Overall, targeted education and training programs, as well as increased access to information and resources, are essential for improving HCPs' knowledge and understanding of HPV and the HPV vaccine. In doing so, we can strive towards reducing the incidence of HPV-related diseases and improving the overall health outcomes of patients in Southern China. Consistent with previous studies [24,32], our study found that the type of license and income level were significant factors influencing knowledge levels of HPV and HPV vaccines among HCPs in Southern China. Specifically, doctors exhibited a higher level of knowledge compared to nurses and other HCPs, and individuals with a higher after-tax annual income had a higher level of knowledge. Other studies also highlighted the importance of effective communication between HCPs and females in raising awareness and acceptance of HPV vaccines [33]. A previous study reported that 78% of female participants expressed interest in receiving more information about HPV from their doctors [34]. Furthermore, another study found that approximately 60% of women who were willing to vaccinate their children against HPV cited their doctor's advice as a critical factor in their decision [35]. In addition, the doctor's advice played an important role in increasing parental willingness to vaccinate their children against HPV. According to the results of this study, 94.7% of the participants recommended the HPV vaccine to their service recipients, and 5.3% did not recommend the HPV vaccine mainly because "vaccine promotion is not my responsibility" and "fear of trouble caused by recommending self-pay vaccines to service recipients". Additionally, HCP with a higher level of knowledge about HPV and HPV vaccines are more likely to recommend the vaccine to their patients. In order to further improve public awareness and the use of the HPV vaccine in the population, training for HCPs involved in the government's HPV vaccination program should not only focus on those with lower levels of knowledge, but also on strengthening HCPs' awareness of publicity and education. This could help to ensure that HCPs are equipped with accurate and up-to-date information about HPV and the HPV vaccine, further enhancing their willingness to recommend the HPV vaccine and increasing their ability to effectively communicate this information with their patients. In addition to this, schools and the general public could also be given information and education about HPV and the vaccine through HCPs and the media. In doing so, we can ensure that people are better informed about HPV-related knowledge and the implications of the HPV vaccine, as well as clear up any misconceptions about HCPs recommending the HPV vaccine. This can ultimately lead to an increase in the rate of HPV vaccination and a reduction in rates of HPV-related diseases in China.

5. Strengths and Limitations

The present study has several strengths that are worth noting. Firstly, it is the first survey conducted in China that specifically explores HPV and HPV vaccine knowledge and attitudes among HCPs involved in the government's HPV vaccination program in Shenzhen. This contributes to the existing literature and fills an important knowledge gap in this field. Secondly, our sample size was relatively large, with 770 HCPs participating in this study. This allowed for a more comprehensive analysis of the knowledge and attitudes of HCPs towards HPV and HPV vaccines. Lastly, we conducted a detailed analysis of the factors influencing HCPs' knowledge levels and recommended behaviors, which could provide valuable insights for improving HCPs' education and training programs in relation to HPV vaccination.

Several limitations of our study should be acknowledged. Firstly, the questionnaire used in this study was only implemented in Shenzhen and was developed based on the national setting of China. Secondly, the findings are restricted to the specific data obtained from Shenzhen. Therefore, caution should be taken when applying these results to other regions where legislative and health-related implementations differ from those in Shenzhen. However, the results are still valuable for promoting the implementation of the free HPV vaccination program in Shenzhen. Lastly, as the study adopted a convenience sample instead of a probability sample, there may be variation in the level of access among participants. Therefore, future studies are recommended to use random sampling and perform rigorous analyses.

6. Conclusions

This study provides an overview of Shenzhen, southern China, where HCPs exhibit a higher level of knowledge and recommended behaviors for the HPV vaccine. The knowledge that HCPs have on HPV infection routes and modes of transmission, as well as some of the reasons for non-recommended behaviors, needs to be improved. The significantly lower scores of HCPs in private CHCs compared to public medical institutions, as well as the factors influencing knowledge levels, indicate that future education and training for HCPs should focus on private CHCs, HCPs whose license type is other than a doctor, and HCPs with a low after-tax annual income.

Author Contributions: Conceptualization: P.L. and D.W.; methodology: D.S., P.L. and D.W.; validation: D.S.; formal analysis: D.S.; resources: all of authors; data curation: D.S., P.L. and D.W.; writing—original draft preparation: D.S.; writing—review and editing: F.Z., Y.W. and Y.Z.; project administration: F.Z., Y.W. and Y.Z. All authors have read and agreed to the published version of the manuscript.

Funding: This study was supported by the Bill & Melinda Gates Foundation [INV-018013], and Cancer Hospital Chinese Academy of Medical Sciences (2021-I2M-1-004). Under the grant conditions of the Foundation, a Creative Commons Attribution 4.0 Generic License was assigned to the Author Accepted Manuscript version that might arise from this submission.

Institutional Review Board Statement: The study was conducted in accordance with the Declaration of Helsinki, and approved by the Ethics Committee of Shenzhen Maternity & Child Healthcare Hospital, Southern Medical University (protocol code SFYL[2021]060 and 3 December 2021 of approval).

Informed Consent Statement: Written informed consent was obtained from the patient(s) to publish this paper.

Data Availability Statement: The data that support the findings of this study are available from the corresponding author.

Conflicts of Interest: The authors declare no conflict of interest.

References

1. Sung, H.; Ferlay, J.; Siegel, R.L.; Laversanne, M.; Soerjomataram, I.; Jemal, A.; Bray, F. Global Cancer Statistics 2020: GLOBOCAN Estimates of Incidence and Mortality Worldwide for 36 Cancers in 185 Countries. *CA Cancer J. Clin.* **2021**, *71*, 209–249. [CrossRef] [PubMed]
2. Zheng, R.; Zhang, S.; Zeng, H.; Wang, S.; Sun, K.; Chen, R.; He, J. Cancer incidence and mortality in China, 2016. *J. Natl. Cancer Cent.* **2022**, *2*, 1–9. [CrossRef]
3. Li, X.; Zheng, R.; Li, X.; Shan, H.; Wu, Q.; Wang, Y.; Chen, W. Trends of incidence rate and age at diagnosis for cervical cancer in China, from 2000 to 2014. *Chin. J. Cancer Res.* **2017**, *29*, 477–486. [CrossRef] [PubMed]
4. Bansal, A.; Singh, M.P.; Rai, B. Human papillomavirus-associated cancers: A growing global problem. *Int. J. Appl. Basic Med. Res.* **2016**, *6*, 84–89. [PubMed]
5. de Martel, C.; Georges, D.; Bray, F.; Ferlay, J.; Clifford, G.M. Global burden of cancer attributable to infections in 2018: A worldwide incidence analysis. *Lancet Glob. Health* **2020**, *8*, e180–e190. [CrossRef]
6. Arbyn, M.; Xu, L.; Simoens, C.; Martin-Hirsch, P.P. Prophylactic vaccination against human papillomaviruses to prevent cervical cancer and its precursors. *Cochrane Database Syst. Rev.* **2018**, *5*, Cd009069. [CrossRef] [PubMed]
7. Wheeler, C.M.; Skinner, S.R.; Del Rosario-Raymundo, M.R.; Garland, S.M.; Chatterjee, A.; Lazcano-Ponce, E.; Struyf, F. Efficacy, safety, and immunogenicity of the human papillomavirus 16/18 AS04-adjuvanted vaccine in women older than 25 years: 7-year follow-up of the phase 3, double-blind, randomised controlled VIVIANE study. *Lancet Infect. Dis.* **2016**, *16*, 1154–1168. [CrossRef]
8. Zhu, F.C.; Hu, S.Y.; Hong, Y.; Hu, Y.M.; Zhang, X.; Zhang, Y.J.; Struyf, F. Efficacy, immunogenicity and safety of the AS04-HPV-16/18 vaccine in Chinese women aged 18–25 years: End-of-study results from a phase II/III, randomised, controlled trial. *Cancer Med.* **2019**, *8*, 6195–6211. [CrossRef]
9. Kjaer, S.K.; Nygård, M.; Dillner, J.; Brooke Marshall, J.; Radley, D.; Li, M.; Saah, A.J. A 12-Year Follow-up on the Long-Term Effectiveness of the Quadrivalent Human Papillomavirus Vaccine in 4 Nordic Countries. *Clin. Infect. Dis.* **2018**, *66*, 339–345. [CrossRef]
10. WHO. Launch of the Global Strategy to Accelerate the Elimination of Cervical Cancer. 2020. Available online: https://www.who.int/news-room/events/detail/2020/11/17/default-calendar/launch-of-the-global-strategy-to-accelerate-the-elimination-of-cervical-cancer (accessed on 1 April 2023).
11. PATH. Available online: https://path.azureedge.net/media/documents/Global_Vaccine_Intro_Overview_Slides_Final_PATHwebsite_2021AUG17_fx7PZjH.pdf (accessed on 1 April 2023).
12. Song, Y.F.; Liu, X.X.; Yin, Z.D.; Yu, W.Z.; Cao, L.; Cao, L.S.; Wu, J. Estimated vaccination rates for human papillomavirus vaccine in women aged 9-45 years in China, 2018–2020. *China Vaccine Immun.* **2021**, *27*, 570–575.
13. Zhang, Y.; Wang, Y.; Liu, L.; Fan, Y.; Liu, Z.; Wang, Y.; Nie, S. Awareness and knowledge about human papillomavirus vaccination and its acceptance in China: A meta-analysis of 58 observational studies. *BMC Public Health* **2016**, *16*, 216. [CrossRef] [PubMed]
14. Zhang, X.; Wang, Z.; Ren, Z.; Li, Z.; Ma, W.; Gao, X.; Zhang, R.; Qiao, Y.; Li, J. HPV vaccine acceptability and willingness-related factors among Chinese adolescents: A nation-wide study. *Hum. Vaccin. Immunother.* **2021**, *17*, 1025–1032. [CrossRef] [PubMed]

15. Ning, Y.E.; Liu, Y.; Xu, X.Y.; Zhang, X.Y.; Wang, N.; Zheng, L.Q. Knowledge of Cervical Cancer, Human Papilloma Virus (HPV) and HPV Vaccination Among Women in Northeast China. *J. Cancer Educ.* **2020**, *35*, 1197–1205. [CrossRef]
16. McRee, A.L.; Gilkey, M.B.; Dempsey, A.F. HPV vaccine hesitancy: Findings from a statewide survey of health care providers. *J. Pediatr. Health Care* **2014**, *28*, 541–549. [CrossRef] [PubMed]
17. Paterson, P.; Meurice, F.; Stanberry, L.R.; Glismann, S.; Rosenthal, S.L.; Larson, H.J. Vaccine hesitancy and healthcare providers. *Vaccine* **2016**, *34*, 6700–6706. [CrossRef] [PubMed]
18. Rosenthal, S.L.; Weiss, T.W.; Zimet, G.D.; Ma, L.; Good, M.B.; Vichnin, M.D. Predictors of HPV vaccine uptake among women aged 19-26: Importance of a physician's recommendation. *Vaccine* **2011**, *29*, 890–895. [CrossRef]
19. Loke, A.Y.; Kwan, M.L.; Wong, Y.T.; Wong, A.K.Y. The Uptake of Human Papillomavirus Vaccination and Its Associated Factors Among Adolescents: A Systematic Review. *J. Prim. Care Community Health* **2017**, *8*, 349–362. [CrossRef]
20. Lubeya, M.K.; Zekire Nyirenda, J.C.; Chanda Kabwe, J.; Mukosha, M. Knowledge, Attitudes and Practices Towards Human Papillomavirus Vaccination Among Medical Doctors at a Tertiary Hospital: A Cross Sectional Study. *Cancer Control* **2022**, *29*, 10732748221132646. [CrossRef]
21. Rosen, B.L.; Ashwood, D.; Richardson, G.B. School Nurses' Professional Practice in the HPV Vaccine Decision-Making Process. *J. Sch. Nurs.* **2016**, *32*, 138–148. [CrossRef]
22. Malo, T.L.; Giuliano, A.R.; Kahn, J.A.; Zimet, G.D.; Lee, J.H.; Zhao, X.; Vadaparampil, S.T. Physicians' human papillomavirus vaccine recommendations in the context of permissive guidelines for male patients: A national study. *Cancer Epidemiol. Biomarkers Prev.* **2014**, *23*, 2126–2135. [CrossRef]
23. Xu, X.; Wang, Y.; Liu, Y.; Yu, Y.; Yang, C.; Zhang, Y.; Hong, Y.; Wang, Y.; Zhang, X.; Bian, R.; et al. A nationwide post-marketing survey of knowledge, attitudes and recommendations towards human papillomavirus vaccines among healthcare providers in China. *Prev. Med.* **2021**, *146*, 106484. [CrossRef]
24. McSherry, L.A.; O'Leary, E.; Dombrowski, S.U.; Francis, J.J.; Martin, C.M.; O'Leary, J.J.; Sharp, L. Which primary care practitioners have poor human papillomavirus (HPV) knowledge? A step towards informing the development of professional education initiatives. *PLoS ONE* **2018**, *13*, e0208482. [CrossRef]
25. Yin, X.; Gong, Y.; Yang, C.; Tu, X.; Liu, W.; Cao, S.; Lu, Z. A Comparison of Quality of Community Health Services Between Public and Private Community Health Centers in Urban China. *Med. Care* **2015**, *53*, 888–893. [CrossRef] [PubMed]
26. Wei, X.; Yang, N.; Gao, Y.; Wong, S.Y.; Wong, M.C.; Wang, J.; Wang, H.H.; Li, D.K.; Tang, J.; Griffiths, S.M. Comparison of three models of ownership of community health centres in China: A qualitative study. *J. Health Serv. Res. Policy* **2015**, *20*, 162–169. [CrossRef] [PubMed]
27. Sherman, S.M.; Bartholomew, K.; Denison, H.J.; Patel, H.; Moss, E.L.; Douwes, J.; Bromhead, C. Knowledge, attitudes and awareness of the human papillomavirus among health professionals in New Zealand. *PLoS ONE* **2018**, *13*, e0197648. [CrossRef] [PubMed]
28. Sherman, S.M.; Cohen, C.R.; Denison, H.J.; Bromhead, C.; Patel, H. A survey of knowledge, attitudes and awareness of the human papillomavirus among healthcare professionals across the UK. *Eur. J. Public Health* **2020**, *30*, 10–16. [CrossRef]
29. Patel, H.; Austin-Smith, K.; Sherman, S.M.; Tincello, D.; Moss, E.L. Knowledge, attitudes and awareness of the human papillomavirus amongst primary care practice nurses: An evaluation of current training in England. *J. Public Health* **2017**, *39*, 601–608. [CrossRef]
30. Nilsen, K.; Aasland, O.G.; Klouman, E. The HPV vaccine: Knowledge and attitudes among public health nurses and general practitioners in Northern Norway after introduction of the vaccine in the school-based vaccination programme. *Scand. J. Prim. Health Care* **2017**, *35*, 387–395. [CrossRef]
31. Leung, S.O.A.; Akinwunmi, B.; Elias, K.M.; Feldman, S. Educating healthcare providers to increase Human Papillomavirus (HPV) vaccination rates: A Qualitative Systematic Review. *Vaccine X* **2019**, *3*, 100037. [CrossRef]
32. Trucchi, C.; Restivo, V.; Amicizia, D.; Fortunato, F.; Manca, A.; Martinelli, D.; Montecucco, A.; Piazza, M.F.; Prato, R.; Tisa, V.; et al. Italian Health Care Workers' Knowledge, Attitudes, and Practices Regarding Human Papillomavirus Infection and Prevention. *Int. J. Environ. Res. Public Health* **2020**, *17*, 5278. [CrossRef]
33. Mullins TL, K.; Griffioen, A.M.; Glynn, S.; Zimet, G.D.; Rosenthal, S.L.; Fortenberry, J.D.; Kahn, J.A. Human papillomavirus vaccine communication: Perspectives of 11-12 year-old girls, mothers, and clinicians. *Vaccine* **2013**, *31*, 4894–4901. [CrossRef]
34. Montgomery, M.P.; Dune, T.; Shetty, P.K.; Shetty, A.K. Knowledge and acceptability of human papillomavirus vaccination and cervical cancer screening among women in Karnataka, India. *J. Cancer Educ.* **2015**, *30*, 130–137. [CrossRef]
35. Madhivanan, P.; Li, T.; Srinivas, V.; Marlow, L.; Mukherjee, S.; Krupp, K. Human papillomavirus vaccine acceptability among parents of adolescent girls: Obstacles and challenges in Mysore, India. *Prev. Med.* **2014**, *64*, 69–74. [CrossRef]

Disclaimer/Publisher's Note: The statements, opinions and data contained in all publications are solely those of the individual author(s) and contributor(s) and not of MDPI and/or the editor(s). MDPI and/or the editor(s) disclaim responsibility for any injury to people or property resulting from any ideas, methods, instructions or products referred to in the content.

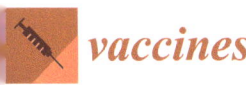

Article

Knowledge of HPV and HPV Vaccination among Polish Students from Medical and Non-Medical Universities

Dominik Pruski [1,*], Sonja Millert-Kalińska [1,2], Jan Haraj [3], Sandra Dachowska [3], Robert Jach [4], Jakub Żurawski [5] and Marcin Przybylski [1]

1. Department of Obstetrics and Gynecology, District Public Hospital in Poznan, 60-479 Poznan, Poland; millertsonja@gmail.com (S.M.-K.); nicramp@poczta.onet.pl (M.P.)
2. Doctoral School of Poznan University of Medical Sciences, 61-701 Poznan, Poland
3. Faculty of Medicine, Poznan University of Medical Sciences, 61-701 Poznan, Poland
4. Department of Gynecological Endocrinology, Jagiellonian University Medical College, 31-008 Cracow, Poland; jach@cm-uj.krakow.pl
5. Department of Immunobiology, Poznan University of Medical Sciences, 60-806 Poznan, Poland; zurawski@ump.edu.pl
* Correspondence: dominik.pruski@icloud.com

Abstract: Human papillomavirus (HPV) is a common sexually transmitted infection that can cause both benign and malignant lesions. HPV vaccines, preferably administered before the onset of sexual activity, have demonstrated remarkable efficacy in preventing HPV-related cancers. The impact of a healthcare provider's recommendation on HPV vaccine acceptance is substantial. Therefore, medical students must undergo thorough training in this domain. This study compares fundamental understanding and viewpoints regarding HPV and anti-HPV vaccines among Polish students pursuing medical and non-medical sciences. This study was based on the authors' questionnaire, and the results were statistically analyzed. The participants in this study were 1025 students (medical sciences students—520 respondents in total; and non-medical sciences students—505 respondents in total). According to the results, medical students' knowledge about the consequences of HPV infection and vaccination against HPV was significantly greater. To date, numerous publications have investigated the understanding of particular social, gender, parental, etc., groups about vaccination, but the knowledge of students at different universities—medical and other—has not been compared. Social awareness is still insufficient, even in groups of medical students. There is much to be done to educate and encourage preventive behavior in those not receiving primary prevention in early childhood.

Keywords: HPV vaccination; healthcare; students' knowledge; medical university education

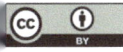

1. Introduction

Human papillomavirus (HPV) is a common sexually transmitted infection that can cause both benign and malignant lesions in the body. According to the newest data, nearly 70% of the population may be exposed to HPV during their lifetime [1]. Human papillomavirus has been linked to around 5% of cancer cases globally [2,3]. To date, scientists have determined more than 200 genotypes of HPV. Of these, HPV DNA of the following genotypes has been determined: 16, 18, 31, 33, 35, 39, 45, 51, 52, 56, 58, 59, 68, 73, and 82, which are are categorized as high-risk genotypes; 26, 53, 66, 70, 73, and 82—probable high-risk genotypes; and 6, 11, 40, 42, 43, 44, 54, 61, 70, 72, 81, and CP6108—low-risk genotypes [4]. High-risk genotypes are typically linked to cervical cancer, vulvar and vaginal cancer, as well as penile, anal, head, and neck cancers. Low-risk genotypes typically result in benign or low-grade cervical lesions, as well as genital warts on various parts of the body, including the cervix, vagina, vulva, penis, scrotum, and anus [5,6].

The most effective means of preventing cervical cancer (cc) is using anti-HPV vaccines. Vaccines protect primarily by stimulating antibody production by the immune system. HPV vaccines use virus-like particles (VLPs) that contain elements from the HPV virus's surface. VLPs do not have viral DNA; therefore, they are not infectious or carcinogenic but closely resemble the natural virus. Antibodies that respond to VLPs also provide immunity against the virus [7,8].

Currently, there are three HPV prophylactic vaccines available commercially in Europe: Gardasil®4 (quadrivalent vaccine against HPV 16, 18, 6, and 11; available from 2006), Cervarix™ (bivalent vaccine against HPV 16 and 18; approved by the EMA in 2007 and FDA in 2009), and Gardasil®9 (nonavalent vaccine against HPV 6, 11, 16, 18, 31, 33, 45, 52, and 58; available from 2014) [9]. Recommended vaccination schedules include two doses for boys and girls between 9 and 14 and three doses for those 15 years or older. The decision about which type of vaccine to use should be made on an individual basis [9,10]. However, in April 2020, the WHO Strategic Advisory Group of Experts on Immunization (SAGE) reviewed evidence indicating that one- or two-dose schedules are as effective as three. The WHO's recommendations will be revised after receiving feedback from all the stakeholders [11].

Anti-HPV vaccines have been shown to decrease the risk of HPV-associated lesions, including cervical intraepithelial neoplasia (CIN), genital warts, anal neoplasia, and recurrent respiratory papillomatosis (RRP); they are often used to lower the chance of disease recurrence [12,13]. There is also evidence that they reduce the risk of the recurrence of high-grade squamous intraepithelial lesions (CIN2+, which means HSIL—CIN 2 + CIN 3 + small invasive cervical cancer), especially in cases involving HPV16 or HPV18, in women who have undergone local excision by administering the vaccine after treatment [14,15].

Research has presented substantial proof that anti-HPV vaccines have played a crucial role in decreasing the incidence of cervical cancer as a significant health concern [16]. By 2030, the World Health Organization aims to ensure that 90% of girls are fully vaccinated by the time they reach the age of 15. Cervical cancer affects many women, with around 570,000 cases and 311,000 deaths occurring yearly. This disease is particularly prevalent in low- and lower-middle-income countries, making it difficult to eliminate [17,18]. Australia is a prime example of a country implementing a nationwide HPV vaccination program, as it did so in 2007 for girls and five years later for boys. As a result, Australia is on a path to eradicate cervical cancer in the next 20 years, with fewer than four new cases per 100,000 women each year by 2028. Other high-income countries that have successfully reduced the number of HPV-related cancers are the United Kingdom, New Zealand, and Sweden [19–21]. Vaccine hesitancy remains a significant issue in European countries despite the implementation of various programs. Developing informational campaigns and encouraging healthcare professionals to be open to listening and discussing vaccine concerns with patients is crucial [22,23].

This study aims to compare fundamental understanding and viewpoints regarding HPV and anti-HPV vaccines among Polish students pursuing medical and non-medical sciences. We aim to identify the differences in knowledge and opinions between the two groups and genders. The findings from this study can shed light on any gaps in knowledge and highlight the need for modifying the approach to educating and disseminating information within the academic setting.

2. Materials and Methods

2.1. Study Design and Participants

The study was carried out between 1 June and 31 July 2023. The Bioethics Committee approved it at the Poznań University of Medical Sciences (540/22), and the survey was based on the authors' questionnaire. In the study, 1025 students (655 women, 361 men, and 9 participants who did not state their gender) at Polish universities completed the questionnaire voluntarily. Participants were divided into two groups: medical sciences students—520 respondents in total; and non-medical sciences students—505 respondents.

This study originally included 1033 students, but all the questionnaires that were completed incorrectly or contained incomplete data were eliminated from the study and were not included in the statistical analysis.

2.2. Questionnaire

A questionnaire was designed specifically for this study by the authors. The survey consisted of 28 questions: 24 were closed, comprising 20 single-choice questions and 4 multiple-choice questions, 4 were semi-open, comprising 2 single-choice questions and 2 multiple-choice questions; 3 were open. The first part of the questionnaire included questions about gender, age, the city of the study, the name of the university, and a question differentiating medical and non-medical sciences students. The second part of the questionnaire consisted of questions referring to the student's knowledge about HPV and HPV vaccination and their vaccination status. The last part of the questionnaire included questions about public health associated with HPV vaccination.

The survey was sent via Google Forms and shared on social media and fora at various universities in Poland. In the introduction to the questionnaire, the respondents were assured that their participation in the survey was completely voluntary and that it was anonymous. If the respondents indicated permanent contraindications to vaccination, the following were considered: an anaphylactic reaction to a previous dose or an allergy to any part of the vaccine.

2.3. Statistical Analysis

Statistical analysis was developed using R software (version R4.1.2). The characteristics of the responses to individual categorical questions were summarized with regard to their number and percentage share in the group. To characterize the age of the responders, we used basic descriptive statistics (mean, standard deviation, median, interquartile range, minimum value, and maximum value). Comparisons between medical students and other respondents were made using Pearson's Chi-square test or Fisher's exact test, depending on the condition of the expected number of observations. All the statistical calculations assumed $\alpha = 0.05$.

3. Results

In the survey, 1025 volunteers participated, of whom 655 (63.9%) were women and 361 (35.2%) were men. Nine subjects did not want to disclose their gender. The demographic data of the respondents are presented in Table 1. Half of the respondents were students at medical universities (50.7%), and the rest were students at other non-medical universities in Poland (49.3%).

When asked about the possible transmission of infection with human papillomavirus, 972/1025 (94.8%) unanimously answered that it was sexual. Less than half of the respondents knew that HPV can cause cancer of the oropharynx or anal cancer (47.9% and 43.8%, respectively). Regarding knowledge about prophylaxis, 853 subjects—which is 83.2% of the study group—had heard of HPV vaccination. To the question "What HPV vaccination is recommended?", 33.7% answered "I do not know", and 16.8% did not respond. Out of all the respondents, 314 (30.6%) declared that they were vaccinated against HPV, 539 (52.6%) said they were not vaccinated, and 172 people did not answer. Arguments supporting the decision not to vaccinate and their percentage distribution (multiple answers possible) are presented in Table 2.

Table 3 presents the respondents' answers divided into fields of study—medical and non-medical. To the question, "How many types of HPV are there?", 57.5% of the medical group answered that there were about 200 types, and another 24.8% answered that there were a dozen, which is a significant difference ($p < 0.001$) compared to the non-medical group (10.7% and 16.2%, respectively). To the question "What is the route of HPV transmission?", both groups most often marked the answer "sexual"—97.7% from the medical group and 91.9% from the non-medical group ($p < 0.001$). Significantly more often, people from the non-medical group also marked the answer "by blood"—38% compared to 22.7% from the medical group. Statistical significance also concerned vertical transmission during labor and droplet transmission.

Table 1. Characteristics of the study group.

Question	n/Mean (SD)	% of the Group/Median (IQR)	Range
N	1025	100.0	-
gender			
woman	655	63.9	-
man	361	35.2	-
do not want to specify	9	0.9	-
Age, years	22.43 ± 2.62	22.00 (21.00; 23.00)	18.00–44.00
medical student			
yes	520	50.7	-
no	505	49.3	-
onset of intercourse			
yes	652	63.6	-
no	219	21.4	-
do not want to answer	154	15.0	-
age of onset of intercourse, years *	18.17 ± 2.07	18.00 (17.00; 19.00)	12.00–25.00

SD is the standard deviation, and IQR is the interquartile range. * n = 652.

Table 2. Vaccination against HPV in the study group.

Question	n	% of the Group
Are you vaccinated against HPV?		
Yes	314	30.6
No	539	52.6
Lack of an answer	172	16.8
If not, why? *		
Lack of knowledge	225	41.7
Lack of financial opportunities	157	29.1
Parents' unwillingness	115	21.3
No vaccine available	106	19.7
Permanent contradictions to HPV vaccination	6	1.1
Other	92	17.1

* n = 539. The total exceeded 100% due to the possibility of selecting more than one answer.

According to the results, medical students' knowledge about the consequences of HPV infection was significantly greater. Almost the entire medical group (98.8%) marked the answer "cervical cancer", whereas 70.3% ($p < 0.001$) marked this answer in the non-medical group. Indeed, fewer non-medical students marked the answer "oropharyngeal cancer"—22.2% (non-medical group) vs. 72.9% (medical group)—or "anal cancer"—21.6% (non-medical group) vs. 65.4% (medical group). Despite significant differences in the results among the groups, the low awareness of the medical group about the consequences of persistent, long-term infection with oncogenic HPV genotypes is noteworthy. In the medical group, 74.2% answered "condylomas", 40%—"smelly discharge, pelvic pain", 39.8%—"bleeding after intercourse", and 37.1%—"hoarseness, cough". Knowledge about the possibility of preventing primary infection varied significantly between the groups of the respondents (91.7% of the medical group believed it was preventable, whereas 68.5% of the non-medical group believed it was preventable). Responses about the cervical cancer prevention program in Poland (85.5% vs. 61.6%) and HPV vaccination (98.3% vs. 67.7%) were similar. Of noteworthy interest is the high percentage of responses among medical students regarding the value of vaccination after starting intercourse (84.4%) and recommending vaccination in men (79.2%). The question "Do you find vaccination against HPV safe?" shows a significant gap in social consciousness. Only half of the non-medical student group agreed with this notion (50.3%), and 91.9% of the medical student group supported it ($p < 0.001$). One should also pay attention to the low rates of vaccination among Polish young people—only 38.7% of the medical students were vaccinated, and the percentage was 22.4% in the non-medical group. The answer to the question "Do you recommend HPV vaccination for your loved ones and/or children in the future?" divided the study group—91.5% of the medical ones recommended it, and in the non-medical group—only 50.3% recommended it.

Table 3. Comparison of answers regarding HPV vaccinations between the medical and non-medical groups.

Question	Group		p
	Medical (n = 520)	Non-Medical (n = 505)	
How many HPV genotypes are there?			
Several	33 (6.3)	72 (14.3)	<0.001
10–20	129 (24.8)	54 (10.7)	
About 200	299 (57.5)	82 (16.2)	
Do not know	59 (11.3)	297 (58.8)	
What is the route of HPV transmission? *			
Sexual	508 (97.7)	464 (91.9)	<0.001
By blood	118 (22.7)	192 (38.0)	<0.001
By saliva	101 (19.4)	127 (25.1)	0.033
Vertical (during labor)	141 (27.1)	72 (14.3)	<0.001
Droplets	23 (4.4)	94 (18.6)	<0.001
It does not spread between people	2 (0.4)	4 (0.8)	0.445 [1]
What are the consequences of HPV infection? *			
Cervical cancer	514 (98.8)	355 (70.3)	<0.001
Oropharyngeal cancer	379 (72.9)	112 (22.2)	<0.001
Anal cancer	340 (65.4)	109 (21.6)	<0.001
No consequences	1 (0.2)	2 (0.4)	0.619 [1]
Do not know	6 (1.2)	152 (30.1)	<0.001
What are the consequences of persistent infection with oncogenic HPV genotypes? *			
Anogenital precancerous lesions	476 (91.5)	240 (47.5)	<0.001
Condylomas	386 (74.2)	211 (41.8)	<0.001
Smelly discharge, pelvic pain	208 (40.0)	92 (18.2)	<0.001
Bleeding after intercourse	207 (39.8)	70 (13.9)	<0.001
Hoarseness, cough	193 (37.1)	34 (6.7)	<0.001
No symptoms	5 (1.0)	7 (1.4)	0.733
Do not know	28 (5.4)	213 (42.2)	<0.001
Can primary HPV infection be prevented?			
Yes	477 (91.7)	346 (68.5)	<0.001
No	11 (2.1)	19 (3.8)	
Do not know	32 (6.2)	140 (27.7)	
Is there a cervical cancer prevention program in Poland?			
Yes	444 (85.4)	311 (61.6)	<0.001
No	27 (5.2)	25 (5.0)	
Do not know	49 (9.4)	169 (33.5)	
Have you ever heard about vaccination against HPV?			
Yes	511 (98.3)	342 (67.7)	<0.001
No	9 (1.7)	163 (32.3)	

Table 3. Cont.

Question	Group		p
	Medical (n = 520)	Non-Medical (n = 505)	
If so, where?			
Social media	58 (11.2)	100 (19.8)	
During studies	149 (28.7)	0 (0.0)	
From family	85 (16.3)	55 (10.9)	
I obtained information on my own	75 (14.4)	53 (10.5)	<0.001
From the school's teacher	58 (11.2)	58 (11.5)	
From a doctor	35 (6.7)	38 (7.5)	
From peers	35 (6.7)	31 (6.1)	
Other	16 (3.1)	7 (1.4)	
No answer	9 (1.7)	163 (32.3)	-
What is the recommended age for HPV vaccination as a primary prevention?			
0–8 (2-doses schedule)	20 (3.8)	2 (0.4)	
9–14 (2-doses schedule)	379 (72.9)	167 (33.1)	
15–20 (3-doses schedule)	75 (14.4)	70 (13.9)	<0.001
over 20 (3-doses schedule)	1 (0.2)	5 (1.0)	
Do not know	36 (6.9)	98 (19.4)	
No answer	9 (1.7)	163 (32.3)	-
Is it worth getting vaccinated after starting sexual intercourse or in an HPV-positive population?			
Yes	439 (84.4)	211 (41.8)	
No	21 (4.0)	13 (2.6)	
Do not know	43 (8.3)	98 (19.4)	<0.001
No opinion	8 (1.5)	20 (4.0)	
No answer	9 (1.7)	163 (32.3)	-
Is HPV vaccination recommended for men?			
Yes	412 (79.2)	159 (31.5)	
No	25 (4.8)	29 (5.7)	<0.001
Do not know	74 (14.2)	154 (30.5)	
No answer	9 (1.7)	163 (32.3)	-
What are the contradictions to HPV vaccination? *			
Allergic reaction (including anaphylaxis) to any component of the vaccine	453 (87.1)	199 (39.4)	<0.001
Allergic reaction (including anaphylaxis) after the first dose of the vaccine	432 (83.1)	148 (29.3)	<0.001
High temperature	374 (71.9)	119 (23.6)	<0.001
Exacerbation of a chronic disease	312 (60.0)	82 (16.2)	<0.001
Pregnancy	181 (34.8)	133 (26.3)	0.004
Breastfeeding	120 (23.1)	97 (19.2)	0.150
No contradictions	6 (1.2)	3 (0.6)	0.506 [1]
Do not know	37 (7.1)	126 (25.0)	<0.001
Are you vaccinated against HPV?			
Yes	201 (38.7)	113 (22.4)	
No	310 (59.6)	229 (45.3)	0.073
No answer	9 (1.7)	163 (32.3)	-
If not, why? *			
Lack of knowledge	105 (20.2)	120 (23.8)	<0.001
Lack of financial opportunities	105 (20.2)	52 (10.3)	0.006
Parents' unwillingness	79 (15.2)	36 (7.1)	0.009
No vaccine available	72 (13.8)	34 (6.7)	0.021
Persistent contradictions to HPV vaccination	1 (0.2)	5 (1.0)	0.088 [1]
Other	51 (9.8)	41 (8.1)	0.744

Table 3. Cont.

Question	Group		p
	Medical (n = 520)	Non-Medical (n = 505)	
Do you plan to vaccinate against HPV in the future?			
Yes	164 (31.5)	74 (14.7)	
No	49 (9.4)	36 (7.1)	<0.001
Do not know	97 (18.7)	119 (23.6)	
No answer	210 (40.4)	276 (54.7)	-
If not, why? *			
No need	37 (7.1)	28 (5.5)	>0.999
No financial opportunities	6 (1.2)	4 (0.8)	>0.999 [1]
Scared of side effects	1 (0.2)	9 (1.8)	0.002 [1]
No vaccine available	5 (1.0)	0 (0.0)	0.070 [1]
Persistent contradictions to HPV vaccination	0 (0.0)	3 (0.6)	0.072 [1]
Other	6 (1.2)	2 (0.4)	0.458 [1]
Do you find vaccination against HPV safe?			
Yes	478 (91.9)	254 (50.3)	
No	4 (0.8)	10 (2.0)	<0.001
No opinion	29 (5.6)	78 (15.4)	
No answer	9 (1.7)	163 (32.3)	-
Do you think information about vaccines against HPV should be better communicated among young people?			
Yes	493 (94.8)	324 (64.2)	
No	6 (1.2)	0 (0.0)	0.011 [1]
No opinion	12 (2.3)	18 (3.6)	
No answer	9 (1.7)	163 (32.3)	-
Do you think the introduction of vaccination programs against HPV is important for fighting HPV-related lesions?			
Yes	505 (97.1)	324 (64.2)	
No	3 (0.6)	4 (0.8)	0.001 [1]
No opinion	3 (0.6)	14 (2.8)	
No answer	9 (1.7)	163 (32.3)	-
Do you recommend vaccination against HPV to your loved ones and future children?			
Yes	476 (91.5)	254 (50.3)	
No	5 (1.0)	6 (1.2)	
Do not know	19 (3.7)	50 (9.9)	<0.001
No opinion	11 (2.1)	32 (6.3)	
No answer	9 (1.7)	163 (32.3)	-

Data are presented as a number of observations (% of the group). Comparisons between medical students and other respondents were made using the Pearson Chi-square test or Fisher's exact test [1]. * The total exceeded 100% due to the possibility of selecting more than one answer.

4. Discussion

Our study compared the fundamental understanding and viewpoints regarding HPV and vaccines against HPV among two groups of Polish students studying medical and non-medical sciences. We aimed to identify the differences in knowledge and opinions between the groups. The findings from this study can shed light on any gaps in knowledge and highlight the need for modifying the approach to educating and disseminating information within an academic setting.

The answers provided highlight the need to conduct social and promotional campaigns addressed to young adults. This is because this is the age group both starting sexual activity and being the most active in this regard, thus being the most exposed to fresh HPV infections. The respondents also stressed the need to better communicate information about HPV vaccination among young people. They believed that the introduction of a cervical cancer prevention program was an essential element in the fight against HPV-related diseases. Perhaps greater social awareness, not only among groups related to medical professions, could contribute to a greater willingness to vaccinate oneself, one's children, and other family members in the future. It is for this reason that we emphasize the value of social campaigns addressed to people caring for children—parents, teachers, and tutors.

So far, there had been numerous publications describing the knowledge of particular social, gender, parental, etc. groups about vaccination, but the knowledge of students at different universities—medical and other—had not been compared prior.

Bednarczyk R., in his study, attempted to explain five myths about HPV vaccination and explain why there was such a low level of knowledge in society in general. He highlighted the fact that, five years ago, the utilization rates for a single dose of the HPV vaccine and the completion of the HPV vaccine series were 66% and 49%, respectively. This contrasts with the adoption rates of the tetanus, diphtheria, and acellular pertussis vaccines (89%) as well as the quadrivalent meningococcal conjugate vaccine (85%). Five prevalent misconceptions were addressed, including the beliefs that HPV vaccination lacked effectiveness in preventing cancer, Pap smears alone were adequate for cervical cancer prevention, HPV vaccination posed safety concerns, HPV vaccination was unnecessary because the immune system naturally clears most infections, and vaccinating at 11–12 years of age was too early [24].

The results of this review from 2020 were worse than the results we received. Still, they showed the factors that conditioned disproportions in knowledge about HPV and the willingness to get vaccinated. This study's findings indicate a lack of comprehensive adolescent knowledge regarding HPV and its preventive vaccine. Adolescents tend to underestimate their susceptibility to HPV infections. To enhance their understanding of HPV and its implications, researchers suggest that information be disseminated through compulsory schooling, primary healthcare channels, and the creation of interactive and informative interventions. The limited understanding and perceived vulnerability observed among adolescents towards HPV infection and related illnesses underscore the urgency of a well-crafted training program aimed at bridging the information gap concerning the HPV virus and promoting the acceptance of the HPV vaccine [25]. A similar study was conducted by Zhang et al. in the Chinese population [26], and, two years ago, scientists from Poland presented the results of an extensive analysis conducted on the knowledge of medical and dental students. They found that 259 (24.41%) of the 1061 medical students were vaccinated against HPV. A notable enhancement in overall knowledge during the later years of education (4–6) was delineated in contrast to the early years (1–3).

Nevertheless, it was shown that, despite advancements in medical education, substantial knowledge gaps persist regarding the connection between HPV infection and HPV-related lesions. We also share these conclusions, although it is worth noting that the vaccination coverage of Polish students in medical schools increased from 24.4 to 38.7%, which is very optimistic [27]. Another interesting study worth mentioning is the testing of knowledge among people closely related to gynecology, including gynecology and obstetrics residents, and this study was undertaken via research conducted by the International Society for the Vulvovaginal Diseases (ISSVD) [28]. Such studies are not comparative among the populations studied but provide a picture of knowledge about rarer diseases. Among other similar studies, other interesting ones focus on knowledge about HPV—among nursing students from Turkey [29] and non-medical students from India or Alabama [30,31]. The former study (the cross-section study among nursing and midwifery students in Turkey) revealed that both nursing and midwifery students knew little about HPV, even when divided into groups. More considerable awareness was observed in midwifery students than in nursing. Additional analysis showed significantly higher knowledge in women than in men, which may probably be due to the belief that HPV-related diseases only affect women. In the past, it was believed that only girls should be vaccinated. However, current standards and increasing social awareness have contributed to an increase in the vaccination rate in society.

5. Conclusions

Many papers lead to the conclusion that the social awareness of HPV and HPV vaccinations is still insufficient. Even medical students, despite increased understanding of the HPV virus, have gaps in their knowledge. However, it is a source of pride that, compared to other analyses, young Polish adults emerge in a favorable light. There is still much to be done to educate and encourage preventive behavior in those not receiving primary prevention in early childhood. We emphasize the need to conduct information campaigns strictly targeting this age group, as well as the need for a more careful dissemination of knowledge by health providers.

Our study has several limitations: first, the data were collected quickly, and second, the analysis was performed using a researcher-designed questionnaire. The last limitation is that some of the questions might have been constructed in language that was too specialized for non-medical recipients.

Author Contributions: Conceptualization, D.P. and S.M.-K.; Methodology, D.P.; Software, S.M.-K.; Formal analysis, D.P., M.P., J.Ż. and S.M.-K.; Investigation, D.P., J.H. and S.D.; Resources, D.P. and M.P.; Data curation, D.P., S.M.-K., J.H. and S.D.; Writing—original draft, D.P., R.J., J.H. and S.D.; Writing—review and editing, D.P. and S.M.-K.; Visualization, S.M.-K.; Supervision, R.J. and J.Ż.; Project administration, D.P., S.M.-K. and M.P.; Funding acquisition, D.P. All authors have read and agreed to the published version of the manuscript.

Funding: This research received no external funding.

Institutional Review Board Statement: The study was conducted in accordance with the Declaration of Helsinki and approved by the Ethics Committee (540/22).

Informed Consent Statement: Informed consent was obtained from all subjects involved in the study.

Data Availability Statement: All the data are available from the corresponding author.

Conflicts of Interest: The authors declare no conflict of interest.

References

1. Sung, H.; Ferlay, J.; Siegel, R.L.; Laversanne, M.; Soerjomataram, I.; Jemal, A.; Bray, F. Global Cancer Statistics 2020: GLOBOCAN Estimates of Incidence and Mortality Worldwide for 36 Cancers in 185 Countries. *CA Cancer J. Clin.* **2021**, *71*, 209–249. [CrossRef] [PubMed]
2. Rosalik, K.; Tarney, C.; Han, J. Human Papilloma Virus Vaccination. *Viruses* **2021**, *13*, 1091. [CrossRef] [PubMed]
3. Williamson, A.L. Recent Developments in Human Papillomavirus (HPV) Vaccinology. *Viruses* **2023**, *15*, 1440. [CrossRef] [PubMed]
4. Mo, Y.; Ma, J.; Zhang, H.; Shen, J.; Chen, J.; Hong, J.; Xu, Y.; Qian, C. Prophylactic and Therapeutic HPV Vaccines: Current Scenario and Perspectives. *Front. Cell Infect. Microbiol.* **2022**, *12*, 909223. [CrossRef] [PubMed]
5. Nowakowski, A.; Jach, R.; Szenborn, L.; Bidzinski, M.; Jackowska, T.; Kotarski, J.; Mastalerz-Migas, A.; Nitsch-Osuch, A.; Pinkas, J.; Sawicki, W.; et al. Recommendations of the Polish Society of Gynaecologists and Obstetricians, Polish Paediatric Society, Polish Society of Family Medicine, Polish Society of Vaccinology, Polish Society of Oncological Gynaecology and Polish Society of Colposcopy and Pathophysiology of the Uterine Cervix on prophylactic vaccinations against infections with human papillomaviruses in Poland. *Ginekol. Pol.* **2022**, *94*, 759–767. [CrossRef]
6. Luria, L.; Cardoza-Favarato, G. Human Papillomavirus. In *StatPearls [Internet]*; StatPearls Publishing: Treasure Island, FL, USA, 2023. Available online: http://www.ncbi.nlm.nih.gov/books/NBK448132/ (accessed on 13 July 2023).
7. Yadav, R.; Zhai, L.; Tumban, E. Virus-like Particle-Based L2 Vaccines against HPVs: Where Are We Today? *Viruses* **2019**, *12*, 18. [CrossRef] [PubMed]
8. Ashique, S.; Hussain, A.; Fatima, N.; Altamimi, M.A. HPV pathogenesis, various types of vaccines, safety concern, prophylactic and therapeutic applications to control cervical cancer, and future perspective. *VirusDisease* **2023**, *34*, 172–190. [CrossRef] [PubMed]
9. Crosbie, E.J.; Kitchener, H.C. Cervarix–a Bivalent L1 Virus-Like Particle Vaccine for Prevention of Human Papillomavirus Type 16- and 18-Associated Cervical Cancer. *Expert Opin. Biol. Ther.* **2007**, *7*, 391–396. [CrossRef]
10. Dilley, S.; Miller, K.M.; Huh, W.K. Human papillomavirus vaccination: Ongoing challenges and future directions. *Gynecol. Oncol.* **2020**, *156*, 498–502. [CrossRef]
11. World Health Organization. One-dose Human Papillomavirus (HPV) vaccine offers solid protection against cervical cancer. *Saudi Med. J.* **2022**, *43*, 538.

12. Di Donato, V.; Caruso, G.; Bogani, G.; Cavallari, E.N.; Palaia, G.; Perniola, G.; Ralli, M.; Sorrenti, S.; Romeo, U.; Pernazza, A.; et al. HPV Vaccination after Primary Treatment of HPV-Related Disease across Different Organ Sites: A Multidisciplinary Comprehensive Review and Meta-Analysis. *Vaccines* **2022**, *10*, 239. [CrossRef] [PubMed]
13. Pruski, D.; Millert-Kalińska, S.; Łagiedo, M.; Sikora, J.; Jach, R.; Przybylski, M. Effect of HPV Vaccination on Virus Disappearance in Cervical Samples of a Cohort of HPV-Positive Polish Patients. *J. Clin. Med.* **2023**, *12*, 7592. [CrossRef]
14. Eriksen, D.O.; Jensen, P.T.; Schroll, J.B.; Hammer, A. Human papillomavirus vaccination in women undergoing excisional treatment for cervical intraepithelial neoplasia and subsequent risk of recurrence: A systematic review and meta-analysis. *Acta Obstet. Gynecol. Scand.* **2022**, *101*, 597–607. [CrossRef] [PubMed]
15. Kechagias, K.S.; Kalliala, I.; Bowden, S.J.; Athanasiou, A.; Paraskevaidi, M.; Paraskevaidis, E.; Dillner, J.; Nieminen, P.; Strander, B.; Sasieni, P.; et al. Role of human papillomavirus (HPV) vaccination on HPV infection and recurrence of HPV related disease after local surgical treatment: Systematic review and meta-analysis. *BMJ* **2022**, *378*, e070135. [CrossRef] [PubMed]
16. Drolet, M.; Bénard, É.; Pérez, N.; Brisson, M.; HPV Vaccination Impact Study Group. Population-level impact and herd effects following the introduction of human papillomavirus vaccination programmes: Updated systematic review and meta-analysis. *Lancet* **2019**, *394*, 497–509. [CrossRef] [PubMed]
17. Toh, Z.Q.; Russell, F.M.; Garland, S.M.; Mulholland, E.K.; Patton, G.; Licciardi, P.V. Human Papillomavirus Vaccination After COVID-19. *JNCI Cancer Spectr.* **2021**, *5*, pkab011. [CrossRef] [PubMed]
18. Hall, M.T.; Simms, K.T.; Lew, J.B.; Smith, M.A.; Brotherton, J.M.; Saville, M.; Frazer, I.H.; Canfell, K. The projected timeframe until cervical cancer elimination in Australia: A modelling study. *Lancet Public Health* **2019**, *4*, e19–e27. [CrossRef]
19. Innes, C.R.; Williman, J.A.; Simcock, B.J.; Hider, P.; Sage, M.; Dempster-Rivett, K.; Lawton, B.A.; Sykes, P.H. Impact of human papillomavirus vaccination on rates of abnormal cervical cytology and histology in young New Zealand women. *N. Z. Med. J.* **2020**, *133*, 72–84.
20. Du, J.; Åhrlund-Richter, A.; Näsman, A.; Dalianis, T. Human papilloma virus (HPV) prevalence upon HPV vaccination in Swedish youth: A review based on our findings 2008–2018, and perspectives on cancer prevention. *Arch. Gynecol. Obstet.* **2021**, *303*, 329–335. [CrossRef]
21. Bralsford, K.J.; Jamieson, E. Following Australia's lead to eradicate cervical cancer. *BMJ* **2019**, *366*, l4955. [CrossRef]
22. Gauna, F.; Verger, P.; Fressard, L.; Jardin, M.; Ward, J.K.; Peretti-Watel, P. Vaccine hesitancy about the HPV vaccine among French young women and their parents: A telephone survey. *BMC Public Health* **2023**, *23*, 628. [CrossRef] [PubMed]
23. Wemrell, M.; Gunnarsson, L. Attitudes Toward HPV Vaccination in Sweden: A Survey Study. *Front. Public Health* **2022**, *10*, 729497. [CrossRef] [PubMed]
24. Bednarczyk, R.A. Addressing HPV vaccine myths: Practical information for healthcare providers. *Hum. Vaccines Immunother.* **2019**, *15*, 1628–1638. [CrossRef]
25. Rebecca, R. Ortiz, Andrea Smith & Tamera Coyne-Beasley A systematic literature review to examine the potential for social media to impact HPV vaccine uptake and awareness, knowledge, and attitudes about HPV and HPV vaccination. *Hum. Vaccines Immunother.* **2019**, *15*, 1465–1475. [CrossRef]
26. Zhang, X.; Wang, Z.; Ren, Z.; Li, Z.; Ma, W.; Gao, X.; Zhang, R.; Qiao, Y. HPV vaccine acceptability and willingness-related factors among Chinese adolescents: A nationwide study. *Hum. Vaccines Immunother.* **2021**, *17*, 1025–1032. [CrossRef]
27. Milecki, T.; Michalak, M.; Milecki, J.; Michalak, M.; Kadziszewski, R.; Kuncman, Ł.; Jarzemski, P.; Milecki, P.; Antczak, A. Polish Medical Students' Knowledge Regarding Human Papillomavirus's Ways of Transmission, Risk of Cancer Development and Vaccination, and Their Intention to Recommend Vaccination. *Vaccines* **2021**, *9*, 776. [CrossRef]
28. Bevilacqua, F.; Selk, A.; Stockdale, C.; Vieira-Baptista, P.; Adedipe, T.; Bohl, T.; Marozio, L.; Borella, F.; Gallio, N.; Pollano, B.; et al. The International Society for the Study of Vulvovaginal Disease (ISSVD) Vulvar Awareness Day Campaign: Knowledge of Vulvovaginal Diseases Among Italian Obstetrics and Gynecology Residents. *J. Low Genit. Tract. Dis.* **2023**, ahead of print. [CrossRef]
29. Güllü, A. Examining HPV knowledge levels of midwifery and nursing undergraduate students: A cross-sectional study in Turkey. *Afr. J. Reprod. Health* **2023**, *27*, 101–109. [CrossRef]
30. Daniel, C.L.; McLendon, L.; Green, C.L.; Anderson, K.J.; Pierce, J.Y.; Perkins, A.; Beasley, M. HPV and HPV Vaccination Knowledge and Attitudes Among Medical Students in Alabama. *J. Cancer Educ.* **2021**, *36*, 168–177. [CrossRef]
31. Rashid, S.; Labani, S.; Das, B.C. Knowledge, Awareness and Attitude on HPV, HPV Vaccine and Cervical Cancer among the College Students in India. *PLoS ONE* **2016**, *11*, e0166713. [CrossRef]

Disclaimer/Publisher's Note: The statements, opinions and data contained in all publications are solely those of the individual author(s) and contributor(s) and not of MDPI and/or the editor(s). MDPI and/or the editor(s) disclaim responsibility for any injury to people or property resulting from any ideas, methods, instructions or products referred to in the content.

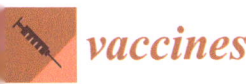

Systematic Review

School Teachers' Perceptions of Adolescent Human Papillomavirus (HPV) Vaccination: A Systematic Review

Jihye Choi [1,2,*], Efrat K. Gabay [2] and Paula M. Cuccaro [1,2]

1. Department of Health Promotion and Behavioral Sciences, School of Public Health, The University of Texas Health Science Center at Houston, 7000 Fannin St., Houston, TX 77030, USA; paula.m.cuccaro@uth.tmc.edu
2. Center for Health Promotion and Preventive Research, School of Public Health, The University of Texas Health Science Center at Houston, 7000 Fannin St., Houston, TX 77030, USA; efrat.k.gabay@uth.tmc.edu
* Correspondence: jihye.choi@uth.tmc.edu

Abstract: School nurses are uniquely positioned to educate students about immunizations, including human papillomavirus (HPV) vaccination, but schools are often without a nurse for different reasons. In lieu of nurses, teachers who closely interact with students and are traditionally well-trusted by parents may be able to communicate about HPV vaccination, alleviating parental vaccine hesitancy. This systematic review explores school teachers' perspectives on adolescent HPV vaccination and factors influencing their willingness to make vaccine recommendations. We searched three databases with appropriate medical subject headings and keywords to identify relevant studies. We reviewed fifteen studies and provided an extensive summary and a comparison of the results across the studies. Teachers had low to moderate levels of HPV knowledge with low self-efficacy to counsel parents about the HPV vaccine and expressed concerns about the vaccine condoning adolescent sexual activity, vaccine side effects, and parental disapproval. Nonetheless, some teachers showed interest in learning about vaccine effectiveness in preventing HPV-associated cancers and wanted guidance on vaccine communication with parents, viewing schools as adequate venues to promote and deliver HPV vaccines. Schools should consider educating teachers on HPV and HPV vaccination, with a focus on effective vaccine communication practices to increase adolescent HPV vaccine uptake.

Keywords: teachers; adolescents; HPV; vaccine; recommendations; attitudes

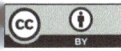

1. Introduction

Cancers associated with human papillomavirus (HPV) are vaccine-preventable, and near elimination of such cancers can be achieved with on-time, gender-neutral, HPV vaccination. Increasing evidence indicates that the HPV vaccine is safe and provides a more potent immune response for maximum protection if it is administered at ages 9 to 14 years, before sexual debut [1]. While some countries have achieved promising HPV vaccine coverage, such as Australia, where 80% of female adolescents and 77% of male adolescents have completed the vaccine series in 2022 [2], these rates continue to be suboptimal in many parts of the world. Globally, only about 17% of girls and 5% of boys were fully vaccinated against HPV, and 21% and 7% of girls and boys, respectively, received at least one dose in 2022 [2]. Low uptake of the HPV vaccine is primarily due to parents' lack of knowledge, negative perceptions of the vaccine, and lack of provider recommendation [3–5]. In addition to little understanding of the importance of the HPV vaccine, parents may have the misconception that vaccination equates with permission for early sexual initiation, skepticism around vaccine side effects, and low perceived risk of HPV, which is common among parents of boys due to the persistent overidentification of HPV with females [6].

Schools, where adolescents spend most of their time, are ideal settings for HPV vaccine promotion especially in those staffed with nurses. Bridging the health and education sectors, school nurses are uniquely positioned to improve adolescents' awareness and understanding of immunizations, including HPV vaccination [7]. School nurse efforts can help parents become well-informed before obtaining vaccination services for their children in clinical settings. However, an ongoing shortage of school nurses worldwide presents a potential gap in providing vaccine recommendations [8,9]. The next decade is likely to reveal a significant school nurse workforce shortage [10], with many countries already experiencing the absence of school nurses [11]. In lieu of school nurses, teachers who regularly and closely interact with students and are traditionally well-trusted by parents may be able to communicate about HPV vaccination to students and parents, thus improving their knowledge of the vaccine and alleviating parental vaccine hesitancy. Given the influential role of teachers, there is value in raising their awareness of the importance of the prophylactic HPV vaccine to facilitate effective vaccine communication in schools.

A plethora of previous research, including a recent review, has examined school nurses' knowledge and perceptions of adolescent HPV vaccination [12–17]. However, fewer studies have engaged school teachers and no review has been conducted to date on this topic. This systematic review aimed to explore the current literature on school teachers' perspectives on adolescent HPV vaccination and factors influencing teachers' willingness to make HPV vaccine recommendations to students and parents.

2. Methods

A systematic review was conducted and reported using the guidelines of the Preferred Reporting Items for Systematic Reviews and Meta-Analyses (PRISMA) 2020 checklist [18]. A detailed protocol for this review was registered a priori with PROSPERO (CRD42023429812), an international database of prospectively registered systematic reviews.

2.1. Search Strategy

We performed a literature search on three major electronic databases (PubMed, Embase, and Medline OVID) in July 2023. The search strategy comprised three categories of keywords: HPV vaccination, school teachers, and vaccine acceptance. The following medical subject heading (MeSH) terms along with relevant keywords or their variants were included in the advanced search process using the conjunction "AND" and the disjunction "OR": human papillomavirus, HPV vaccine, HPV vaccination, school teacher, teacher, school staff, knowledge, awareness, attitude, belief, perception, acceptability, intention, and refusal. Reference lists of eligible articles were also manually checked to retrieve other potentially relevant articles and all "related to" or similar articles of the identified articles were followed.

2.2. Inclusion and Exclusion Criteria

This review included peer-reviewed articles in the scientific literature that constituted original research. To understand recent research trends, articles had to be published within the last decade between 1 January 2013 and 30 June 2023, and the publication language was restricted to English. The review included articles that specifically reported on school teachers' and staff's knowledge and perceptions of adolescent HPV vaccination, willingness to recommend the vaccine to students and parents, and perspectives on HPV vaccine delivery or promotion in school settings. No restriction was placed on the type of school or geographic region. Articles were excluded from the review if they focused on only school nurses or teachers' HPV vaccination status and personal determinants of vaccination without any reference to their attitudes towards student vaccination. Articles were also excluded if they were systematic or scoping reviews, meta-analyses, project protocols, conference proceedings, briefing reports, or publications from non-indexed journals.

2.3. Selection Process and Data Synthesis

Upon obtaining the search results, all duplicated articles across the databases were removed using Endnote, followed by a manual verification. Titles and abstracts of the remaining articles were independently screened by the authors against the inclusion and exclusion criteria. Articles of the selected abstracts were retrieved and full-text reviewed. Articles were eliminated if their full-text versions were not available. Full-text reviewed articles that adhered to the eligibility criteria were included in the final synthesis and qualitatively analyzed. This qualitative analysis entailed an extensive summary of the eligible studies and a risk of bias assessment of their methodological quality, followed by a comparison of the results across the studies.

2.4. Quality Assessment

The methodological quality and risk of bias for the included studies were appraised using three validated instruments. The quality of the quantitative studies was assessed using the 7-item Joanna Briggs Institute (JBI) Critical Appraisal Checklist with three response options (yes, no, unclear) [19]. The qualitative studies were assessed on the level of risk of bias (i.e., low risk, high risk, or unclear) using the 10-item Critical Appraisal Skills Programme (CASP) Checklist [20]. The quality of the mixed-methods studies was assessed using the 5-item Mixed Methods Appraisal Tool (MMAT) with three response options (yes, no, can't tell) [21]. An overview of the three assessment tools is included in Supplementary Table S1.

3. Results

3.1. Search Results

The literature search and review process are shown in Figure 1. After the removal of duplicates within and across databases (Embase, Medline, and PubMed), titles and abstracts of 136 unique articles were screened to identify whether they adhered to the eligibility criteria and qualified for full-text review. We full-text reviewed 59 articles and excluded 44 articles for the following reasons: lack of focus on school teachers (n = 19), not focused on perceptions of adolescent HPV vaccination (n = 5), unavailability of full-text article (n = 2), focus on vaccination program evaluation (n = 14), narrative only (n = 2), and not peer-reviewed (n = 2). We selected a total of 15 studies published between 1 January 2013 and 30 June 2023 as the final set of records for the review. No additional eligible articles were identified.

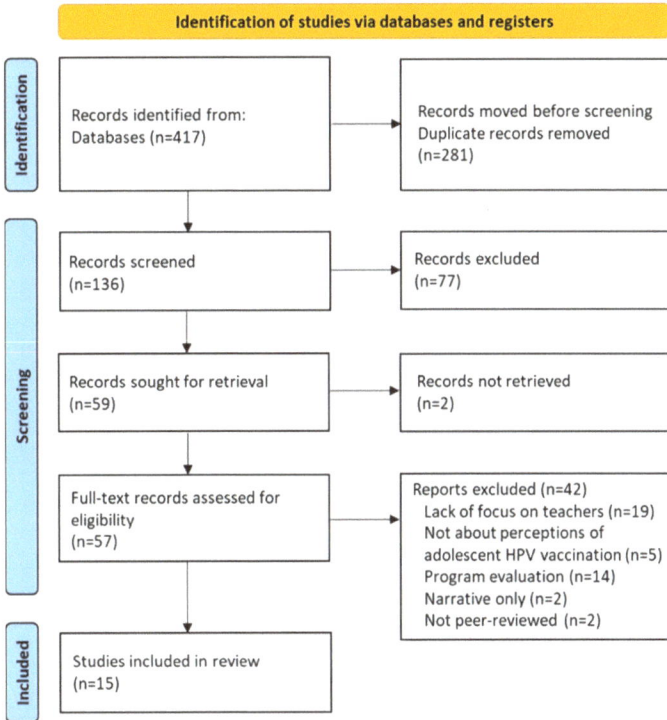

Figure 1. PRISMA flow diagram.

3.2. Study Characteristics

Table 1 shows the characteristics of the included studies [22–36]. Studies were conducted in various geographic settings: five studies from Asia (Hong Kong, Japan, the Republic of Korea, and Uzbekistan), two studies from North and South America (Canada and Peru), five studies from Africa (Kenya, Nigeria, and Tanzania), and three studies from Europe (France and Scotland). Five studies focused on teachers from elementary/primary schools, six studies involved teachers from secondary schools (middle or high schools), two studies included teachers from both primary and secondary schools, and two studies did not specify the type of school for their participants. Four studies specified the subject taught by the teachers. As for primary study outcomes, seven studies examined teachers' support for and acceptance of adolescent HPV vaccination, five studies assessed their willingness to communicate and recommend the HPV vaccine to students and parents, and three studies included both acceptance of and willingness to recommend the vaccine. Factors affecting these primary outcomes were categorized as either barriers or drivers of teachers' acceptance of adolescent HPV vaccination. Barriers were teachers' lack of HPV knowledge, negative vaccine attitudes (low perceived need for the HPV vaccine, distrust towards the HPV vaccine, and perceived burden of HPV vaccine promotion), and fear of parents' HPV vaccine disapproval. Drivers were teachers' perceived benefits of adolescent HPV vaccination, HPV awareness and desire for more HPV education, and perception of schools and teachers as important avenues for HPV vaccine promotion. Table 2 shows a detailed summary of each study.

Table 1. Characteristics of the included studies, 2013–2023 (n = 15).

Study Characteristics		n (%)
Region	Asia	5 (33.3%)
	North America	1 (6.7%)
	South America	1 (6.7%)
	Africa	5 (33.3%)
	Europe	3 (20.0%)
Region income level	High	7 (46.7%)
	Upper-middle	2 (13.3%)
	Lower-middle	6 (40.0%)
School level	Elementary/primary school	5 (33.3%)
	Secondary (middle/high) school	6 (40.0%)
	Both primary and secondary school	2 (13.3%)
	Not specified	2 (13.3%)
Teacher type	Health/Health Sciences	2 (13.3%)
	Sciences/Life Sciences	1 (6.7%)
	Arts and Math	1 (6.7%)
	Not specified	11 (73.3%)
Study design	Quantitative	6 (40.0%)
	Qualitative	6 (40.0%)
	Mixed methods	3 (20.0%)
Primary outcome measure	Acceptance of HPV vaccination	7 (46.7%)
	Willingness to recommend HPV vaccination	5 (33.3%)
	Both acceptance of and willingness to recommend HPV vaccination	3 (20.0%)

Table 2. Summary of the included studies.

Study	Aim	Country	Study Design and Size	School Level	Gender-Neutral HPV Vaccination ‡	Key Findings
High income region †						
Choi et al., 2013 [22]	To identify factors associated with Korean health teachers' intention to recommend the HPV vaccine	Republic of Korea	Quant N = 119	Elementary, Middle, High	No, female-only	Less than 12% of teachers reported having recommended HPV vaccination to students and parents. The mean score of the intention to recommend the HPV vaccine was 5.29 out of 10. Teachers had the highest intention to recommend the vaccine to high school students or their parents (6.12), followed by middle school students or their parents (5.32) and elementary school students or their parents (4.45). Teachers did not consider themselves responsible for promoting the vaccine due to having a heavy workload. *
Spratt et al., 2013 [23]	To examine secondary school teachers' views of their roles as partners in a school-based HPV vaccination program	Scotland	Qual N = 32	Secondary	Yes	Teachers were concerned about the impact of vaccination on students' current understanding of sex and sexuality. They showed unease that vaccination could potentially compromise childhood innocence. Some teachers feared negative publicity or parental complaints if they were seen to promote adolescent HPV vaccination. *
Rosberger et al., 2014 [24]	To explore the effect of a workshop intervention designed to provide the most up-to-date information among educators and counselors about their knowledge, attitudes, and beliefs about HPV and the HPV vaccine	Canada	Quant N = 37	Not stated	Yes	Most teachers knew that HPV is sexually transmitted (86.5%) and that the HPV vaccine prevents cervical cancer (83.8%). Teachers reported low levels of confidence (M = 2.8/7) in discussing HPV vaccination with parents. Willingness to recommend the HPV vaccine was not significantly associated with knowledge nor confidence in providing accurate HPV vaccine information. Common types of additional information requested were regarding HPV vaccination in males and the long-term side effects of the vaccine.

Table 2. Cont.

Study	Aim	Country	Study Design and Size	School Level	Gender-Neutral HPV Vaccination ‡	Key Findings
High income region †						
Kamada et al., 2018 [25]	To determine the ways to increase teachers' willingness to encourage the use of the HPV vaccine	Japan	Quant N = 247	Not stated	No, female-only	While 63% knew that the HPV vaccine prevents cervical cancer, 36% knew that HPV causes cervical cancer. Seventy-seven percent of the teachers feared vaccine side effects and 69% would not recommend the vaccine to their daughters and students. The information they most wanted was a proof of the HPV vaccine's preventive effect.
Ishiwada et al., 2020 [26]	To identify the current status, issues, and barriers regarding HPV vaccination among health science teachers	Japan	Quant N = 37	High	No, female-only	Teachers were initially uncertain (51.3%) and fearful (30.8%) about HPV vaccination. Teachers were significantly more inclined to recommend the HPV vaccine to students ($p < 0.05$) once they were more informed about HPV and became less fearful of HPV vaccine side effects.
Bocquier et al., 2023 [27]	To identify barriers, facilitators, and needs of the different school professionals involved in the implementation of HPV vaccination promotion interventions in French middle schools	France	Mixed N = 315	Middle (94% public schools, 5% private schools)	Yes	Eighty percent of teachers knew that HPV is sexually transmitted, but less than half knew that HPV can cause genital warts, and oral and cervical cancers. Seventy-six percent knew that the HPV vaccine protects against HPV-related cancers, and 56% knew that the vaccine is recommended for boys. Teachers had positive attitudes towards the benefits of HPV vaccination (mean score > 5 on a scale of 1–7). Teachers had mixed views about providing HPV education at school; focus groups agreed that offering HPV vaccination does not fall within the school's role. Perceived barriers included teachers' additional workload and fear of parents' negative reactions.

Table 2. Cont.

Study	Aim	Country	Study Design and Size	School Level	Gender-Neutral HPV Vaccination ‡	Key Findings
High income region †						
Ailloud et al., 2023 [28]	To evaluate knowledge, perceptions, beliefs, facilitators, and barriers to HPV vaccination among school staff from middle schools	France	Qual N = 14	Middle	Yes	Teachers lacked HPV knowledge and saw HPV as a women's issue. Teachers considered that children are too young to receive a sexually-related vaccine. HPV discussion in school was hindered because of sexuality being a taboo and a difficult topic for school staff. Some teachers believed that teachers are a legitimate means to conduct awareness sessions on HPV but felt burdened to do so at the same time. Teachers mentioned that the role of schools could be more important in transmitting information on HPV to students and parents.
Upper-middle income region †						
Siu et al., 2019 [29]	To investigate how school teachers in primary and secondary schools perceive HPV and HPV vaccines	Hong Kong	Qual N = 35	Primary, secondary	No, female-only	Teachers believed that cervical cancer protection and HPV vaccination were difficult concepts for their students who were too young to be considered vulnerable. Schools would oppose HPV vaccine promotion, and it was not prioritized compared to other health education topics (e.g., influenza). Teachers worried that HPV vaccine promotion could convey a negative message on sex attitudes. Parents' attitudes affected teachers' motivation. Without parental support, teachers could not justify school-based HPV vaccine promotion.
Llavall et al., 2021 [30]	To understand teachers' perceived barriers and facilitators to implementing HPV vaccination program, HPV knowledge and attitudes, and recommendations on strategies to increase vaccination rates	Peru	Qual N = 10	Primary	No, female-only	While teachers pointed out a necessity for their students to be protected against cervical cancer, there was distrust towards the HPV vaccine and fear generated in terms of harming adolescents' fertility. Teachers thought parents were not informed about HPV and the vaccine. Teachers also reported that parents rejected the vaccine because it would lead to sexual initiation among children. Teachers reported perceived parents' fear of serious side effects such as infertility.

Table 2. *Cont.*

Study	Aim	Country	Study Design and Size	School Level	Gender-Neutral HPV Vaccination ‡	Key Findings
High income region †						
Lower-middle income region †						
Ajah et al., 2015 [31]	To describe the knowledge and attitude of secondary school teachers towards HPV vaccination; to explore the feasibility of enlisting teachers towards promoting vaccine uptake	Nigeria	Quant N = 412	Middle, High	No, female-only	About 80% of teachers who were aware of cervical cancer knew that HPV caused cervical cancer. Among these, less than 40% knew the availability and benefits of the HPV vaccine, and 70% were willing to accept and recommend the vaccine to their daughters and students. Knowledge was significantly associated with HPV vaccine acceptability.
Masika et al., 2015 [32]	To assess primary school teachers' knowledge and acceptability of HPV vaccine	Kenya	Mixed N = 339	Primary (34 public schools, 3 private schools)	No, female-only	Teachers had low to moderate levels of knowledge about HPV and the HPV vaccine (mean score of 48%), especially men's susceptibility to HPV infection (mean score of 8%). However, vaccine acceptability was high (89%). One-third of all teachers indicated insufficient vaccine information and fear of vaccine side effects as the main barriers. Nearly all respondents (98%) expressed interest to know more about the HPV vaccine, and 93% supported school-based vaccine delivery.
Vermandere et al., 2015 [33]	To verify teachers' awareness of and support for HPV vaccination programs; to assess barriers in HPV vaccine promotion	Kenya	Qual N = 43	Not stated	No, female-only	When asked about causes of cervical cancer, HPV was rarely mentioned as a primary cause. Teachers showed distrust towards the HPV vaccine. While protecting a girl's fertility was a driver for HPV vaccine acceptance, the same vaccine generated fear in terms of harming the girl's fertility. At least three teachers described perceived parental fear that vaccination would enhance sexual activity among children. Some were keen to provide information and promote the vaccine given their daily contact with the children. *

Table 2. Cont.

Study	Aim	Country	Study Design and Size	School Level	Gender-Neutral HPV Vaccination ‡	Key Findings
High income region †						
Keehn et al., 2021 [34]	To assess primary school teachers as key informants when assessing barriers to parent acceptance of the HPV vaccine	Tanzania	Mixed N = 155	Primary	No, female-only	While 95% had heard of cervical cancer, only 37% and 29% of participants had heard of HPV and the HPV vaccine, respectively. Teachers from all seven schools included in this study mentioned parental lack of HPV knowledge as the main barrier but were willing to promote the vaccine to parents. Common questions from focus groups included: inquiries about vaccine side effects and why boys are not being vaccinated at this time.
Enebe et al., 2021 [35]	To determine the level of awareness, acceptability and uptake of HPV vaccine among female secondary school teachers	Nigeria	Quant N = 377	Secondary	No, female-only	Less than half (41.9%) of the teachers had high knowledge of cervical cancer, and 48.3% knew that HPV vaccination can prevent cervical cancer. Only 14.6% indicated having taught their students about cervical cancer or HPV vaccine. Acceptability was high among teachers who were aware of the vaccine, as the majority of teachers (93.6%) would recommend the vaccine to their children and students if the vaccine were given for free by the government.
Warsi et al., 2023 [36]	To understand barriers and drivers to general and HPV vaccination among key target groups (teachers) in Uzbekistan	Uzbekistan	Qual N = 32	Elementary	No, female-only	Teachers' vaccine hesitancy stemmed from knowledge gaps on vaccine safety. Few participants were aware of HPV, its relation to cervical cancer, and the HPV vaccine.* The primary anxieties of the teachers were any potential negative effects of the vaccine on students' future fertility. Teachers highlighted the need for clear and credible information on the safety of the HPV vaccine to be confident in their support for the vaccine.

† Source: The World Bank, using gross national income (GNI) per capita data in U.S. dollars, converted from local currency using the World Bank Atlas method. ‡Federal approval for gender-neutral HPV vaccination at the time of publication. * Data were not quantified.

3.3. Quality Assessment of the Included Studies

All six quantitative studies [22,24–26,31,35] provided a detailed description of their study setting and participants, measured variables of interest in a valid and reliable way, and used appropriate statistical analyses. Non-compliance to quality criteria for the quantitative studies was mostly due to limited or unclear reporting of confounding factors and how they were managed in the analysis. All six qualitative studies [23,28–30,33,36] stated the research aims, used appropriate qualitative methods, reported ethics approval, and clearly explained the value of their findings. Four studies [23,28,29,33] did not adequately address the recruitment strategy and had minor concerns about the small sample size, which may have incurred selection bias. Five studies [23,28,29,33,36] had unclear reporting of whether the relationship between the researcher and participants had been adequately considered during the interviews. All three mixed-methods studies [27,32,34] were compliant with the quality criteria except for the item regarding adequate rationale for using a mixed-methods design to address the research question (only one study [27] met this criterion). Overall, the included studies were relevant to the topic, presented their data and research findings coherently, and reflected on their methodological limitations. Figure 2 illustrates the quality assessment of the included studies in detail.

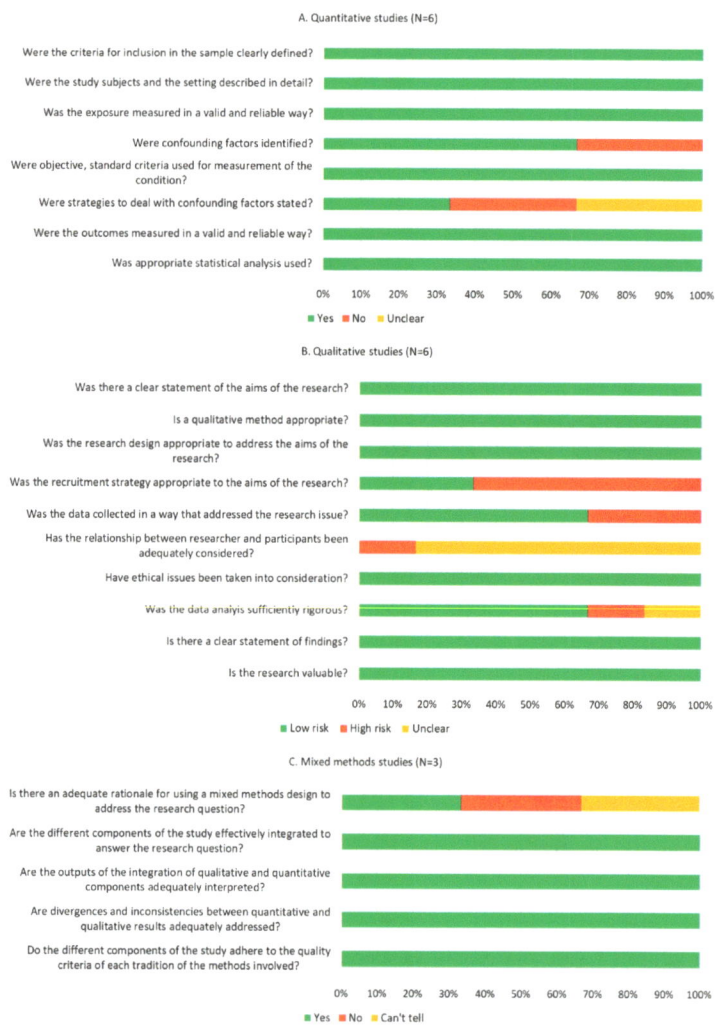

Figure 2. Quality assessment of the included studies.

3.4. Synthesis of Evidence

3.4.1. Lack of Knowledge

Ten studies [25,27–29,31–36] described teachers' overall lack of knowledge regarding the etiology of HPV-associated diseases, the availability of the HPV vaccine and its effectiveness in preventing HPV-associated cancers, and boys' eligibility for HPV vaccination. Less than 50% of primary, middle, and high school teachers in six studies conducted in Nigeria, Kenya, Japan, Tanzania, and France knew that HPV causes genital warts and cancer and had heard of the HPV vaccine and its benefits in preventing cervical cancer [25,27,31,32,34,35]. Less than 5% of teachers in Kenya knew that the vaccine can prevent vulvar and anal cancers in addition to cervical cancer [32], and 23% of teachers in a French study responded correctly that HPV can cause oral cancer [27]. In one qualitative study from Kenya, when teachers were asked about the causes of cervical cancer, HPV was rarely mentioned as a primary cause among many possibilities, such as not practicing self-hygiene [33]. Two qualitative studies from Hong Kong and Uzbekistan provided evidence that teachers across all school levels lacked knowledge regarding the HPV vaccine and who should receive it, as well as vaccine safety, which led to their vaccine hesitancy [29,36]. The disconnect between HPV risk and males was clear. For example, 8% and 71% of primary and middle school teachers in Kenya and France, respectively, answered correctly that HPV infects both men and women [27,32]. Another qualitative study of middle school teachers in France, a country that promoted gender-neutral HPV vaccination, reported that teachers regarded HPV as an infection concerning females and was irrelevant to males, commonly labeling the vaccine as the "cervical cancer vaccine" [28]. At least one teacher in each of the four focus group studies [27,28,32,34] questioned the importance or benefits of the HPV vaccine for boys. Lack of knowledge about HPV and HPV vaccination was observed among teachers regardless of the grade levels they served in a mix of high- and lower-income regions.

3.4.2. Negative Attitudes towards HPV Vaccines

Twelve studies reported on teachers' negative attitudes towards promoting HPV vaccination to their students [22–30,32,33,36]. Six studies from the Republic of Korea, Kenya, Hong Kong, and France delineated low perceived susceptibility to HPV as reasons for teachers' non-acceptance of HPV vaccination [22,27–29,32,33]. HPV vaccination was not prioritized compared to other health education topics, such as influenza vaccination, especially at the primary school level, based on the belief that students were too young to be considered vulnerable to sexually transmitted diseases [27–29,33]. The concept of preventing cervical cancer with a vaccine associated with risky sexual behavior was perceived to be superfluous and difficult to understand for young students. Teachers also demurred from providing younger students with "too much" information about sexual health [23]. Distrust towards the HPV vaccine was common among teachers who claimed that insufficient research has been conducted on the vaccine and who were concerned about vaccine side effects [25,26,30,32,33,36]. In two qualitative studies from Peru and Uzbekistan, primary school teachers believed that the HPV vaccine may harm girls' reproductive health and future fertility and would first wait to see how others fared before making HPV vaccine recommendations [30,36]. In another qualitative study from Kenya, in which the school level was not reported, teachers had mixed views pertaining to fertility; while protecting a girl's fertility was a driver for HPV vaccine acceptance, the same vaccine generated fear in terms of harming the girl's fertility [33]. Four studies from the Republic of Korea, Scotland, Kenya, and Hong Kong reported on teachers' concerns about seemingly condoning or encouraging adolescents' sexual promiscuity by promoting the vaccine [22,23,29,32]. They expressed discomfort that early HPV vaccination could potentially compromise students' childhood innocence and that students would misinterpret the vaccine as permission for premarital sexual initiation [23,29]. In one study conducted in France, sexuality being a cultural taboo made it difficult for school staff to discuss sexually transmitted infections in class [28]. Teachers from the Republic of Korea, Scotland, Kenya, France, and Uzbekistan were also reluctant to promote HPV-related prevention behaviors because they saw health and education as separate silos; across all school levels, HPV vaccine promotion was not considered teachers' responsibility but rather seen as a substantial burden added to their work [22,23,27,28,33,36].

3.4.3. Fear of Parents' HPV Vaccine Disapproval

Teachers identified anticipated negative reactions from parents as a significant barrier to discussing the HPV vaccine with parents due to its association with sexuality, which hindered teachers' willingness to make vaccine recommendations [23,24,27–30,33,34,36]. One qualitative study of primary and middle school teachers in Hong Kong articulated that parents are the predominant partners of schools according to the home-school-doctor model, and teachers could not justify HPV vaccine promotion in school settings without the support of parents [29]. Given the possible controversy around HPV vaccination, teachers across school levels from Scotland, Uzbekistan, and France feared parental complaints if they were seen to promote the vaccine and did not want to be held responsible by parents for any potentially adverse health outcomes in children due to vaccination [23,27,28,36]. Qualitative studies of primary and middle school teachers from Hong Kong and Peru found that parents' lack of knowledge and interest in HPV vaccination as well as their disapproval of the vaccine diminished teachers' self-efficacy and willingness to recommend the vaccine to students [29,30]. Teachers in a Canadian study also reported low levels of confidence (M = 2.8/7) in discussing HPV vaccination with parents of school-aged children [24]. Convincing parents to vaccinate their child against HPV was challenging for teachers if parents did not believe in scientific evidence for HPV vaccine efficacy and if teachers themselves did not have formal education about the vaccine. To that end, a qualitative study from Kenya found that parents' persistent mistaken beliefs that HPV vaccination encourages sexual initiation among young children dampened teachers' willingness to communicate about the vaccine [33]. Similar to the other barriers described in this review, teachers' fear of parental vaccine disapproval was documented in studies from regions with varying degrees of income levels.

3.4.4. Drivers of Teachers' Acceptance of Adolescent HPV Vaccination

Despite low HPV knowledge and skepticism towards the HPV vaccine—variables most dominant across the studies—teachers across school levels expressed interest in knowing about HPV and HPV vaccination before making vaccine recommendations. In seven studies from the Republic of Korea, Japan, Kenya, Tanzania, Canada, and France, teachers across varying school levels demonstrated positive attitudes towards HPV vaccine promotion as they sought more education about HPV and the vaccine, coupled with accurate and up-to-date information [22,24,25,28,32,34,36]. For example, 89.1% of Korean teachers expressed a desire to know more about HPV and the HPV vaccine [22]. The information that Canadian, Japanese, and Tanzanian teachers most wanted to obtain was about HPV vaccination in males, long-term vaccine side effects, and proof of the vaccine's preventive effect [24,25,34]. Two studies from Canada and Japan, in which HPV education was provided to teachers as part of their research, found that willingness to recommend the vaccine significantly improved following the educational intervention compared to their baseline results ($p < 0.05$) [24,26]. Knowing that parents place great trust in them, teachers were willing to take on a role in communicating with parents about the HPV vaccine. For example, two qualitative studies of primary school teachers from Peru and Uzbekistan requested guidance on effective communication with parents about HPV vaccination and cancer prevention [30,36]. Finally, in five studies from Kenya, Tanzania, Nigeria, and France, primary and middle school teachers acknowledged that schools are appropriate venues for the education, promotion, and delivery of HPV vaccination given their daily contact with children [27,28,33–35].

4. Discussion

The growing recognition of the global scarcity of school nurses has shed light on school teachers' potential to provide students and parents with HPV vaccine recommendations. This systematic review revealed that while there was an inclination to accept and promote adolescent HPV vaccination, teachers confronted predominantly barriers to making HPV vaccine recommendations. These barriers can be mitigated by implementing educational interventions and providing tailored vaccine communication training to increase teachers' HPV knowledge and self-efficacy for HPV vaccine communication.

The lack of knowledge about HPV and HPV vaccination among teachers is not surprising given that explicit vaccination education is not part of their employment mandate [37]. In the absence of school nurses in low-resource schools, however, teachers may be required to serve overlapping roles in the classroom as educators and health managers [38]. These circumstances indicate the need for teachers' increased access to health-related information, including HPV immunization. Previous research found that school staff were not aware of specifically the prevalence and age distribution of HPV infection [39]. Our results show teachers across school levels, especially those in African regions, have a limited understanding of the connection between HPV and noncervical HPV-associated cancers and the effectiveness of HPV vaccination. They seemed to heavily focus on the prevention of cervical cancer compared with other HPV-associated cancers, such as oral, anal, and oropharyngeal cancers. The mere focus on cervical cancer prevention in countries that have yet to adopt gender-neutral HPV vaccination may have hindered teachers from recognizing the necessity of vaccinating boys, despite the growing burden of noncervical HPV-associated cancers for males [40]. In fact, studies in this review were conducted in countries without gender-neutral HPV vaccination at the time of publication, except for Canada, France, and Scotland, although French teachers had little awareness of male eligibility for HPV vaccination [27,28]. School districts and healthcare providers should consider investing in concerted efforts to provide teachers with short, web-based continuing education to maximize reach and improve content knowledge [41]. This education should be designed to inform teachers about HPV consequences to increase the perceived severity of HPV and defeminize HPV by highlighting the importance of vaccinating all genders. Importantly, primary teachers from three different regions all worried that the HPV vaccine may harm fertility as its side effect [30,33,36], a concern often raised by caregivers [42]. Therefore, educators should prioritize providing accurate, evidence-based information pertaining to vaccine side effects to allay distrust towards HPV vaccine safety for teachers of younger children.

Health problems and risk-taking behavior such as unsafe sexual activity are associated with low scholastic performance in adolescents [43]. However, it was evident that teachers tend to perceive health and education as separate silos and that becoming embroiled in HPV vaccine promotion would equate to unwanted additional work. For example, two studies from France and Uzbekistan conveyed teachers' argument that HPV vaccine promotion should involve health workers and general practitioners, rather than school staff, in which case parents would be more receptive and consider vaccinating their children [27,36]. These perceptions deterred teachers' willingness to make vaccine recommendations. Additional professional development may be necessary to inculcate teachers with their role in helping students safely transition into adulthood, and the value in ensuring students' academic achievement as well as primary prevention practices. For teachers, recognizing themselves as influential figures in protecting adolescents from adverse behavioral outcomes may be a stronger priority predictor of making HPV vaccine recommendations than having HPV knowledge [15]. School-based vaccination is considered the most efficient means of reaching high vaccine coverage for adolescents, especially given reduced visits to healthcare providers as youth transition from childhood to adolescence [44]. As earlier studies have emphasized the effective use of schools for HPV vaccine programs in successfully adopting HPV vaccination in low-resource settings, our review also confirmed that teachers from various geographic regions, regardless of the grade levels they serve, view schools as an appropriate venue for the education, promotion, and delivery of HPV vaccines. Teachers' sensitization to HPV and adequate levels of commitment and engagement in school-based HPV vaccination programs are important facilitators of vaccine uptake among students [37,45].

Finally, we observed that teachers were less willing to recommend the HPV vaccine due to its association with sexually transmitted diseases and concerns about negative reactions from parents. Initiating conversations about HPV vaccination becomes even more difficult for teachers when parents are reluctant about the vaccine based on unverified assumptions. Teachers working in schools that implement school-based HPV vaccination programs have reported typically not feeling comfortable about the vaccine or promoting its use [46]. In another study, school staff appeared disinclined to accept adolescent HPV vaccination because of concerns about generating antagonism between parents and the school [47]. Although initial challenges may arise, enlisting school teachers can be a promising strategy to attenuate parents' vaccine hesitancy and promote the less-recognized HPV vaccine. Teachers' attitudes will be crucial, especially when discussing difficult subjects with parents [48]. In this review, almost half of the studies (46.7%) affirmed teachers' desires for additional HPV information and guidance on effective communication with parents regarding the vaccine, for which they had low self-confidence. A "train-the-trainer" approach may be a feasible option, where teachers are formally trained on how to deliver HPV vaccine recommendations and address caregivers' questions and concerns about vaccine safety using research-tested messages [49]. A recent US study on increasing adolescent HPV vaccination corroborated that healthcare providers' attendance in training on counseling hesitant parents was associated with increased motivation to routinely recommend the vaccine as well as increased positive vaccine attitudes and self-efficacy, which also led to a small increase in adolescents' vaccine uptake [50]. Other studies have noted that formal scientific training was associated with increased vaccine confidence among teachers [37,51]. These findings suggest that a public health partnership opportunity with teachers may be successful in increasing not only their vaccine confidence but also their self-efficacy for vaccine communication.

Strengths and Limitations

This review has a few limitations. First, we excluded studies that mainly discussed the design and implementation of school-based or community-based HPV vaccination programs, but such studies may have assessed vaccine attitudes of school staff. Second, imposing a restriction on the publication year may have limited inclusion of other relevant research conducted outside of the specified publication years. The rationale for choosing a ten-year window was to stay current with the growing HPV literature and shifts in HPV vaccination considerations regarding gender, schedules, and recommendations. Lastly, the findings of this review may not be applicable to private or religiously affiliated schools and schools in all countries, especially the US, as no study from the US was included. The significance of our review is that it provides insights into teachers' perceptions of adolescent HPV vaccination compared to other reviews that have focused on school nurses. Another strength is that this review presents data from low-, middle-, and high-income countries. Schools can refer to this review to prepare training that addresses teachers' concerns and equips them with the needed knowledge before implementing school-based HPV vaccination programs.

5. Conclusions

This systematic review highlights school teachers' perspectives on adolescent HPV vaccination and factors influencing their willingness to recommend the vaccine to students and parents. We observed that some teachers were cognizant of the importance of HPV vaccination and held positive vaccine attitudes. However, overall lack of HPV knowledge, skepticism of the HPV vaccine, and fear of disapproval from parents were substantial barriers to teachers' willingness to recommend the vaccine to students and parents. These findings suggest that schools, especially those without nurses, should seek opportunities to offer teachers education on HPV and HPV vaccination as well as formal training on HPV vaccine communication practices on the road to increased HPV vaccine uptake among adolescents, both females and males.

Supplementary Materials: The following supporting information can be downloaded at: https://www.mdpi.com/article/10.3390/vaccines12040361/s1, Table S1: Overview of the quality assessment tools.

Author Contributions: Conceptualization, J.C., E.K.G. and P.M.C.; methodology, J.C., E.K.G. and P.M.C.; formal analysis, J.C.; writing—original draft preparation, J.C.; writing—review and editing, J.C., E.K.G. and P.M.C. All authors have read and agreed to the published version of the manuscript.

Funding: This research did not receive any specific grant from funding agencies in the public, commercial, or not-for-profit sectors.

Institutional Review Board Statement: Not applicable.

Informed Consent Statement: Not applicable.

Data Availability Statement: No new data were created or analyzed in this study. Data sharing is not applicable to this article.

Conflicts of Interest: The authors declare no conflicts of interest.

References

1. Shapiro, G.K. HPV vaccination: An underused strategy for the prevention of cancer. *Curr. Oncol.* **2022**, *29*, 3780–3792. [CrossRef] [PubMed]
2. World Health Organization. Human Papillomavirus (HPV) Vaccination Coverage. 2022. Available online: https://immunizationdata.who.int/pages/coverage/hpv.html (accessed on 13 October 2023).
3. Hendry, M.; Lewis, R.; Clements, A.; Damery, S.; Wilkinson, C. "HPV? Never heard of it!": A systematic review of girls' and parents' information needs, views and preferences about human papillomavirus vaccination. *Vaccine* **2013**, *31*, 5152–5167. [CrossRef] [PubMed]
4. Ortiz, R.R.; Smith, A.; Coyne-Beasley, T. A systematic literature review to examine the potential for social media to impact HPV vaccine uptake and awareness, knowledge, and attitudes about HPV and HPV vaccination. *Hum. Vaccines Immunother.* **2019**, *15*, 1465–1475. [CrossRef] [PubMed]
5. Garbutt, J.; Wang, R.; Graham, S.; McKay, V.; Haire-Joshu, D.; Barker, A.; Liu, L. Provider and Practice Factors Associated With On-Time HPV Vaccination in Primary Care. *Acad. Pediatr.* **2023**, *23*, 800–807. [CrossRef] [PubMed]
6. Daley, E.M.; Vamos, C.A.; Thompson, E.L.; Zimet, G.D.; Rosberger, Z.; Merrell, L.; Kline, N.S. The feminization of HPV: How science, politics, economics and gender norms shaped US HPV vaccine implementation. *Papillomavirus Res.* **2017**, *3*, 142–148. [CrossRef] [PubMed]
7. White, L.S.; Maulucci, E.; Kornides, M.; Aryal, S.; Alix, C.; Sneider, D.; Gagnon, J.; Winfield, E.C.; Fontenot, H.B. HPV Vaccination Rates of 7th Grade Students After a Strong Recommending Statement from the School Nurse. *J. Sch. Nurs.* **2022**, 10598405221118824. [CrossRef] [PubMed]
8. Duffy, B.; Fotinatos, N.; Smith, A.; Burke, J. Puberty, health and sexual education in Australian regional primary schools: Year 5 and 6 teacher perceptions. *Sex Educ.* **2013**, *13*, 186–203. [CrossRef]
9. Galemore, C.A.; Marion, S.; Moran Fossile, K.; O'Toole, S.; Ragan, K.; Robertson, B. Leading during a pandemic: A school nurse administrator roundtable. *NASN Sch. Nurse* **2022**, *37*, 155–164. [CrossRef]
10. Galemore, C.; Alattar, H.Y.; Fatica, K.; Huey, A.; Schulz, K. Millennial school nurses: A roundtable discussion. *NASN Sch. Nurse* **2019**, *34*, 329–334. [CrossRef]
11. Szefler, S.J.; Fitzgerald, D.A.; Adachi, Y.; Doull, I.J.; Fischer, G.B.; Fletcher, M.; Hong, J.; García-Marcos, L.; Pedersen, S.; Østrem, A.; et al. A worldwide charter for all children with asthma. *Pediatr. Pulmonol.* **2020**, *55*, 1282–1292. [CrossRef]
12. Gottvall, M.; Tydén, T.; Larsson, M.; Stenhammar, C.; Höglund, A.T. Challenges and opportunities of a new HPV immunization program: Perceptions among Swedish school nurses. *Vaccine* **2011**, *29*, 4576–4583. [CrossRef] [PubMed]
13. Rosen, B.L.; Goodson, P.; Thompson, B.; Wilson, K.L. School nurses' knowledge, attitudes, perceptions of role as opinion leader, and professional practice regarding human papillomavirus vaccine for youth. *J. Sch. Health* **2015**, *85*, 73–81. [CrossRef] [PubMed]
14. Rosen, B.L.; Ashwood, D.; Richardson, G.B. School nurses' professional practice in the HPV vaccine decision-making process. *J. Sch. Nurs.* **2016**, *32*, 138–148. [CrossRef] [PubMed]
15. Rosen, B.L.; DiClemente, R.; Shepard, A.L.; Wilson, K.L.; Fehr, S.K. Factors associated with school nurses' HPV vaccine attitudes for school-aged youth. *Psychol. Health Med.* **2017**, *22*, 535–545. [CrossRef] [PubMed]

16. Grandahl, M.; Larsson, M.; Tydén, T.; Stenhammar, C. School nurses' attitudes towards and experiences of the Swedish school-based HPV vaccination programme–A repeated cross sectional study. *PLoS ONE* **2017**, *12*, e0175883. [CrossRef] [PubMed]
17. McNally, K.; Roess, A.; Weinstein, A.; Lindley, L.; Wallin, R. School Nurses' Experiences and Roles in Promoting and Administering the HPV Vaccine: A Systematic Review Using the Socioecological Framework. *J. Sch. Nurs.* **2023**, *40*, 43–57. [CrossRef] [PubMed]
18. Page, M.J.; McKenzie, J.E.; Bossuyt, P.M.; Boutron, I.; Hoffmann, T.C.; Mulrow, C.D.; Shamseer, L.; Tetzlaff, J.M.; Akl, E.A.; Brennan, S.E.; et al. The PRISMA 2020 statement: An updated guideline for reporting systematic reviews. *Int. J. Surg.* **2021**, *88*, 105906. [CrossRef] [PubMed]
19. The Joanna Briggs Institute. *JBI Critical Appraisal Checklist for Analytical cross Sectional Studies*; The Joanna Briggs Institute: Adelaide, Australia, 2016.
20. Long, H.A.; French, D.P.; Brooks, J.M. Optimising the value of the critical appraisal skills programme (CASP) tool for quality appraisal in qualitative evidence synthesis. *Res. Methods Med. Health Sci.* **2020**, *1*, 31–42. [CrossRef]
21. Hong, Q.N.; Fàbregues, S.; Bartlett, G.; Boardman, F.; Cargo, M.; Dagenais, P.; Gagnon, M.P.; Griffiths, F.; Nicolau, B.; O'Cathain, A.; et al. The Mixed Methods Appraisal Tool (MMAT) version 2018 for information professionals and researchers. *Educ. Inf.* **2018**, *34*, 285–291. [CrossRef]
22. Choi, K.B.; Mo, H.S.; Kim, J.S. Factors associated with the intention to recommend human papillomavirus vaccination among Korean school health teachers. *J. Spec. Pediatr. Nurs.* **2013**, *18*, 297–310. [CrossRef]
23. Spratt, J.; Shucksmith, J.; Philip, K.; McNaughton, R. Active agents of health promotion? The school's role in supporting the HPV vaccination programme. *Sex Educ.* **2013**, *13*, 82–95. [CrossRef]
24. Rosberger, Z.; Krawczyk, A.; Stephenson, E.; Lau, S. HPV vaccine education: Enhancing knowledge and attitudes of community counselors and educators. *J. Cancer Educ.* **2014**, *29*, 473–477. [CrossRef] [PubMed]
25. Kamada, M.; Inui, H.; Kagawa, T.; Mineda, A.; Tamura, T.; Fujioka, T.; Motoki, T.; Hirai, H.; Ishii, E.; Irahara, M. What information can change the attitude of teachers toward the human papillomavirus vaccine? *J. Obstet. Gynaecol. Res.* **2018**, *44*, 778–787. [CrossRef] [PubMed]
26. Ishiwada, N.; Suzuki, C.; Hasebe, S.; Tsuchiya, A.; Takeuchi, N.; Hishiki, H.; Sato, Y.; Sugita, K. The effects of health education on health science teachers' intention to recommend adolescent HPV vaccine for female students in Japan. *Hum. Vaccines Immunother.* **2020**, *16*, 2752–2757. [CrossRef] [PubMed]
27. Bocquier, A.; Branchereau, M.; Gauchet, A.; Bonnay, S.; Simon, M.; Ecollan, M.; Chevreul, K.; Mueller, J.E.; Gagneux-Brunon, A.; Thilly, N.; et al. Promoting HPV vaccination at school: A mixed methods study exploring knowledge, beliefs and attitudes of French school staff. *BMC Public Health* **2023**, *23*, 486. [CrossRef] [PubMed]
28. Ailloud, J.; Branchereau, M.; Fall, E.; Juneau, C.; Partouche, H.; Bonnay, S.; Oudin-Doglioni, D.; Michel, M.; Gagneux-Brunon, A.; Bruel, S.; et al. How can we improve the acceptability of vaccination against Human Papillomavirus (HPV) in France? An original qualitative study with focus groups comprising parents and school staff, interviewed separately. *Vaccine* **2023**, *41*, 4594–4608. [CrossRef] [PubMed]
29. Siu JY-m Lee, A.; Chan, P.K. Schoolteachers' experiences of implementing school-based vaccination programs against human papillomavirus in a Chinese community: A qualitative study. *BMC Public Health* **2019**, *19*, 1514.
30. Clave Llavall, A.; de Wildt, G.; Meza, G.; Tattsbridge, J.; Jones, L. Nurses' and teachers' perceived barriers and facilitators to the uptake of the Human Papilloma Virus (HPV) vaccination program in Iquitos, Peru: A qualitative study. *PLoS ONE* **2021**, *16*, e0255218. [CrossRef] [PubMed]
31. Ajah, L.; Iyoke, C.; Ezeonu, P.; Ugwu, G.; Onoh, R.; Ibo, C. Association between knowledge of cervical cancer/screening and attitude of teachers to immunization of adolescent girls with human papilloma virus vaccine in Abakaliki, Nigeria. *Am. J. Cancer Prev.* **2015**, *3*, 8–12.
32. Masika, M.M.; Ogembo, J.G.; Chabeda, S.V.; Wamai, R.G.; Mugo, N. Knowledge on HPV vaccine and cervical cancer facilitates vaccine acceptability among school teachers in Kitui County, Kenya. *PLoS ONE* **2015**, *10*, e0135563. [CrossRef]
33. Vermandere, H.; Naanyu, V.; Degomme, O.; Michielsen, K. Implementation of an HPV vaccination program in Eldoret, Kenya: Results from a qualitative assessment by key stakeholders. *BMC Public Health* **2015**, *15*, 875. [CrossRef] [PubMed]
34. Keehn, D.C.; Chamberlain, R.M.; Tibbits, M.; Kahesa, C.; Msami, K.; Soliman, A.S. Using key informants to evaluate barriers to education and acceptability of the HPV vaccine in Tanzania: Implications for cancer education. *J. Cancer Educ.* **2021**, *36*, 1333–1340. [CrossRef] [PubMed]
35. Enebe, J.T.; Enebe, N.O.; Agunwa, C.C.; Nduagubam, O.C.; Okafor, I.I.; Aniwada, E.C.; Aguwa, E.N. Awareness, acceptability and uptake of cervical cancer vaccination services among female secondary school teachers in enugu, nigeria: A cross-sectional study. *Pan Afr. Med. J.* **2021**, *39*, 62. [CrossRef] [PubMed]
36. Warsi, S.K.; Nielsen, S.M.; Franklin, B.A.; Abdullaev, S.; Ruzmetova, D.; Raimjanov, R.; Nagiyeva, K.; Safaeva, K. Formative Research on HPV Vaccine Acceptance among Health Workers, Teachers, Parents, and Social Influencers in Uzbekistan. *Vaccines* **2023**, *11*, 754. [CrossRef] [PubMed]
37. Racey, C.S.; Donken, R.; Fox, E.; Porter, I.; Bettinger, J.A.; Mark, J.; Bonifacio, L.; Dawar, M.; Gagel, M.; Kling, R.; et al. Characterization of vaccine confidence among teachers in British Columbia, Canada: A population-based survey. *PLoS ONE* **2023**, *18*, e0288107. [CrossRef] [PubMed]
38. Clay, D.L.; Cortina, S.; Harper, D.C.; Cocco, K.M.; Drotar, D. Schoolteachers' experiences with childhood chronic illness. *Child. Health Care* **2004**, *33*, 227–239. [CrossRef]

39. Reiter, P.L.; Stubbs, B.; Panozzo, C.A.; Whitesell, D.; Brewer, N.T. HPV and HPV vaccine education intervention: Effects on parents, healthcare staff, and school staff. *Cancer Epidemiol. Biomark. Prev.* **2011**, *20*, 2354–2361. [CrossRef] [PubMed]
40. Schmeler, K.M.; Sturgis, E.M. Expanding the benefits of HPV vaccination to boys and men. *Lancet* **2016**, *387*, 1798–1799. [CrossRef]
41. Rhodes, D.; Visker, J.D.; Cox, C.; Sas, A.; Banez, J.C. Effects of an online educational module on school nurses' knowledge of HPV vaccination. *J. Contin. Educ. Nurs.* **2017**, *48*, 431–436. [CrossRef]
42. Adeyanju, G.C.; Sprengholz, P.; Betsch, C.; Essoh, T.-A. Caregivers' willingness to vaccinate their children against childhood diseases and human papillomavirus: A cross-sectional study on vaccine hesitancy in Malawi. *Vaccines* **2021**, *9*, 1231. [CrossRef]
43. Knopf, J.A.; Finnie, R.K.; Peng, Y.; Hahn, R.A.; Truman, B.I.; Vernon-Smiley, M.; Johnson, V.C.; Johnson, R.L.; Fielding, J.E.; Muntañer, C., et al. School based health centers to advance health equity: A community guide systematic review. *Am. J. Prev. Med.* **2016**, *51*, 114–126. [CrossRef]
44. Davies, C.; Marshall, H.S.; Zimet, G.; McCaffery, K.; Brotherton, J.M.; Kang, M.; Garland, S.; Kaldor, J.; McGeechan, K.; Skinner, S.R.; et al. Effect of a School-Based Educational Intervention About the Human Papillomavirus Vaccine on Psychosocial Outcomes Among Adolescents: Analysis of Secondary Outcomes of a Cluster Randomized Trial. *JAMA Netw. Open* **2021**, *4*, e2129057. [CrossRef] [PubMed]
45. Batista Ferrer, H.; Trotter, C.L.; Hickman, M.; Audrey, S. Barriers and facilitators to uptake of the school-based HPV vaccination programme in an ethnically diverse group of young women. *J. Public Health* **2016**, *38*, 569–577. [CrossRef] [PubMed]
46. Dubé, E.; Gagnon, D.; Clément, P.; Bettinger, J.A.; Comeau, J.L.; Deeks, S.; Guay, M.; MacDonald, S.; MacDonald, N.E.; Mijovic, H.; et al. Challenges and opportunities of school-based HPV vaccination in Canada. *Hum. Vaccines Immunother.* **2019**, *15*, 1650–1655. [CrossRef] [PubMed]
47. Audrey, S.; Ferrer, H.B.; Ferrie, J.; Evans, K.; Bell, M.; Yates, J.; Roderick, M.; MacLeod, J.; Hickman, M. Impact and acceptability of self-consent procedures for the school-based human papillomavirus vaccine: A mixed-methods study protocol. *BMJ Open* **2018**, *8*, e021321. [CrossRef] [PubMed]
48. Leenders, H.; De Jong, J.; Monfrance, M.; Haelermans, C. Building strong parent–teacher relationships in primary education: The challenge of two-way communication. *Camb. J. Educ.* **2019**, *49*, 519–533. [CrossRef]
49. Ahmed, D.; VanderEnde, K.; Harvey, P.; Bhatnagar, P.; Kaur, N.; Roy, S.; Singh, N.; Denzongpa, P.; Haldar, P.; Loharikar, A. Human papillomavirus (HPV) vaccine introduction in Sikkim state: Best practices from the first statewide multiple-age cohort HPV vaccine introduction in India–2018–2019. *Vaccine* **2022**, *40*, A17–A25. [CrossRef]
50. Brewer, N.T.; Mitchell, C.G.; Dailey, S.A.; Hora, L.; Fisher-Borne, M.; Tichy, K.; McCoy, T. HPV vaccine communication training in healthcare systems: Evaluating a train-the-trainer model. *Vaccine* **2021**, *39*, 3731–3736. [CrossRef]
51. Frayon, S. New Caledonian biology teachers' opinions about vaccination: Preliminary findings. *Health Educ. J.* **2020**, *79*, 594–606. [CrossRef]

Disclaimer/Publisher's Note: The statements, opinions and data contained in all publications are solely those of the individual author(s) and contributor(s) and not of MDPI and/or the editor(s). MDPI and/or the editor(s) disclaim responsibility for any injury to people or property resulting from any ideas, methods, instructions or products referred to in the content.

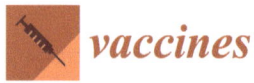

Article

"You Don't Know If It's the Truth or a Lie": Exploring Human Papillomavirus (HPV) Vaccine Hesitancy among Communities with Low HPV Vaccine Uptake in Northern California

Julie H. T. Dang [1,*], Alexandra Gori [2], Lucy Rios [3,4], Angelica M. Rolon [2], Jingwen Zhang [5] and Moon S. Chen, Jr. [3]

1. Division of Health Policy and Management, Department of Public Health Sciences, School of Medicine, University of California, Davis, CA 95816, USA
2. Comprehensive Cancer Center, University of California, Davis, CA 95816, USA; acgori@ucdavis.edu (A.G.); amiperez@ucdavis.edu (A.M.R.)
3. Division of Hematology and Oncology, Department of Internal Medicine, School of Medicine, University of California, Davis, CA 95817, USA; lucrios@ucdavis.edu (L.R.); mschenjr@ucdavis.edu (M.S.C.J.)
4. Department of Public Health Sciences, University of California, Davis, CA 95817, USA
5. Department of Communication, Department of Public Health Sciences, University of California, Davis, CA 95616, USA; jwzzhang@ucdavis.edu
* Correspondence: jtdang@ucdavis.edu; Tel.: +1-916-734-5222

Citation: Dang, J.H.T.; Gori, A.; Rios, L.; Rolon, A.M.; Zhang, J.; Chen, M.S., Jr. "You Don't Know If It's the Truth or a Lie": Exploring Human Papillomavirus (HPV) Vaccine Hesitancy among Communities with Low HPV Vaccine Uptake in Northern California. *Vaccines* **2024**, *12*, 372. https://doi.org/10.3390/vaccines12040372

Academic Editor: Francesco Vitale

Received: 26 February 2024
Revised: 25 March 2024
Accepted: 29 March 2024
Published: 1 April 2024

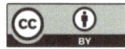

Copyright: © 2024 by the authors. Licensee MDPI, Basel, Switzerland. This article is an open access article distributed under the terms and conditions of the Creative Commons Attribution (CC BY) license (https://creativecommons.org/licenses/by/4.0/).

Abstract: Background: Vaccine hesitancy, delaying or refusing to vaccinate despite the availability of vaccines, impedes the progress of achieving optimal HPV vaccine coverage. Little is known about the sources of human papillomavirus (HPV) vaccine hesitancy among racially/ethnically and geographically diverse communities. The purpose of this paper is to explore HPV vaccine hesitancy among rural, Slavic, and Latino communities that reside in counties with low HPV vaccine uptake rates. Methods: Key informant interviews and focus groups were conducted with rural, Slavic, and Latino communities that reside within counties in California that have low HPV vaccine up to date rates (16–25%). Qualitative data were transcribed verbatim and analyzed using inductive and deductive thematic analysis. Results: A total of seven focus groups and 14 key informant interviews were conducted with 39 individuals from seven California counties. Salient themes that contributed to HPV vaccine hesitancy included the following: social media and the anti-vaccination movement; a strong belief in acquiring immunity naturally; prior vaccine experiences; and vaccine timing concerns. Participants suggested the provision of culturally appropriate, in-language, in-person easy to understand HPV vaccine education to mitigate HPV vaccine hesitancy. Conclusions: Our findings can inform future interventions to increase HPV vaccine uptake among hesitant communities.

Keywords: human papillomavirus (HPV) vaccine hesitancy; key informant interviews; focus groups; qualitative research; racially/ethnically diverse communities; rural

1. Introduction

The World Health Organization (WHO) considers vaccine hesitancy as one of the top threats to global health [1]. Vaccine hesitancy, defined as a "reluctance or refusal to vaccinate despite the availability of vaccines", impedes the progress of achieving optimal HPV vaccine coverage [2]. While vaccine hesitancy is not a new phenomenon, greater access to and more rapid dissemination of vaccine misinformation via social media and the Internet, coupled with a lower prevalence of vaccine-preventable diseases, an extensive childhood vaccination schedule, and rising public skepticism, have all contributed to human papillomavirus (HPV) vaccine hesitancy [3,4]. Since its introduction in 2006, the HPV vaccine has experienced public distrust and criticism [5,6]. This hesitancy has been attributed to a lack of confidence in the vaccine's safety, misinformation, perceived low risks of vaccine-preventable diseases, and perceptions that the vaccine does not work [3,7,8]. In recent years, deploying strategies to mitigate the effects of vaccine hesitancy has proven to be challenging, especially because of the COVID-19 pandemic. The pandemic created postponement of routine health care, including HPV vaccination [9], and ignited new vaccine hesitancies [10].

A study analyzing data from the CDC's National Immunization Survey (NIS)-Teen Survey from 2012 to 2018 found that despite a provider recommendation, 60.6% of unvaccinated adolescents had no intention to initiate the HPV vaccine series [11]. Over the six-year study period, parental reluctance to initiate the HPV vaccine series for girls increased from 54.1% to 60.1%, and for boys, parental reluctance for the vaccine rose from 44.4% to 59.2% [11]. Despite the HPV vaccine being a highly effective public health intervention, in 2022, only 62.6% of U.S adolescents aged 13–17 were up to date with HPV vaccine (UTD HPV) [12], which continues to remain below the Healthy People 2030 goal of 80% [13]. While HPV vaccination rates have begun to steadily increase, studies have reported disparities in HPV vaccination rates and in HPV-associated cancers among rural communities [14–16] and among racial and ethnic groups [17,18]. The goal of this paper is to investigate sources of HPV vaccine hesitancy among rural, Latino, and Slavic communities. Additionally, we sought to gain insight from these individuals on strategies and recommendations to improve HPV vaccine acceptance in their respective communities.

2. Materials and Methods

2.1. Study Sample and Recruitment

We recruited parents, health professionals, and community members from rural inland northern California counties with lower UTD HPV rates than the U.S. (16–25% compared to 62.6%) [12–19] and from Latino and Slavic communities located in the University of California, Davis Comprehensive Cancer Center's catchment area to participate in semi-structured focus groups and key informant interviews. We did not include the counties with the lowest HPV vaccination rates in the catchment area in this study as another study has been published that focused on those rural counties and Native American adolescents [20]. Participants were recruited from Nevada, Placer, Yolo, El Dorado, Sacramento, San Joaquin, and Merced Counties. Eligibility included being at least 18 years of age and residing or working in one of the above seven counties. We define rural as having a Rural-Urban Community Area Codes (RUCA) classification of 4–10 [21]. While all seven counties have RUCA zip codes that are designated as rural, for the purpose of our study, participants from Nevada and El Dorado Counties were considered rural. The majority of individuals who identify as Slavic are from countries located mostly in Eastern Europe and Western Asia and speak Polish, Russian, and Ukrainian. We purposively targeted Sacramento, Placer, and Yolo counties for Slavic participants as the majority reside there; and for Hispanic/Latino participants, we targeted the counties of San Joaquin and Merced. We utilized StudyPages, an online participant-facing platform, to recruit and register participants to the study [22]. Through flyers, listservs, outreach to past research participants, social media advertisement, engagement with community partners, and a media release, participants were directed to our StudyPages website to screen for study eligibility, register, provide language preference, and specify whether they wanted to participate in a focus group or interview. Eligible participants were contacted by the study team to coordinate a date and time.

As an alternative to StudyPages, the participants were also provided with the study team's phone number and email for direct contact. Focus groups and interviews were conducted during the period of February 2021 to September 2021. Verbal informed consent from each participant was obtained at the beginning of each session and the participants received a USD 20 gift card for their time. Data collection continued until saturation was reached with no new themes emerging from additional interviews and or focus groups. Focus groups and interviews lasted between 30 and 60 min. This study was approved by the University of California, Davis Institutional Review Board.

2.2. Focus Group and Interview Guide

Focus groups and interviews were conducted in English, Spanish, Russian, and were conducted in person and virtually, using Zoom. Each focus group or interview was conducted by a trained facilitator and in the language of preference of the participant. Focus group and interview questions came from the Vaccine Hesitancy Determinants Matrix (VHDM) and a survey tool developed by the Strategic Advisory Group of Experts (SAGE) Working Group on Vaccine Hesitancy [2,23]. The matrix organizes factors that contribute to vaccine hesitancy into three main categories: contextual, individual and group, and vaccine/vaccination-specific influences. See Table 1 for determinants, constructs, and general focus/interview guide questions. In our introduction, we told participation we were interested in both their personal experiences and perspectives about general vaccinations and the human papillomavirus (HPV) vaccine. For participants who were not familiar with the HPV vaccine, we provided a brief explanation of the vaccine. To begin, we asked participants what their current thoughts were on vaccinations and if they were familiar with the HPV vaccine. Questions were tailored and adapted based on the participants' familiarity of the HPV vaccine. Additionally, we asked all participants what they thought would be successful strategies that can help with increasing the uptake of the HPV vaccine within their community.

Table 1. General interview/focus group vaccine hesitancy determinant matrix.

Determinant	Construct	Interview/Focus Group Question
Contextual Influences	Communication and media environment	Who do you trust the most for information about vaccines and why?
		Who do you trust the least and why?
		Where do you go for trusted information about vaccinations and why?
		Do you share information related to vaccination within your own social media network? Probe: What type of information do you share and on what platform?
	Influential leaders, gatekeepers, and anti- or pro-vaccination lobbies	Are you practicing [religion] if so which religion? Does ____ your place of worship, have any recommendations/thoughts on vaccines?
		What is your religion/philosophy/culture's stance on vaccination? Probe: If positive/negative: Which vaccines? What is the reason [religion, philosophy, or culture]? Probe: Has your community in the past refused to accept certain vaccines which ones and why?
		What have leaders (religious, political, teachers, health care workers) in your community said about childhood vaccinations? How about the HPV vaccine? Probe: [If advice was given] Did you follow this advice?
	Historical influences	Do you remember any events in the past that would discourage you from getting a vaccine for yourself or your child/children (if you have kids)? Probe: Have reports you heard/read in the media/on social media made you reconsider the choice to have to yourself or your child vaccinated? Probe: If yes, do you remember the source of that information? Who posted that information?

Table 1. *Cont.*

Determinant	Construct	Interview/Focus Group Question
Contextual Influences	Politics or policies	Do you trust (or distrust) that our government is making decisions in your best interest with respect to what vaccines are available? Probe: What about vaccines that are required (list these: if needed) Probe: Do you disagree with the choice of vaccine or vaccination recommendation by the government?
	Geographic barriers	[Only if they have kids] Has distance, clinic hours, time needed to get to clinic or clinic wait time and/or vaccine costs prevented you from getting your child immunized? Probe: If yes, which ones were the biggest factors?
Individual and Group Influences	Immunization as a social norm vs. not needed/harmful	Do you think that most parents have their children vaccinated with all the recommended vaccines? What about the HPV vaccine?
	Health system and providers' trust and personal experience	Do you feel able to openly discuss your concerns about vaccines with your doctor? Probe: Do you trust the information you receive about vaccines your provider? Probe: Do you feel that your health care provider cares about what is best for your child?
Vaccine or Vaccination Specific Issues	Introduction of new vaccine	Are you familiar with the HPV vaccine? If yes, no what do you know about it?
	Risk/benefit	Has your child been vaccinated against HPV, yes or no? Probe: Concerns
		Do you believe vaccines are safe for yourself, for your child [remember if they have kids or not], for those in your community?
	Vaccination schedule	Have you ever delayed vaccinating your child with a newly introduced/recommended vaccine, if so why?

2.3. Data Analysis

All focus groups and interviews were transcribed verbatim, uploaded onto Dedoose [24], and analyzed using inductive and deductive thematic analysis [25,26]. For the Spanish and Russian focus groups and interviews, the recordings were transcribed from the native language audio file to English by bilingual study team members. A team of three coders reviewed and analyzed all transcripts first using an inductive coding approach, allowing for themes and codes to emerge from the raw data. After this initial coding, a deductive approach was used to group similar themes and codes into categories based on the domains and constructs of the VHDM. The first author (principal investigator for the study) read all transcripts and randomly coded ten interviews to ensure consistency. The coders and the PI met weekly to review, reconcile, refine, and define themes, codes, and categories, and to resolve disagreements. Representative quotes were identified to support categories. After salient themes were determined, a post-study focus group was conducted with a group of prior participants to confirm preliminary data analysis.

3. Results

A total of seven focus groups (five in English, one in Spanish, and one in Russian) and fourteen key informant interviews (nine in English, one in Spanish, and four in Russian) were conducted with 39 individuals from the Nevada ($n = 7$), Placer ($n = 2$), Yolo ($n = 3$), El Dorado ($n = 2$), Sacramento ($n = 8$), San Joaquin ($n = 8$), and Merced ($n = 9$) counties. Most participants were female (87.2%) and identified as being a parent (82.1%). About a quarter of the participants were from the Latino/Hispanic community (25.6%); 17.9% were from the rural non-Hispanic White community; 15.4% were from the Slavic community; a little over a third (35.9%) represented multiple communities (e.g., worked with all communities,

Latino/Hispanic, and/or rural); and 5.1% represented other communities (e.g., urban non-Hispanic White, Hmong). See Table 2 for a description of the participants.

Table 2. Description of focus group and key informant participants.

Residential County	Method (I/FG) *	Conduct Language	Population	Gender	Number and Type of Participants
El Dorado	I	English	Rural—non-Hispanic White	Female	1 (community)
El Dorado	I	English	Rural—non-Hispanic White	Female	1 (parent)
Nevada	I	English	Rural—non-Hispanic White	Male	1 (health professional/parent)
Nevada	I	English	Rural—non-Hispanic White	Female	1 (health professional)
Nevada	FG	English	Rural—non-Hispanic White	2—Female 1—Male	3 (parents/health professionals)
Nevada	I	Spanish	Latino/Hispanic	Female	1 (community health worker/parent)
Merced	I	English	Hmong	Male	1 (parent)
Merced	FG	English	Hispanic, Hmong, and Rural	All female	5 (parents and school staff)
Merced	FG	English	Hispanic, Hmong, and Rural	All female	4 (parents and school staff)
Sacramento	I	English	non—Hispanic white	Female	1 (community)
Sacramento	I	English	All	Female	1 (parent/cancer organization)
Sacramento	I	English	All	Female	1 (parent/cancer organization)
Sacramento	I	Russian	Slavic	Female	1 (parent)
Sacramento	I	Russian	Slavic	Female	1 (parent)
Sacramento	FG	Russian	Slavic	Both female	2 (parents)
San Joaquin	FG	English	Latino/Hispanic	2—Female 1—Male	3 (parents and community)
San Joaquin	FG	English	Latino/Hispanic	4—Female 1—Male	5 (parents and community)
Placer	I	Russian	Slavic	Female	1 (parent)
Placer	I	Russian	Slavic	Female	1 (parent)
Yolo	I	English	Latino/Hispanic	Female	1 (parent)
Yolo	FG	English	All	All female	3 (parents and community)

* I = Interview and FG = Focus Group.

We organized our findings into the three categories of the Working Group on Vaccine Hesitancy Determinants Matrix, and within each category, we describe the themes we found to be the most salient. Under contextual influences, we report on the role of communication and media environment, as well as the antivaccination movement, in contributing to HPV vaccine hesitancy. The antivaccination movement can be explained as a combination of several determinants under contextual influences (e.g., anti-vaccination lobby, religion/culture, politics/policies, and perceptions of the pharmaceutical industry); thus, below, we have it listed as its own determinant. Under individual and group influences, we describe participants vaccination beliefs, and attitudes about health and prevention; risk perceptions; and how their personal, family and/or community members' experience with vaccination are sources of HPV vaccine hesitancy. For vaccine/vaccination-specific influences, we discuss the participants' views on the timing of administering the HPV vaccine. Since late 2016, only Gardasil-9 is distributed to the U.S.; thus, we assumed all discussions regarding the HPV vaccine were in reference to the 9-valent vaccine.

3.1. Contextual Influences

All participants shared that contextual influences contributed to both their HPV vaccine and overall vaccine hesitancy. The research team identified two constructs within this determinant as themes that were most salient in the focus groups and interviews: (1) communication, and media environment; and (2) the anti-vaccination movement.

3.1.1. Communication and Media Environment

Social media coverage of the HPV vaccine was identified as a major source of HPV vaccine hesitancy among participants. Participants shared examples of how easy it is to post vaccine information (regardless of accuracy and validity) on social media platforms such as Facebook, Instagram, TikTok, and YouTube. One participant said, "On Facebook [you] can put any information out and anyone can say what they want, and no one can know if it's the truth or lie" (Participant 1, Interview, Nevada County). When asked if they can recall having seen anything on social media that may have made them reconsider vaccinating their child against HPV, one participant recalled, "...on TikTok people really follow really quickly [in reference to how people can quickly amass followers and with videos going vial] then there could be a lot of misinformation through Tik Tok because anybody can post whatever and make it sound a certain way" (Participant 2, Focus Group #1, San Joaquin County). This impression of how effectively individuals can create and post sensualized HPV vaccine messaging on social media and the reoccurrence of these videos is explained by this participant:

"If I'm watching some like YouTube thing like they'll have some educational stuff on vaccines. But you look on the side of whatever you're watching the next thing that pops up will be something like the signs of why you should not get the HPV vaccine. People easily get sucked into these videos and the videos will just play automatically. It's like oh my gosh, this story is crazy and the only thing that happened was this vaccine. I think it's these lived experience stories even if you don't know the person or remotely know the person, it could be actors for all you know, but the story itself stands out" (Participant 5, Focus Group, Nevada County).

In terms of what they can remember reading and or seeing on social media, the majority reported that the information was always negative. Participants recalled that the main take-away messages from the vaccine information they have heard on social media focused on the notion that vaccines can cause autism, as well as an emphasis on severe and not necessarily correct adverse effects. One participant shared, "I have seen groups on Facebook of mothers that are against the vaccinations [HPV] and that also did say that it could cause autism and that it did certain things to their kids" (Participant 3, Focus Group #1, Merced County). Another participant disclosed, "I see a lot of people sharing [on YouTube] their vaccine horror stories of how bad their reaction was, or they know someone who had a horrible reaction and those are really easy to find and they're the first things that pop up when you research vaccines" (Participant 4, Interview, El Dorado County). A participant shared that, similarly, she receives social media videos from her friends that spread HPV vaccine misinformation. She described a video in which the main point of the story was how a study came out in Spain that talked about how the HPV vaccine affected adolescents over there, she said "...that friend of mine [who shared the video] said, no don't be putting the vaccine [HPV] to your kids, you are going to provoke a reaction or they become sterile" (Participant 1, Interview, Nevada County).

3.1.2. Anti-Vaccination Movement

Participants discussed the influence of the anti-vaccination movement and named public figures who have spoken out against vaccination when asked what contributed to not only their HPV vaccine hesitancy, but hesitancy among their family, friends, and community. One participant recalled Jenny McCarthy, an American actress, model, and television personality, publicizing that her child became autistic after receiving a vaccine, "I don't remember which vaccine it was, but that was- that got me thinking that, hey maybe vaccines are actually not really good for you" (Participant 6, Interview, Sacramento County). Another participant spoke about how she was a part of an online mom's group and when conversations around vaccination come up, she shared, "there's a whole string of people with their conspiracy theories that the government is involved, that they don't feel that they're safe, that there's mercury in them, that it causes autism..." (Participant 7, Interview, Nevada County). Participant 5 summarized how vocal and persistent the anti-vaccination movement has been around spreading their message against vaccination:

> "They kind of suck people in easily because their message is so strong and out there. It seems really well organized whereas pro-vaccine seems a little bit more, I don't know, not as robust...I rarely see a pro-vaccine posting and when I do, there's like 20 other comments about, 'Why are you doing that? Why are you posting this pro-vaccine?' It just gets buried in this anti-vaccine sentiment."

Another participant shared a similar response when describing how the anti-vaccination movement has created a culture of intimidation in which individuals are afraid to ask questions about vaccines for fear of backlash from the movement. This participant stated, "I know a lot of people don't want to voice their opinions or comment their concerns about the vaccines because of anti-vax or whatever or just be made fun of." (Participant 15, Interview, Yolo County).

3.2. Individual and Group Influences

All participants described how their own personal perceptions of vaccines, as well as those of their family, community and social networks, have contributed to their HPV vaccine hesitancy. The research team identified three constructs within this determinant: (1) personal beliefs and attitudes about health and prevention; (2) risk perceptions; and (3) personal, family and community members' experiences with vaccination.

3.2.1. Personal Beliefs and Attitudes about Health and Prevention

The participants discussed how their personal attitudes and beliefs about vaccines have contributed to their vaccine hesitancy. The participants shared that they believed that children should develop immunity from vaccine-preventable diseases naturally. As explained by one participant, "Sometimes, protecting them a little too much from getting sick ends up being worse than putting them out there and letting them get sick is basically how I see it" (Participant 8, Focus Group, Merced County). When asked to elaborate on this notion of natural immunity, participants expressed that they believe kids need to be exposed to germs to stimulate their immune system and as a result their immune system will become stronger. Several other participants referenced this natural health philosophy as "letting kids eat dirt", an expression that suggests that kids need to be exposed to soil, dust, bacteria, germs, etc. As one parent stated, "how I see it, let them eat dirt. It's okay, it won't kill them" (Participant 11, Focus Group #1, Merced County). While another one said "...or they [kids] could just eat some dirt and get some immunity to bacteria" (Participant 12, Interview, Sacramento County). Similarly, another participant shared, "... you should just let your kids eat dirt because that, in fact, creates a lot of immunity" (Participant 9, Interview, Nevada County). Among participants, the belief that kids can develop immunity by being exposed to nature was commonly cited as an alternative to vaccination. A participant summarized:

> "I think just getting dirty and letting them be kids and eventually the immunity will increase based on the environment that we actually grew up with. I think that's just one way kids would be able to grow their immunity by making sure that they're exposed to any type of environment as possible, I mean outdoors" (Participant 10, Interview, Merced County).

In addition to letting kids be exposed to the environment, another participant explained that her mother would always tell her that kids need to also be exposed to other kids, "...human interaction is going to be important for us to develop, you know strong not just muscles but also internally" (Participant 3, Focus Group #1, San Joaquin County).

3.2.2. Risk Perceptions

The participants described how their lack of confidence in vaccine safety and lack of perceived benefits of vaccination contributed to their HPV vaccine hesitancy. The participants shared that they felt that taking the HPV vaccine is a risk as they are concerned with what is inside the vaccine, as well as whether they believed the side effects are worth it. As one participant explains, "Taking a risk of injecting something into your body that may not be necessary and you're introducing ingredients that are not really organic." (Participant 6, Interview, Sacramento County). Another participant shares, "Vaccine components are complicated, some consist of heavy metals and regardless, it is still not good for brain cells" (Participant 15, Interview, Placer County). When describing the decision to vaccinate a child, one participant disclosed that the decision weighs heavily on the parent, "Vaccination does not guarantee that we will not get sick...there are a lot of side effects so it should be weighed.... if it is a child then his parents should take responsibility because it happens that children do not tolerate vaccination very well..." (Participant 17, Interview, Placer County). Another participant shared that they thought the HPV vaccine was unnecessary as they did not perceive the benefits of vaccination, "I feel that it's really unnecessary unless somebody does or they are high risk then they may want to discuss it with their doctor and weigh the pros and cons, but there may be girls out there that are really not at risk and may never get that cancer, so why bother getting the vaccine because it's not really necessary." (Participant 6, Interview, Sacramento County). When asked what were the major factors that contributed to HPV vaccine hesitancy, participants cited that safety concerns were one of the main reasons why parents are not getting the HPV vaccine for their children. One focus group participant explained, "I think it comes down to parents being concerned that it's not safe, those who aren't getting it" (Participant 5, Focus Group, Nevada County). Another focus group participant echoed similar sentiments, stating "I do think that if people believe these vaccines are safe and effective, they will get them" (Participant 16, Focus Group, Nevada County).

3.2.3. Personal, Family, or Community Members' Experiences with Vaccination

Participants described how their personal, family or community members' experiences with vaccination have greatly influenced their HPV vaccination decision. This theme was particularly salient among participants who immigrated to the U.S. from another country. These participants shared how their experiences growing up in another country and their culture have influenced their vaccine hesitancy. One participant described, "I noticed here [in the U.S] the difference is that they exaggerate with the babies, and they want to disinfect everything...You know the kids there [Mexico] didn't even get sick. So, I think the best way for a child to create [immunity] so they can fight against it is to create antibodies so that his own body can fight" (Participant 13, Focus Group #2, San Joaquin County). Slavic participants shared that many members of their community do not believe in vaccinations and these participants recounted vaccine stories that occurred in their home country. One participant shared that her sister had a bad reaction to getting a vaccine, "After about an hour after the injection, her body was having a reaction, her face started swelling, her ears were swelling, and she started turning blue. This happened in Moscow...After that event, no one in my family got vaccinated against anything" (Participant 15, Interview, Yolo County). Another participant shared that the fear of adverse effects is something her community is very concerned with, "...for instance Russia as a whole, many mothers are scared to vaccinate due to the possibility of adverse effects, some may not have had personal experiences [with adverse effects] in their family, but they are scared from hearing about stories and that happen to their children if they give them a vaccine" (Russian Interview 5_23). Another interviewee explained that while some vaccines were acceptable to administer to children to prevent severe diseases, they felt that children in America are being given too many vaccines, "...A lot of young mothers that are here for a while now, we came from Ukraine two years ago, we are used to vaccinating our children because no one wanted their children to be sick with smallpox, mumps, or chickenpox. But here a lot of moms say that NO, in America they administer too many vaccines, it's very bad for the children, children become stupid, slow, develop autism..." (Participant 16, Interview, Sacramento County). Stories of adverse reactions coupled with the notion that too many vaccines are being administered was stated as the main reasons why participants felt that their community did not vaccinate. One participant stated, "From my Russian friends and people that I know, no one vaccinates." (Participant 17, Focus Group, Yolo County). Additionally, from that same focus group, another participant concurred, "Here in the U.S. the people I am around are very anti vaccine, any vaccine... [and] yes, it's mostly neighbors [Russian] or such who advocate against [vaccination]." (Participant 18, Focus Group, Yolo County).

3.3. Vaccine/Vaccination-Specific Influences

The participants discussed how the timing of when the HPV vaccine is recommended to their child from their doctor during a medical appointment and the number of vaccines administered at one time were contributing factors to their vaccine acceptance or resistance.

Vaccine Timing

The participants expressed how children are receiving too many vaccines during one medical visit and how the timing of the vaccine conversation contributed to their hesitancy. The participants described how important it is to recommend the HPV vaccine at the right time rather than at every office visit. As one participant states:

"For comparison, in Moldova, before getting vaccinated, the patient must pass a urine test and a chemical blood test... If one of the indicators in these tests does not correspond to standards or indicates that there is some kind of infection in the body or some aspect of this analysis is bad, then now is not the time to get vaccinated. In America you get vaccinated just because it's time. And often children with runny noses, with screams, are vaccinated and then there are a lot of such cases that we hear out there. Maybe the vaccination is good but because it was not done at the right time, it played a bad role. So for me it's so strange" (Participant 16, Interview, Yolo County)

In addition to the timing of the vaccine conversation between parents and providers, the participants also discussed their preference of spacing out the vaccines as to not give children too many vaccines at one time. One participant shared "...I did lean towards spacing out the vaccines...we don't want to give too many vaccines at once. Let your body respond accordingly and then move on to the next one..." (Participant 18, Interview, Sacramento County). A participant summarized the reason they split up the vaccines was because of fear of the reaction:

"So, when my kids were little, I would always split their vaccinations up because I would call it a martini drink or martini mix because it be so many in one. So, they would get a 3-in-1, so I would always- they were always behind because I would split them up because of reaction that I heard people would have..." (Participant 19, Focus Group, Merced County)

3.4. Strategies and Recommendations

The participants stressed the importance of providing culturally appropriate, in-language, in-person, easy-to-understand HPV vaccine education that is tailored to the concerns of their community. As expressed by one participant, "I think there needs to be intentional education out there, outreach, and people that speak their language and understand a little bit about the purpose why people need to get those vaccine" (Participant 10, Interview, Merced County). Specifically, for the Russian community, the participants felt that more education is needed. One participant stated, "I think that for the Russian community, we need to be giving more explanation and education for what a vaccine is needed, what are the goals, so people can understand..." When asked about the mode of delivery for intervention strategies, the participants preferred in-person engagement. As expressed by one participant, "Mail, no. Telephone, no. Face to face is best" (Participant #20, Interview, Nevada County). The participants also reminded the research team that language barriers and health literacy were important factors to consider. As identified by one participant, "...you want to make sure that interpretation or translation is also available to people because not everyone can read English or understand big words" (Participant #21, Interview, Yolo County). One participant summarized:

> "...making sure that one's reading the material that is culturally responsive and you know culturally appropriate because we're not all the same, so just making sure that whatever materials are being done and whatever's being distributed, that there is that checking in with the different cultures and making sure that it's appropriate for their culture..." (Participant #22, Focus Group #1, San Joaquin County)

The participants also suggested removing logistical barriers to vaccination by providing the vaccine at community locations. One participant shared, "...the only way I got it [the HPV vaccine] was because there was like this van that would go to low income apartments and they would give free flu shots and stuff like that...My mom went to go get her flu shot and I went with her to translate and that's when the nurse that was there was talking to my mom and she brought up the HPV vaccine. That's how I got—I got my first dose there...the only reason I got it was because I was there at that moment." (Participant #19, Focus Group, Merced County). In addition to clinicians and nurses, the participants also suggested using trusted community leaders as HPV vaccine advocates. One participant shared, "some of our families really do listen to what their leaders in their faith community talk about and then from that also work with teachers because teachers are considered to be trusted sources with information" (Participant #8, Focus Group, Merced County).

4. Discussion

This study broadly examined sources of vaccine hesitancy and described how these sources influenced HPV vaccine decision making among populations who have expressed vaccine hesitancy in counties with low HPV vaccine uptake. To the best of our knowledge, this is the first study to explore HPV vaccine hesitancy from the perspectives of rural, Latino/Hispanic, and Slavic communities. The geographic and ethnic/racial diversity of our participants provides unique insights into these understudied populations that highlight gaps in the existing literature and includes community-recommended strategies for building HPV vaccine confidence. Within these communities, we sought to understand the contextual, individual and group, and vaccine/vaccination-specific influences that the participants discussed as reasons for HPV vaccine hesitancy among themselves and their community.

Utilizing both focus groups and key informant interviews, we were able to elicit salient factors contributing to HPV vaccine hesitancy in these communities and how these factors influenced their vaccine decision making. Six main themes were identified from the focus groups and interviews: (1) The use of social media in spreading easily accessible negative vaccine-related content regardless of editorial and scientific oversight. (2) The tactics used by the anti-vaccination movement to instill HPV vaccine hesitancy by spreading

HPV vaccine misinformation and disinformation, and intimidation. (3) The participants' vaccination beliefs and attitudes stemming from their personal health philosophies. (4) The participants' lack of confidence in the safety of the vaccine and how that has contributed to their perceptions of the risk and benefits of HPV vaccination. (5) The vaccine experiences of their family, friends, and community members. (6) The timing of when the HPV vaccine conversation occurs between doctors and parents/patients as well as the number of vaccines administered to children at the same time.

The participants described the influence of social media on contributing to HPV vaccine hesitancy and how challenging it is to distinguish whether the media content being shared is factual (e.g., "you don't know if it's the truth or a lie") because of how powerful the messaging is. The participants interchangeably discussed social media and the anti-vaccination movement within the same context as social media is one of the main modes the movement utilizes to disseminate their information. The participants shared how social media content on the HPV vaccine consists mostly of HPV vaccine information related to potentially false adverse health effects and claims related to vaccine safety. Supporting our findings, in a prior study assessing the HPV vaccine, Facebook posts from local health agencies and groups within the same geographic region as this study provoked more positive emotion, more negative emotion and more anger than the posts with concerns mostly focused on vaccine safety, risks, and injury [27]. Additionally, prior studies have documented that HPV vaccine misinformation and disinformation spread through social media is a major driver of vaccine hesitancy [27]. Social media usage, particularly among parents, has been growing over the past few decades. A cross-sectional survey was conducted among a group of parents, and the analysis found that nearly all (96%) claimed to use some form of social media; 68% reported using it to obtain health-related information [28]. Even among our racially/ethnically and geographically diverse participants, social media was overwhelmingly mentioned. Promising research shows that HPV vaccine misinformation on social media can be countered with social media messaging that addresses and corrects the misinformation [29,30]. More research is needed on how to develop and implement culturally tailored in-language social media messaging that can combat HPV vaccine misinformation. Interestingly, among our participants who were born in another country, the participants described how the vaccination experiences and health beliefs they held growing up in their native country have contributed to their HPV vaccine hesitancy. This is consistent with a literature review by Daniels et al. that reported refugees, immigrants and migrants had a negative cultural bias towards vaccination because of cultural norms, practices, or beliefs [31]. In another study, 35.3% of surveyed Latina immigrant mothers of 9–12-year-old daughters in Alabama reported HPV vaccine hesitancy despite their physician recommending the vaccine [32]. Tankwanchi et al. suggested that HPV vaccine hesitancy among immigrant populations in the U.S. may be attributed to limited knowledge regarding cervical cancer and HPV vaccination and religion. In our study, while we also found limited knowledge regarding cervical cancer and the HPV vaccine, religion was not cited as a main source of vaccine hesitancy [33]. Within our Hispanic/Latino and Slavic participants, the main reasons described as contributing to their vaccine hesitancy related to their home country were the beliefs that, in the U.S., there is a tendency to over vaccinate children and that not all vaccines are necessary. These participants expressed greater concern for adverse reactions to vaccines and a lower general HPV vaccine knowledge. More research is needed to develop effective HPV vaccination educational materials that would resonate with these communities.

Additionally, the participants explained that personally and within their social networks and community, a major source of HPV vaccine hesitancy is the belief that HPV vaccination is unnecessary because children should develop immunity naturally. The participants repeatedly stated we should "let children eat dirt." While we know participants are not literally stating that we should let children eat dirt and are merely suggesting that we let children develop immunity naturally through direct exposure to germs and pathogens, it is still alarming that this belief resonated with so many of our participants. Reich describes this dichotomy as parents perceiving the differences in natural and artificial immunity, with vaccination being seen as artificial and inferior to immunity occurring from infection with the disease [34]. Other studies have reported similar findings when exploring parental reasoning for incomplete and/or a lack of childhood vaccinations [35–37]. The participants also perceived the vaccine as being high risk with low benefits. The participants described having low confidence in the safety of the vaccine. Consistent with a systematic review of 71 studies on the beliefs around childhood vaccines in the U.S., the participants in our study described that their HPV vaccine hesitancy was influenced by the beliefs that vaccines contain harmful ingredients; natural immunity is better than vaccine acquired immunity; receiving a vaccine can cause illnesses; and that receiving too many vaccines at one time can overwhelm a child's immune system. [36]

While fear about the safety and efficacy of the HPV vaccine has been widely reported in the literature [38], our findings regarding a desire for children to develop immunity naturally due to how children are raised in the participants' native country, coupled with the belief that the U.S. is too fixated on vaccines and cleanliness, adds a unique perspective to the literature. More research is needed to understand the role of social networks and cultural norms among refugee, immigrant, migrant, and rural communities when assessing HPV vaccine uptake. Additionally, educational messaging that provides a clear rationale for vaccination that emphasizes the importance of herd immunization may resonate with these collective communities, as well as an open conversation recognizing that while there are some benefits to natural immunity, vaccines are necessary for the overall health of the population. Interventions targeting these communities should consider including a community strategy as social networks appear to be a significant source of HPV vaccine hesitancy.

Strengths and Limitations

The results reported here are the views of a specific group of individuals and their experiences are not representative of the entire U.S. population nor of the counties and racial/ethnic groups where we recruited participants, but rather provide a broad overview of sources of HPV vaccine hesitancy among vaccine-hesitant communities that can be used as a starting point for future research inquires seeking generalizability. Additionally, our convenience sample size of seven focus groups and 14 key informant interviews with 39 individuals may be considered modest, thus further limiting the generalizability of our findings. However, prior studies have reported that code saturation for interviews can be reached within the first 12 interviews, with basic themes emerging as early as within six interviews [39,40]. In their study, Guest et al. found that 94% of high frequency codes were identified within the first 6 interviews and 97% were identified after 12 interviews [36]. Chen et al. reported that focus group data saturation, with 84% of themes generated, can be reached within the first three focus groups [41]. Our analysis followed a similar pattern in which we were able to reach data saturation within the first 12 interviews and within the first four focus groups. Our findings were further validated as we found other studies have found similar perspectives on HPV vaccine hesitancy to those we determined. Although we felt our sample size was adequate, additional recruitment of more participants within each strata (e.g., rurality, occupation, race/ethnicity, place of residence, occupation) could strengthen our conclusions and increase the generalizability of our findings. However, generalizability is not the goal of qualitative inquiry, and our intent was to obtain an in-depth understanding and gain insight into the nuances of HPV vaccine hesitancy, including uncovering the reasons behind why and how these communities became hesitant, to develop effective interventions to increase HPV vaccination in these communities. Additionally, our recruitment methods, coupled with the monetary compensation participants received, could have also resulted in a selection bias. We also acknowledge that HPV vaccine hesitancy is influenced by a multitude of factors such as social demographics, adolescent gender, and health care usage, which were not assessed in this study. The inclusion of prevalence and characteristics of HPV vaccine hesitancy is beyond the scope of this qualitative study; thus, a quantitative follow-up study that can assess statistically significant determinants of HPV vaccine hesitancy is needed to validate our findings.

Despite these limitations, the strengths of this study include purposeful recruitment of individuals from underrepresented communities (e.g., Slavic, Latino, and rural) and being able to solicit in-depth responses regarding their views on vaccinations. This study can be used to further research determining factors associated with HPV vaccine hesitancy in these communities, which will result in effective interventions to combat HPV vaccine hesitancy within these communities.

5. Conclusions

Among our diverse group of participants that included rural and racial/ethnic diverse foreign-born individuals, we found that the sources of HPV vaccine hesitancy existed across all three determinants of the Vaccine Hesitancy Determinant Matrix. While our findings are consistent with prior studies, our study contributes to the growing literature on understanding local sources of HPV vaccine hesitancy as the factors that influence vaccine hesitancy are unique to each community, especially among Hispanic/Latino, Slavic, and rural communities. This qualitative study allowed participants to describe in their own words and in their language of choice what those factors were and how these have shaped their beliefs and, ultimately, their HPV vaccine decision-making process. Our findings can help inform future interventions to increase HPV vaccine uptake by addressing factors most likely contributing to HPV vaccine hesitancy in these communities.

Author Contributions: Design, J.H.T.D., J.Z. and M.S.C.J.; Conceptualization, J.H.T.D., A.G., L.R., J.Z. and M.S.C.J.; Data Curation, J.H.T.D., A.G. and A.M.R.; Formal Analysis, J.H.T.D., A.G., L.R. and A.M.R.; Funding Acquisition, J.H.T.D. and J.Z.; Investigation, J.H.T.D. and A.M.R.; Methodology, J.H.T.D.; Project Administration, J.H.T.D.; Resources, J.H.T.D. and A.G.; Supervision, J.H.T.D.; Validation, J.H.T.D., A.G. and L.R.; Writing—Original Draft, J.H.T.D.; Writing—Review and Editing, J.H.T.D., A.G., L.R., A.M.R., J.Z. and M.S.C.J.; Final Approval, J.H.T.D., A.G., L.R., A.M.R., J.Z. and M.S.C.J. All authors have read and agreed to the published version of the manuscript.

Funding: This research was funded by the National Cancer Institute, grant number 3P30CA093373-18S5, and by the Christine and Helen S. Landgraf Memorial Fund. J.H.T.D. is supported by the following grants: 1K01CA258956-01A1, 5K12HD051958-17, and P30CA93373. M.S.C. is also supported by P30CA93373.

Institutional Review Board Statement: This study was conducted according to the guidelines of the Declaration of Helsinki and approved by the Institutional Review Board of University of California, Davis (IRB # 1656830-3, approved 18 November 2020).

Informed Consent Statement: Participant consent was received from all the participants prior to conducting this study.

Data Availability Statement: The deidentified data underlying the results presented in this study may be made available upon reasonable request from the corresponding author, Julie HT Dang (jtdang@ucdavis.edu).

Conflicts of Interest: The authors declare no conflicts of interest.

References

1. World Health Organization [Internet]. Ten Threats to Global Health in 2019. Available online: https://www.who.int/news-room/spotlight/ten-threats-to-global-health-in-2019 (accessed on 25 February 2024).
2. MacDonald, N.E.; Eskola, J.; Liang, X.; Chaudhuri, M.; Dube, E.; Gellin, B.; Goldstein, S.; Larson, H.; Manzo, M.L.; Reingold, A.; et al. Vaccine hesitancy: Definition, scope and determinants. *Vaccine* **2015**, *33*, 4161–4164. [CrossRef] [PubMed]
3. Patel, P.R.; Berenson, A.B. Sources of HPV vaccine hesitancy in parents. *Hum. Vaccines Immunother.* **2013**, *9*, 2649–2653. [CrossRef] [PubMed]
4. Szilagyi, P.G.; Albertin, C.S.; Gurfinkel, D.; Saville, A.W.; Vangala, S.; Rice, J.D.; Helmkamp, L.; Zimet, G.D.; Valderrama, R.; Breck, A.; et al. Prevalence and characteristics of HPV vaccine hesitancy among parents of adolescents across the US. *Vaccine* **2020**, *38*, 6027–6037. [CrossRef] [PubMed]

5. Lee, C.; Whetten, K.; Omer, S.; Pan, W.; Salmon, D. Hurdles to herd immunity: Distrust of government and vaccine refusal in the US, 2002–2003. *Vaccine* **2016**, *34*, 3972–3978. [CrossRef] [PubMed]
6. Larson, H.J.; Cooper, L.Z.; Eskola, J.; Katz, S.L.; Ratzan, S. Addressing the vaccine confidence gap. *Lancet* **2011**, *378*, 526–535. [CrossRef] [PubMed]
7. McRee, A.-L.; Gilkey, M.B.; Dempsey, A.F. HPV vaccine hesitancy: Findings from a statewide survey of health care providers. *J. Pediatr. Health Care* **2014**, *28*, 541–549. [CrossRef] [PubMed]
8. Thompson, E.L.; Rosen, B.L.; Vamos, C.A.; Kadono, M.; Daley, E.M. Human Papillomavirus Vaccination: What Are the Reasons for Nonvaccination Among U.S. Adolescents? *J. Adolesc. Health* **2017**, *61*, 288–293. [CrossRef] [PubMed]
9. Saxena, K.; Marden, J.R.; Carias, C.; Bhatti, A.; Patterson-Lomba, O.; Gomez-Lievano, A.; Yao, L.; Chen, Y.-T. Impact of the COVID-19 pandemic on adolescent vaccinations: Projected time to reverse deficits in routine adolescent vaccination in the United States. *Curr. Med. Res. Opin.* **2021**, *37*, 2077–2087. [CrossRef]
10. Coustasse, A.D.; Kimble, C.P.; Maxik, K.M. COVID-19 and Vaccine Hesitancy: A Challenge the United States Must Overcome. *J. Ambul. Care Manag.* **2021**, *44*, 71–75. [CrossRef]
11. Sonawane, K.; Zhu, Y.; Lin, Y.-Y.; Damgacioglu, H.; Lin, Y.; Montealegre, J.R.; Deshmukh, A.A. HPV Vaccine Recommendations and Parental Intent. *Pediatrics* **2021**, *147*, e2020026286. [CrossRef]
12. Pingali, C.; Yankey, D.; Elam-Evans, L.D.; Markowitz, L.E.; Valier, M.R.; Fredua, B.; Crowe, S.J.; DeSisto, C.L.; Stokley, S.; Singleton, J.A. Vaccination Coverage Among Adolescents Aged 13–17 Years—National Immunization Survey–Teen, United States, 2022. *MMWR. Morb. Mortal. Wkly. Rep.* **2023**, *72*, 912–919. [CrossRef] [PubMed]
13. Health People 2030 [Internet]. Washington, DC: U.S. Department of Health and Human Services, Office of Disease Preven-tion and Health Promotion. Available online: https://health.gov/healthypeople/objectives-and-data/browse-objectives/vaccination/increase-proportion-adolescents-who-get-recommended-doses-hpv-vaccine-iid-08 (accessed on 25 February 2024).
14. Vanderpool, R.C.; Stradtman, L.R.; Brandt, H.M. Policy opportunities to increase HPV vaccination in rural communities. *Hum. Vaccines Immunother.* **2019**, *15*, 1527–1532. [CrossRef] [PubMed]
15. Swiecki-Sikora, A.L.; Henry, K.A.; Kepka, D. HPV Vaccination Coverage Among US Teens Across the Rural-Urban Continuum. *J. Rural. Health* **2019**, *35*, 506–517. [CrossRef] [PubMed]
16. Pingali, C.; Yankey, D.; Elam-Evans, L.D.; Markowitz, L.E.; Valier, M.R.; Fredua, B.; Crowe, S.J.; Stokley, S.; Singleton, J.A. National Vaccination Coverage Among Adolescents Aged 13–17 Years—National Immunization Survey-Teen, United States, 2021. *MMWR Morb. Mortal. Wkly. Rep.* **2022**, *71*, 1101–1108. [CrossRef] [PubMed]
17. Buskwofie, A.; David-West, G.; Clare, C.A. A Review of Cervical Cancer: Incidence and Disparities. *J. Natl. Med. Assoc.* **2020**, *112*, 229–232. [CrossRef] [PubMed]
18. Zahnd, W.E.; James, A.S.; Jenkins, W.D.; Izadi, S.R.; Fogleman, A.J.; Steward, D.E.; Colditz, G.A.; Brard, L. Rural–Urban Differences in Cancer Incidence and Trends in the United States. *Cancer Epidemiol. Biomark. Prev.* **2018**, *27*, 1265–1274. [CrossRef] [PubMed]
19. Warren, B.R.; Gillette-Walch, H.; Adler, J.; Arias, R.; Klausner, J.D.; Ashing, K.T.; Villa, A. Assessment of human papillomavirus vaccination rates of adolescents in California, 2018–2019. *Prev. Med. Rep.* **2023**, *32*, 102144. [CrossRef] [PubMed]
20. Dang, J.H.T.; McClure, S.; Gori, A.C.T.; Martens, T.; Mojadedi, A.; Smith, U.; Austin, C.J.; Chen, M.S. Implementation and evaluation of a multilevel intervention to increase uptake of the human papillomavirus vaccine among rural adolescents. *J. Rural. Health* **2023**, *39*, 136–141. [CrossRef]
21. United States Department of Agriculture [Internet]. Economic Research Service. Rural-Urban Commuting Area Codes. Available online: https://www.ers.usda.gov/data-products/rural-urban-commuting-area-codes (accessed on 25 February 2024).
22. StudyPages © 2024 Yuzu Labs PBC. Available online: https://studypages.com/ (accessed on 29 March 2024).
23. Larson, H.J.; Jarrett, C.; Schulz, W.S.; Chaudhuri, M.; Zhou, Y.; Dubé, E.; Schuster, M.; MacDonald, N.E.; Wilson, R.; The SAGE Working Group on Vaccine Hesitancy. Measuring vaccine hesitancy: The development of a survey tool. *Vaccine* **2015**, *33*, 4165–4175. [CrossRef]
24. *Dedoose Version 9.0.17, Cloud Application for Managing, Analyzing, and Presenting Qualitative and Mixed Method Research Data (2021)*; SocioCultural Research Consultants, LLC: Los Angeles, CA, USA, 2021.
25. Vaismoradi, M.; Jones, J.; Turunen, H.; Snelgrove, S. Theme development in qualitative content analysis and thematic analysis. *J. Nurs. Educ. Prac.* **2016**, *6*, 100–110. [CrossRef]
26. Fereday, J.; Muir-Cochrane, E. Demonstrating rigor using thematic analysis: A hybrid approach of inductive and deductive coding and theme development. *Int. J. Qual. Methods* **2006**, *5*, 80–92. [CrossRef]
27. Zhang, J.; Xue, H.; Calabrese, C.; Chen, H.; Dang, J.H.T. Understanding Human papillomavirus vaccine promotions and hesitancy in Northern California through examining public Facebook pages and groups. *Front. Digit. Health* **2021**, *3*, 683090. [CrossRef]
28. Bryan, M.A.; Evans, Y.; Morishita, C.; Midamba, N.; Moreno, M. Parental Perceptions of the Internet and Social Media as a Source of Pediatric Health Information. *Acad Pediatr.* **2020**, *20*, 31–38. [CrossRef]
29. Li, L.; Wood, C.E.; Kostkova, P. Vaccine hesitancy and behavior change theory-based social media interventions: A systematic review. *Transl Behav Med.* **2022**, *12*, 243–272. [CrossRef] [PubMed]
30. Limaye, R.J.; Holroyd, T.A.; Blunt, M.; Jamison, A.F.; Sauer, M.; Weeks, R.; Wahl, B.; Christenson, K.; Smith, C.; Minchin, J.; et al. Social media strategies to affect vaccine acceptance: A systematic literature review. *Expert Rev. Vaccines.* **2021**, *20*, 959–973. [CrossRef]

31. Daniels, D.; Imdad, A.; Buscemi-Kimmins, T.; Vitale, D.; Rani, U.; Darabaner, E.; Shaw, A.; Shaw, J. Vaccine hesitancy in the refugee, immigrant, and migrant population in the United States: A systematic review and meta-analysis. *Hum. Vaccines Immunother.* **2022**, *18*, 2131168. [CrossRef]
32. Khodadadi, A.B.; Redden, D.T.; Scarinci, I.C. HPV Vaccination Hesitancy Among Latina Immigrant Mothers Despite Physician Recommendation. *Ethn. Dis.* **2020**, *30*, 661–670. [CrossRef] [PubMed]
33. Tankwanchi, A.S.; Bowman, B.; Garrison, M.; Larson, H.; Wiysonge, C.S. Vaccine hesitancy in migrant communities: A rapid review of latest evidence. *Curr. Opin. Immunol.* **2021**, *71*, 62–68. [CrossRef]
34. Reich, J.A. Of natural bodies and antibodies: Parents' vaccine refusal and the dichotomies of natural and artificial. *Soc. Sci. Med.* **2016**, *157*, 103–110. [CrossRef] [PubMed]
35. Gross, K.; Hartmann, K.; Zemp, E.; Merten, S. 'I know it has worked for millions of years': The role of the 'natural' in parental reasoning against child im-munization in a qualitative study in Switzerland. *BMC Public Health* **2015**, *15*, 373. [CrossRef]
36. Gidengil, C.; Chen, C.; Parker, A.M.; Nowak, S.; Matthews, L. Beliefs around childhood vaccines in the United States: A systematic review. *Vaccine* **2019**, *37*, 6793–6802. [CrossRef] [PubMed]
37. Dubé, E.; Vivion, M.; Sauvageau, C.; Gagneur, A.; Gagnon, R.; Guay, M. "Nature Does Things Well, Why Should We Interfere?": Vaccine Hesitancy Among Mothers. *Qual. Health Res.* **2016**, *26*, 411–425. [CrossRef] [PubMed]
38. Zheng, L.; Wu, J.; Zheng, M. Barriers to and Facilitators of Human Papillomavirus Vaccination Among People Aged 9 to 26 Years: A Systematic Review. *Sex. Transm. Dis.* **2021**, *48*, e255–e262. [CrossRef]
39. Guest, G.; Bunce, A.; Johnson, L. How Many Interviews Are Enough? An Experiment with Data Saturation and Variability. *Field Methods* **2006**, *18*, 59–82. [CrossRef]
40. Hennink, M.M.; Kaiser, B.N.; Marconi, V.C. Code Saturation Versus Meaning Saturation: How Many Interviews Are Enough? *Qual. Health Res.* **2017**, *27*, 591–608. [CrossRef]
41. Namey, E.; Guest, G.; McKenna, K.; Chen, M. Evaluating bang for the buck: A cost-effectiveness comparison between individual interviews and focus groups based on thematic saturation levels. *Am. J. Eval.* **2016**, *37*, 425–440. [CrossRef]

Disclaimer/Publisher's Note: The statements, opinions and data contained in all publications are solely those of the individual author(s) and contributor(s) and not of MDPI and/or the editor(s). MDPI and/or the editor(s) disclaim responsibility for any injury to people or property resulting from any ideas, methods, instructions or products referred to in the content.

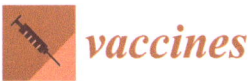

Article

Human Papillomavirus Vaccination Acceleration and Introduction in Sub-Saharan Africa: A Multi-Country Cohort Analysis

Gbadebo Collins Adeyanju [1,2,3,*], Tonè-Alima Essoh [4], Annick Raïssa Sidibe [5], Furaha Kyesi [6] and Muyi Aina [7]

[1] Center for Empirical Research in Economics and Behavioural Science (CEREB), University of Erfurt, 99089 Erfurt, Germany
[2] Psychology and Infectious Disease Lab (PIDI), University of Erfurt, 99089 Erfurt, Germany
[3] Media and Communication Science, University of Erfurt, 99089 Erfurt, Germany
[4] Agence de Médecine Préventive (AMP) Afrique, Abidjan 08 BP 660, Côte d'Ivoire; tae@aamp.org
[5] National Immunization Technical Advisory Groups (NITAGs), Ouaga 06, Ouagadougou 06 BP 9096, Burkina Faso; annickraissa_s@yahoo.fr
[6] Ministry of Health, S.L.P. 743, Dar es Salaam P.O. Box 9283, Tanzania; furahakyesi@hotmail.com
[7] Executive Secretary, National Primary Healthcare Development Agency (NPHCDA), Area 11, Abuja P.O. Box 123, Nigeria
* Correspondence: gbadebo.adeyanju@uni-erfurt.de; Tel.: +49-15216381976

Citation: Adeyanju, G.C.; Essoh, T.-A.; Sidibe, A.R.; Kyesi, F.; Aina, M. Human Papillomavirus Vaccination Acceleration and Introduction in Sub-Saharan Africa: A Multi-Country Cohort Analysis. *Vaccines* **2024**, *12*, 489. https://doi.org/10.3390/vaccines12050489

Academic Editor: Christian Napoli

Received: 25 March 2024
Revised: 24 April 2024
Accepted: 27 April 2024
Published: 1 May 2024

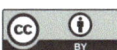

Copyright: © 2024 by the authors. Licensee MDPI, Basel, Switzerland. This article is an open access article distributed under the terms and conditions of the Creative Commons Attribution (CC BY) license (https://creativecommons.org/licenses/by/4.0/).

Abstract: Background: Cervical cancer, caused by human papillomavirus (HPV) infection, is the second-largest cancer killer of women in low- and middle-income countries. The brunt of the global burden is borne predominantly in Sub-Saharan Africa. In 2020 alone, 70,000 of the 100,000 infected women in Africa died from it, thereby making up 21% of global cervical cancer mortality. The introduction of the HPV vaccine into the National Immunization Program was expected to change the trajectory. However, uptake of the vaccination has been poor, especially for the second dose. Only about half of the countries in Africa currently provide the vaccine. Without urgent intervention, the 2030 global cervical cancer elimination targets will be undermined. The study aims to understand the key challenges facing the HPV vaccine and to develop a roadmap to accelerate the uptake. Method: Fourteen countries were purposively included using a cohort design methodology and the investigation spanned March–July 2023. The Africa region was stratified into three focus-group discussion cohorts (Abidjan, Nairobi and Dar es Salaam), comprising pre-selected countries that have already and those about to introduce the HPV vaccine. In each country, the EPI manager, the NITAG chair or representatives and an HPV-focal researcher were selected participants. The methods involved a collaborative and knowledge-sharing format through regional and country-specific discussions, plenary discussions, and workshop-style group missions. Results: The study reached a total of 78 key stakeholders, comprising 30 participants in cohort one, 21 in cohort two and 27 in cohort three. Key outcomes included the prevalence of declining HPV2 vaccination across all countries in the region; country-specific barriers impeding uptake were identified and strategy for accelerating vaccination demand initiated, e.g., utilizing investments from COVID-19 (e.g., electronic registry and multisector coordination); individual countries developing their respective HPV vaccination recovery and acceleration roadmaps; the identification and inclusion of a zero-dose catch-up strategy into the vaccination roadmaps; support for a transition from multiple-doses to a single-dose HPV vaccine; the incorporation of implementation science research to support the decision-making process such as vaccine choices, doses and understanding behavior. Conclusion: Beyond research, the study shows the significance of scientific approaches that are not limited to understanding problems, but are also solution-oriented, e.g., development of roadmaps to overcome barriers against HPV vaccination uptake.

Keywords: HPV; Africa; Sub-Saharan Africa; girls; women; cervical cancer; vaccination; human papillomavirus; vaccine hesitancy

1. Introduction

Human papillomavirus (HPV) is gender-neutral, as both men and women have a 50% risk of being infected at least once in their lifetime [1]. Cervical cancer, caused by HPV infection, is the fourth most frequently diagnosed cancer and the fourth leading cause of cancer-related death among women globally [2,3]. Low-resource countries including those in Sub-Saharan Africa (SSA) have the highest infection burden of the disease with an estimate of 84% and related deaths at 88% [1,4]. In 2020, the number of new global cervical cancer cases stood at over 600,000 with 340,000 deaths, with 90% of these new infections and deaths occurring in low- and middle-income countries (LMIC) [5]. In the same year, in the Africa region alone, 100,000 women were infected, of whom about 70,000 died, making up 21% of global cervical cancer mortality [6]. Therefore, the brunt of the global HPV burden by region is borne predominantly by SSA, at an average of 24% [1,2]. HPV infects basal keratinocytes of the mucosal and cutaneous epithelia, as well as being the common cause of dermatologic diseases, in addition to other variances of cancers including cervical [7].

HPV vaccination has been scientifically trusted to be effective in reducing HPV-induced cancers, especially cervical [2]. With the introduction of the HPV vaccine into National Immunization Programs (NIPs), it is expected to change the trajectory of the disease and also the burden, especially in the SSA region. Unfortunately, compared to other regions, SSA has made limited progress in the implementation of the HPV vaccination program [8–10]. In countries within SSA where the vaccine has been introduced, coverage for the last dose averages at 20% (95% CI: 5–39%) [11]. Only about half of the countries in Africa currently provide the HPV vaccine through the NIPs [5]. Similarly, data for cervical cancer screening in SSA show only 19% of women attend screening programs, i.e., from as low as 0.7% in Benin to 46% in Namibia [12]. Without urgent intervention, the current HPV vaccination status of SSA will undermine the 2030 cervical cancer-elimination target.

Since the introduction of the vaccine against HPV and consequently its introduction into NIPs, its uptake has been below expectation, compounded by the COVID-19 pandemic. Furthermore, studies in 13 SSA countries show that decreased access to healthcare facilities is a barrier to HPV vaccination uptake [13]. However, besides access issues, even in countries where the HPV vaccine is available, the uptake has remained abysmally low [8–10,14,15]. Of course, the COVID-19 pandemic further added to the challenges. Thus, the already limited healthcare resources were diverted to the pandemic response. Also, due to the COVID-19 lockdown, access to eligible girls dropped and has not returned to the pre-pandemic level [16–18]. Similarly, in countries where the HPV vaccination program was to be introduced, misinformation associated with the COVID-19 pandemic, including the COVID-19 vaccine, has hindered such efforts [19–22], while in others, where it has been introduced, the earlier gains have been eroded [23–26].

The World Health Organization (WHO) Cervical Cancer Elimination Strategy set a target of 90% HPV vaccination coverage (for girls, by the age of 15) to be achieved by 2030 [27,28]. However, as reiterated above, uptake or introduction of the HPV vaccine has been challenging in some African countries, and further negatively impacted by the COVID-19 pandemic. The WHO position paper on HPV vaccines issued in December 2022 gave countries the possibility to reduce the dosing schedule and extend the cohorts to be vaccinated up to the age of 20, so as to remove some of the logistical and financial barriers to HPV vaccination introduction into their NIPs and to improve vaccination coverage rates (VCRs) [29,30]. Understanding the barriers and the key enablers of HPV vaccine coverage and/or introduction is crucial to achieving the 2030 agenda of cervical cancer elimination.

HPV vaccination uptake in the region has not been as successful as was expected, with the second dose performing even worse in most of the SSA countries, as seen in Figure 1 [31–33]. In this context, and taking lessons from previous stand-alone symposia on HPV vaccination held in Africa, stakeholders in collaboration with the WHO Regional Office for Africa, regional partners and the countries' Ministries of Health have organized this regional knowledge-sharing focus group study on HPV vaccination acceleration and/or introduction. The primary target groups were the countries' Expanded Program on Immunization (EPI) managers, the National Immunization Technical Advisory Group (NITAG) chairs or representatives and HPV researchers/focal persons, among other state and non-state actors.

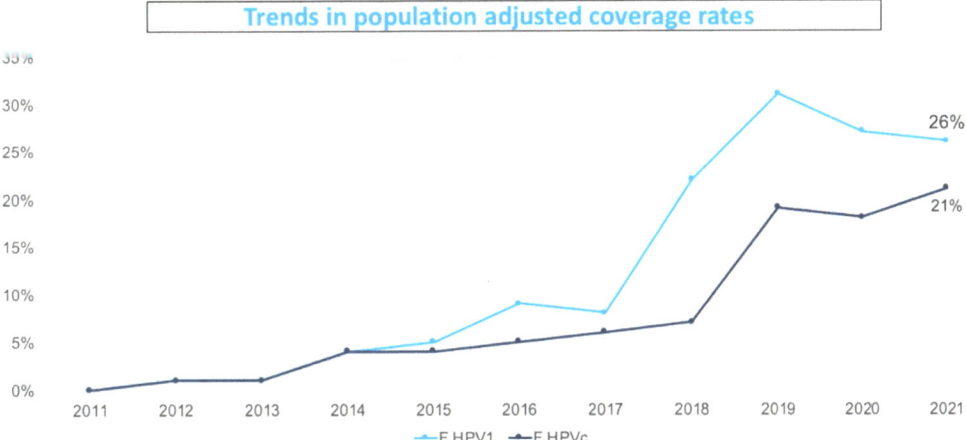

Figure 1. Population-adjusted coverage in Africa (2011–2021) [31].

The goal of the study was to understand the country-specific statuses and challenges facing HPV vaccination uptake and/or introduction in the respective SSA countries, and to proffer strategies for maximizing uptake. The primary outcome was to mentor state actors towards developing country-specific post-COVID-19 recovery roadmap for accelerating HPV vaccination and/or its introduction into SSA. The specific objectives include: providing scientific updates to stakeholders on HPV vaccination in SSA; sharing experiences of enablers of the challenges facing HPV vaccination uptake or introduction in the SSA countries; and developing country-specific roadmaps to accelerate HPV vaccination in SSA countries.

2. Methods

Figure 2 highlights the methodological design frame. A cohort-design method was the implementation technique used [34]. The SSA region was stratified into focus-group discussion (FGD) cohorts and pre-selected countries were included based on high and low HPV coverage, and also countries that have just introduced (e.g., Eswatini and Burkina Faso) HPV vaccination into the NIPs and those that are about to do so (e.g., Nigeria). A total of 14 countries were included in the FGDs. The stratification generated three cohorts. Cohort one took place in Nairobi (Kenya) on 23–24 May 2023 and comprised Kenya, Nigeria, Ethiopia and Rwanda. Cohort two met in Abidjan (Côte d'Ivoire) on 30–31 May 2023 and comprised Côte d'Ivoire, Senegal, Cameroon and Burkina Faso. Cohort three took place in Dar es Salaam (Tanzania) on 6–7 July 2023 and comprised Zambia, Eswatini, Uganda, Tanzania, Malawi and South Africa.

These FGDs adopted a collaborative and interactive knowledge-sharing format using regional and country presentations, plenary discussions, and workshop-style group missions. The regional overview was guided by facilitators from the WHO Regional Office for Africa, the Solina Centre for International Development and Research, the Dose-Reduction Immunobridging and Safety Study (DoRIS), Jhpiego, Merck Sharpe & Dohme (MSD) and Agence de Médicine Préventive (AMP) Afrique, among others. The country-specific overviews (strengths, weaknesses, opportunities and threats (SWOT) analysis) were presented by the EPI managers for each country, where the HPV vaccination status and challenges faced were reported. Participants were mentored in workshop-style sessions to develop a country-specific post-COVID-19 recovery roadmap using pre-defined tools.

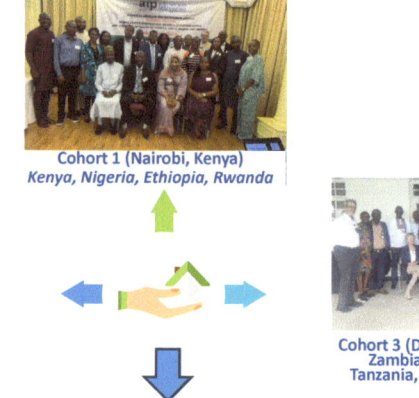
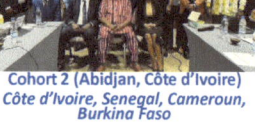

Figure 2. Focus-group discussion cohorts.

The FGDs focused on the importance of HPV vaccination in preventing cervical cancer, given that 75–90% of sexually active women will be exposed to HPV infection during their lifetime and, even more, and more so that vaccination is essential to reduce persistent diseases and associated cancers [35]. The goal of eliminating cervical cancer was reiterated, with an incidence threshold set at less than 4 cases per 100,000 women [36].

An integrated part of the focus group was the workshops designed to help each country develop a recovery plan or an HPV vaccination acceleration or introduction plan, which would be implementable upon return home. The workshop outcomes, which were presented by each country, involved a SWOT analysis of the HPV vaccination program or introduction plans of each country, defining the strategic vision/goal and then mapping into categories the priority strategies envisaged for achieving set goals, such as health policy, demand generation, surveillance, implementation research and vaccine logistics. The priority strategies were backed-up with actionable activities, timelines, and expected outcomes/impacts. The finalized roadmaps were presented at plenary of each cohort for feedback and input from other countries.

Key eligibility criteria for inclusion in the Africa HPV vaccination focus-group discussion cohorts: at least two countries from each regional bloc of SSA (East, West, Central and Southern Africa); a mix of countries with high and low HPV coverage (i.e., those below and above 50%); the EPI manager for the selected countries; the chair or member of NITAG for the selected countries; an HPV researcher/country focal person for the selected countries; representatives from the WHO Regional Office for Africa and country offices of selected countries; and representatives of strategic development partners in the selected countries.

The data were analyzed using a thematic and cohort-based approach, which sought to summarize the data in a cohort or stepwise fashion and assess the themes based on topics. Convergence and divergence of views in each of the cohorts were identified after analyzing each individual submission and categorized them based on the aggregation of the cohort subject outcomes. The participants were coded based on the numbering of the cohorts and an identifier was given (e.g., cohort one as C1_01–30, cohort two as C2_01–21 and cohort three as C3_01–27). The transcribed data were coded and structured along the study objectives, cohort format and themes explored. The coding and themes development were inductively generated.

3. Results

The focus group discussions reached a total of 78 participants (key stakeholders), comprising 30 participants in cohort one (Nairobi, Kenya), 21 in cohort two (Abidjan, Cote d'Ivoire) and 27 in cohort three (Dar es Salaam, Tanzania). The focus groups revealed significant disparities in vaccination coverage as well as differences in the contexts of the implementation of HPV vaccination in the SSA region.

3.1. Key Outcomes: Cohort One

The cohort one stakeholders delved into a series of themes including cervical cancer burden and the introduction of the HPV vaccine in Sub-Saharan Africa. The cohort expanded on the new Strategic Advisory Group of Experts on Immunization (SAGE) recommendation ("WHO Position and SAGE Recommendation for HPV Vaccination"), stressing that HPV vaccines should be introduced early in a coordinated manner and highlighted that the single-dose HPV vaccine offers substantial protection comparable to multiple doses [29,30,37]. Table 1 highlighted the key outcomes.

Table 1. Key Strategies for Maximizing Coverage.

- "There is need for school-based strategies, community outreach, and health facility delivery to optimize coverage and reach out-of-school girls"–C1_01-.
- "We must integrate HPV vaccination with other health services (e.g., Rwanda, Ethiopia, Kenya and Nigeria)"–C1_02.
  - "…Ethiopia: Merge HPV vaccination with COVID-19 and Routine Immunization (RI)"–C1_04.
  - "…Rwanda: Full integration of HPV vaccination into routine immunization and cancer prevention"–C1_02.
  - "…Kenya: Strengthened linkages between health facilities and schools"–C1_05.
  - "…Nigeria: Drawing from prior experiences with new vaccine introductions. In addition, integrating critical outcomes of this discussions into the 2023–2027 National Cancer Control Plan, because 7,968 annual cervical cancer deaths in Nigeria is alarming"–C1_03.
- "…the need for strong governmental commitment. (e.g., Rwanda with over 90% vaccination coverage)"–C1_25.
- "…focus improvement on facility-based HPV vaccination delivery (e.g., Kenya, achieving 75% for HPV1 and 40% for HPV2)"–C1_09.
- "…essentials of rigorous data monitoring (e.g., Ethiopia)"–C1_29.
- "Emphasizing single-dose recommendation for cost and logistical efficiency. Although, there is need for more scientific evidence supporting the single dose's benefits for individual country decisions. While Ethiopia is still considering a single-dose option, Nigeria and others has chosen this route after advice from their NITAGs"–C1_01.
- "Every country recognized the importance of collaboration with various stakeholders, including educational authorities in Ethiopia, religious and tribal leaders in Kenya, and governmental figures in Rwanda and so on"–C1_30.
- "…the importance of research on vaccine's immune-response and efficacy to boost and sustain uptake in high-risk populations"–C1_06.
- "The four nations shared core principles in their HPV vaccination initiatives, such as community engagement, school-based methods, and confronting challenges like funding constraints and misinformation. Yet, they exhibited differences in performance metrics, precise strategies, integration with other health initiatives, and future planning"–C1_23.
- "Rwanda's triumphant efforts provide valuable insights, while Nigeria's introduction added a novel dimension. The discussions here underline that common strategies exist, but the success of each country's approach is intricately linked to its unique circumstances, opportunities, and obstacles"–C1_10.

Challenges and Common Hurdles:
- "…Ethiopia: The country's contention with local political unrest and shaky administrative data"–C1_13.
- "…Kenya: Struggling with sustainable financing for school-based initiatives"–C1_23.
- "…Nigeria: Anticipating challenges during the introduction phase and learning from regional peers"–C1_03.
- "…Rwanda: Reported fewer challenges, indicative of a well-grounded program"–C1_02.
- "Common to all (except Rwanda): "Budget constraints, data quality, and misconceptions leading to vaccine hesitancy"–C1_01.

3.2. Key Outcomes: Cohort Two

The experiences and initiatives of the four pioneering francophone countries (Senegal, Cameroon, Burkina Faso and Côte d'Ivoire) during this study offered invaluable insights (see Table 2), in addition to serving as a roadmap to guide other francophone African countries in the planning and successful implementation of HPV vaccination programs.

Table 2. Key Strategies for Maximizing Coverage.

- "Implementation of field-based research on HPV circulating serotypes is essential"–C2_05
- "Assessment of the clinical, histological and immunological efficacy of single-dose HPV vaccination is still insufficient for strong country-level decision-making on the matter"–C2_21.
- "Extension to new target population such as boys (Burkina Faso, Cameroon) and girls aged 9 to 18 years old (Burkina Faso) could impact general HPV vaccine uptake"–C2_15, C2_19, C2_01, C2_20.
- "Implementation of the single dose vaccination as recommended by WHO (e.g., Burkina Faso, Cameroon, Côte d'Ivoire)"–C2_02, C2_19, C2_03.
- "Improvement of NIP micro-planning (e.g., Côte d'Ivoire)"–C2_03.
- "Strengthen communication activities involving community leaders and mobilizing local partners"–C2_20.
- "Integration of HPV vaccine into the NIPs (e.g., Cameroon)"–C2_19.
- "Vaccine coverage and demand disparities across Francophone Africa region underscore the need to strengthen communication, awareness and community engagement efforts in each country"–C2_21.
- "The focus group discussions allowed key stakeholders to engage on HPV vaccination performance, key challenges and opportunities, thereby opening the need for tailored country specific strategies"–C2_01.

Unique Challenges and Common Hurdles:
- "…Burkina Faso: Striving to meet ambitious targets, i.e., her target is unrealistic"–C2_02.
- "…Côte d'Ivoire: Insufficient communication, poor awareness, and vaccine hesitancy–C2_03.
- "…Cameroon: Strong opposition from religious leaders, communication gaps, and weak leadership commitment"–C2_19.
- "…Senegal: Rumors, misinformation, and insufficient community activities leads to decline in demand"–C2_11.
- Common to all: "Concerns about lack of implementation science research on HPV circulating serotypes and assessing the clinical, histological and immunological efficacy of single-dose HPV vaccination"–C2_21.

Senegal holds the distinction of being the first Gavi-supported francophone African and West African country to introduce the HPV vaccine into her NIP [38]. However, by 2022, the coverage stood at just about 22%, and the COVID-19 pandemic contributed partly to this [39]. Her aim to eliminate cervical cancer as a public health crisis by 2035 seems a bit shaky unless drastic actions are taken. In Côte d'Ivoire, HPV vaccination coverage has stagnated between 34% and 41% since its introduction in 2020 [40]. The low rates are due to vaccine hesitancy among others: insufficient communication, low engagement with HPV vaccination by certain health workers, poor communication on cancers in general, and lack of micro-planning for routine HPV activities [2,41]. Cameroon introduced the HPV vaccine in 2020, alongside COVID-19 vaccination, but faced mass refusal, particularly among religious leaders, leading to a mere 5% coverage rate in 2021 [42,43]. Other challenges identified included gaps in communication, weak leadership commitment, and insufficient partner mobilization [42,43]. In 2022, Burkina Faso launched the HPV vaccination in response to growing demand, with a twofold plan ensuring 95% of 9-year-old girls and boys receiving an HPV vaccine dose by the end of 2024 and achieving at least 95% vaccination among girls aged 10–18 during a catch-up campaign [44].

3.3. Key Outcomes: Cohort Three

The cohort collectively brainstormed on some fundamental pull and push factors driving low HPV vaccine uptake in the region and how to address them (see Table 3). They included the inadequate resources needed to manage cervical cancer in SSA, such as human resources (specialists); infrastructure (vaccine, screening services and treatment), finance (insufficient domestic and donor funding) and cancer registry (limited availability of population-based cancer registries); prevalence of late presentation leading to delayed treatment and then poor health outcome, which are associated with limited awareness and knowledge combined with fear and stigmatization. In addition, there are weak monitoring and evaluation (M&E) systems in the NIP structures; and poor adherence to guidelines, among others.

Table 3. Key Strategies for Maximizing Coverage.

- "Increasing awareness and knowledge of HPV vaccine (e.g., Tanzania, Zambia, Malawi and Uganda)"–C3_03; C3_07, C3_19, C3_24.
- "…Effective monitoring and evaluation systems in the NIPs (e.g., Uganda, South Africa)"–C3_23; C3_27.
- "…Promote transition to single-dose vaccination to help overcome costs and simplify delivery (e.g., Malawi, Eswatini, Tanzania)"–C3_17; C3_30, C3_01.
- "…Legislative advocacy (mandate) of HPV vaccine for 9–14 years old girls (e.g., Malawi)"–C3_19.
- "Relaunching of HPV vaccination campaigns (e.g., in Malawi where coverage declined to 14% for HPV1 and 7% for HPV2 in 2022. Also, for South Africa)"–C3_18; C3_28.
- "Strengthen of HPV vaccination coverage improvement plan (2023–2025) for districts with the highest number of zero dose and under-vaccinated girls (e.g., Tanzania)"–C3_01.
- "Inclusion of implementation science research in NIPs to understand behavioral and contextual factors driving declining HPV vaccination (especially HPV2…e.g., in Malawi, Tanzania, South Africa, Zambia)"–C3_18; C3_02, C3_28, C3_05.
- "…incorporation of teachers as HPV vaccination program partners (e.g., Uganda)"–C3_23; C3_01, C3_30.
- "Strengthening of social mobilization and engagements activities targeting parents (e.g., Uganda, Zambia, Eswatini)"–C3_24; C3_05, C3_29.
- "Strengthen coordination with the Department of Basic Education to incorporate private schools, mitigate turnover of HCWs and improving social mobilization activities (e.g., South Africa, Eswatini)"–C3_28; C3_30.
- "…Increasing mobile services for out-of-school eligible girls in hard-to-reach communities (e.g., Eswatini, Uganda)–C3_30; C3_23.
- "…Identify and use of HPV champions (e.g., Zambia)"–C3_04.
- "Transition to digitalization of data collection and reporting (e.g., Eswatini, Zambia)"–C3_29; C3_05.
- "Inclusion of HPV Vaccine in School Health Guidelines and School Health Policy (e.g., Tanzania)"–C3_02.
- "Mapping of vaccine hesitant groups and providing tailored messaging (e.g., Zambia and others)"–C3_07; C3_24.
- Common to all: "Multi-sectoral collaboration, especially between ministries of health and education is essential"–C3_01.

Unique Challenges and Common Hurdles:
- "…Uganda: Prevalence (57%) of HIV among target group and inadequate human and material capacities to meet needs of school outreaches"–C3_25.
- "…South Africa: Inadequate capacity to provide HPV vaccination beyond public schools and high HCWs turnover"–C3_26; C3_27.
- "…Eswatini: Significant communication gap between parents and school authorities"–C3_30.
- "…Malawi: Rumors and misconception of HPV vaccine as COVID-19 vaccine"–C3_18.
- "…Tanzania: Exclusion of out-of-school girls due to inadequate outreach activities"–C3_03.
- "…Zambia: Frequent school change among eligible girls thereby distorting HVP2 and supply chain issues"–C3_07.
- Common to all: "Poor collaboration between ministries of education and health, global HPV vaccine glitch/shortage, data quality issues"–C3_30.

Malawi introduced the HPV vaccine into the NIP in 2019 in a single-age cohort of 9-year-old girls; however, since the coverage peaked at 83% in 2019, it has rapidly declined to 14% for HPV1 and 12% for HPV2 [45,46]. For Tanzania, following a successful pilot program, Tanzania scaled-up and introduced the HPV vaccine into the NIP in April 2018 for 14-year-old girls, using the routine immunization delivery strategy, and not via campaigns or other point-in-time delivery strategies. In Zambia, the HPV vaccine introduction was in June 2019, and vaccination coverage since then has dropped significantly from 75% in 2019 to 39% in 2021 [47]. The stakeholders attributed the decline essentially to vaccine hesitancy and misinformation. Uganda was among the first countries in SSA to introduce HPV vaccine targeting 10-year-old girls. However, the burden of cervical cancer is still high, with new cases at 6,959, and 4,607 deaths; and with 57% HIV prevalence (adults 15–49 years) [48]. Although the intervention approach was both school-based and community outreach, and stakeholders cited "early engagement of teachers as partners was helpful"–(C3_03, C3_13, C3_19, C3_21), nevertheless, Uganda still struggles with problems of rumors and misconceptions about the HPV vaccine. In South Africa, the high level of commitment and the multi-sectoral involvement of government ministries and civil society organizations played important roles in the successful introduction and implementation of the program. However, the coverage for the first dose has been consistently declining from above 80% in 2014 to 3% in 2022, although affected partly by the COVID-19 pandemic [11,49]. Also, the HPV vaccination point of entry has not been able to move beyond the public schools in South Africa. Meanwhile, Eswatini, who recently launched an HPV vaccination program during the period of this study (June 2023), had a lot to share including resource mobilization and the planning processes. The Manzini district vaccinated the highest number of girls across all ages out of the 9–14 cohort targeted, while 11-year-old girls received the highest number of doses of the first shot in the country.

3.4. The Single-Dose Efficacy

The study on Dose-Reduction Immunobridging and Safety (DoRIS) as presented in the focus group roundtable by DoRIS showed that the single-dose HPV vaccine could reduce cost and simplify delivery; increase the accessibility and sustainability of HPV vaccination programs especially for LIMCs; increase acceptability by girls; high seropositivity (>98%) for HPV16/18 at M36 with one dose of Cervarix® and Gardasil9®; stabilize antibody levels and trajectories over time from M12 and consistent across studies; and avidity [29]. The DoRIS study showed that there is no difference in terms of efficacy between one, two, or three doses of the HPV vaccine as seen Figure 3. For the targeted ages of 9–14-year-old girls, the one dose (1D) immune response in DoRIS was non-inferior compared with three different studies where 1D efficacy was observed. Therefore, the DoRIS study alongside the majority of participants supported the single-dose recommendation in this age group in SSA.

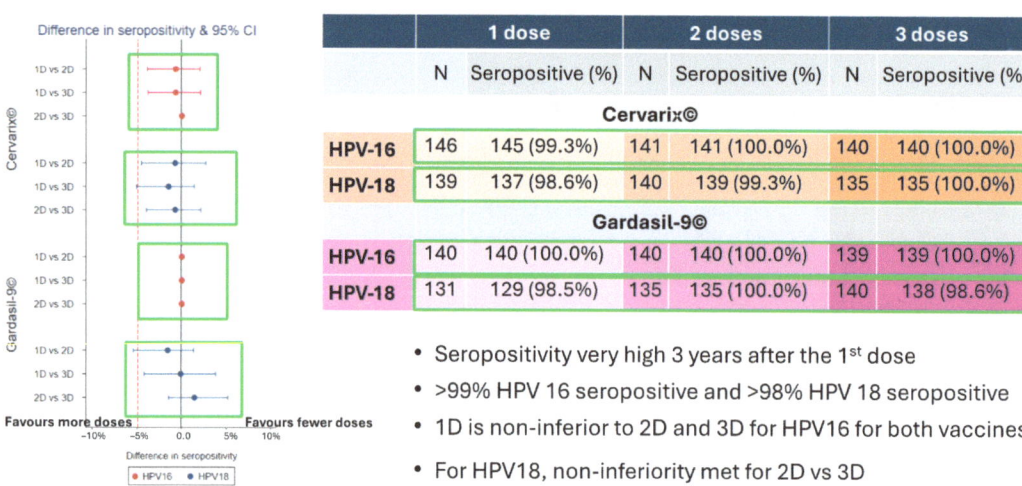

Figure 3. DoRIS study efficacy of single-dose versus multiple doses [29].

3.5. Development of Country-Specific Roadmaps

Each cohort's FGD ended up with a workshop, where each country developed a roadmap after the SWOT analysis of their current HPV vaccination program. The relationships that have been established through this study and between the participating countries were crucial to achieving the common goals of increasing HPV vaccination post-COVID-19 and thus reducing mortality and morbidity associated with cervical cancer in SSA. Figure 4 displays a summary template or sample of the developed country's roadmap.

HPV Vaccination Acceleration Roadmap

Goal: To ensure every child and high risk group is fully vaccinated with high quality and effective vaccines against targeted diseases accorded to recommended strategies

Strategies	Priority activities	Time of implementation	Desired impact on vaccination
Priority Strategies (Health Policy, Demand generation)	Review of evidence to support decision making on the switch to single dose and template review/update of National Cervical Cancer Elimination Strategy	By September 2023 Feb. 2024	Sustained high HPV2 coverage Updated CecX elimination strategy
	Conduct national stakeholders coordination meetings to harmonize on the strategy	Biannual 2023/2024	Improve coordination
	Finalize school health guidelines and print and distribute school health guidelines	2024	Improve coordination
	Review, translate and disseminate IEC material and communication strategy and routinizing advocacy, e.g., airing of messages on different channels	2023 2023-2025	Updated HPV messages Improved awareness
	Develop and pilot mother/daughter pair service package	2024-2025	Improved awareness and access to services
	Facilitate implementation of national catch-up vaccination (campaign) and sensitization of parents on HPV vaccination	2024-2025 On-going	Sustained coverage Improved awareness
	Reorient district leadership, teachers and health workers on the strategy	2023-2025	Improved awareness
Priority Strategy (Surveillance)	Introduce digitization of HPV vaccination data capture	2023/2024	Improve data quality
	Procuring technical assistance for digitizing HPV data (ride on COVID-19)	2023	Improve data quality
	Facilitate CSOs to support in monitoring performance for action AEFI surveillance		Improve coverage for HPV2
Priority strategies (Operations Research, Logistics)	Conduct research on the incidence of the targeted HPV types	2023-2025	HPV impact assessment
	Mobilize funds for operational research	2023-2024	Funds available
	Conduct supportive supervision	2023-2025	
	Conduct trial studies; cancer survivors as drivers of uptake		

Figure 4. HPV Vaccination acceleration roadmap template.

4. Discussion

The goal of the study was to understand the barriers facing HPV-vaccine demand and to leverage stakeholder-led strategies to maximize uptake in SSA. Beyond the impressive participation by the 78 most important stakeholders in the region across 14 countries, the key outcomes included the following: the prevalence of declining HPV2 vaccination across all countries in the region; country-specific barriers impeding uptake were identified and a strategy for accelerating vaccination demand was advanced, e.g., utilizing investments from COVID-19 (e.g., electronic registry and multisector coordination); individual countries developed their respective HPV vaccination recovery and acceleration roadmaps; the identification and inclusion of a zero-dose catch-up strategy into the vaccination roadmap; support for a transition from multiple-to-single-dose HPV vaccine; incorporation of implementation research to support the decision-making process for vaccine choices, doses and understanding behavior.

As part of strengthening communication and demand-generation activities, it is important to focus on information and community awareness to improve knowledge around the HPV vaccine using negative framing, by regularly linking it to a consequence, which is cervical cancer. Constant community mobilization is important for improving vaccination coverage and countering misinformation. Seizing all awareness opportunities that a country's EPIs can find is important. Among the 14 countries, Tanzania, Malawi and Uganda need to do more in this area.

The M&E activities to enhance program-performance tracking need adjustments across all the programs in the region. The study showed weak M&E systems in the EPI or NIPs of countries. A supportive M&E system should be integrated properly into the EPI program plans and decentralized to sub-national levels as well. To this end, it is critical that a budgetary cap of a certain percentage be placed on a country's HPV program, specifically dedicated to M&E.

Promoting the transition to a single-dose vaccination will help countries in SSA overcome the burden of costs and help to simplify vaccine delivery, especially in the post-Gavi-support era. Multidose vaccine schedules are expensive and complex to deliver, and the logistics associated with the vast and scattered population peculiar to the SSA region make it less likely that the region will achieve the elimination target of 2030 unless a new approach (e.g., single-dose strategy) is explored. While this is becoming very popular among countries especially after the WHO recommendation, some others such as Ethiopia, Rwanda, Uganda are still not there, hence a more evidence-based study on single-dose efficacy is required. NITAGs have a lot of work to do here in terms of recommendations to their respective countries EPI.

The expansion of education and HPV vaccination to a broader target population including boys will have a positive impact on the girls as well. Also, it would demystify the conspiracy theories and the talking-points of anti-vaxers around the suspicion of the HPV vaccine, especially being a vaccine for "girls only" in the region [50,51]. Similarly, a critical component of the priority strategies should include the mapping of vaccine-hesitant groups in order to provide tailored messaging to this unique demographic or population. Hesitant groups need to be identified using population-based research and a tailored intervention implemented, primarily with a unique messaging strategy.

Continuous implementation research either as stand-alone or part of the M&E framework of a country's EPI is essential. It will provide data on vaccine effectiveness and the changing or consistent nature of community behavior, all aimed at using evidence to improve the HPV vaccination program at national and sub-national levels. Also, it will be important that all countries strengthen their HPV vaccination plan after the peak of the COVID-19 pandemic, especially for those with high numbers of zero-dose and under-vaccinated girls (e.g., Tanzania and others).

Most of the HPV vaccination interventions are school-based, hence not comprehensive enough to cover out-of-school girls, especially in hard-to-reach communities. The creation of outreach vaccination campaigns for out-of-school-girls using mobile teams and mobile campaigns similar to the polio strategy would be effective in the region. Similarly, the inclusion of the HPV vaccine in the School Health Guidelines and School Health Policy could help normalize the familiarization of adolescent boys and girls with knowledge of HPV and its prevention using a vaccine. There is a need for synergy between the Ministries of Health and Education in the SSA countries.

In francophone Africa, the introduction of the HPV vaccine is progressing at a slow pace, with coverage significantly lagging behind other regions. Among the 54 African countries, only four francophone nations—Burkina Faso, Côte d'Ivoire, Cameroon, and Senegal—have adopted the vaccine. This situation underscores a considerable disparity between Anglo- and Francophone African countries within the region. The slower pace of adoption may mirror underlying challenges tied to communication, cultural acceptance, infrastructure, political commitment, and resource allocation. To accelerate the pace and broaden the vaccine coverage in the Francophone African region, it might be essential to collaborate efforts, develop tailored strategies, and leverage shared learnings from countries that have successfully introduced the vaccine.

The focus groups created a vital platform for the comprehension of the severe impact of cervical cancer and helped lay specific emphasis on the SSA countries, thereby facilitating vibrant and interactive discussions centered on cervical cancer epidemiology, country-specific elimination plans, and the crucial role of HPV vaccination in preventing cervical cancer. The discussions revisited the global goal of eradicating cervical cancer, delineating an ambitious yet attainable target of fewer than four cases per 100,000 women. This target effectively framed the discussion, steering it towards tangible actions and measurable progress.

Strategic Discussions for Improving HPV Vaccine Uptake in SSA

The focus-group cohorts were a big trove of data for experience-sharing and lesson-drawing between the countries to scale up HPV vaccination or introduction into their NIPs. The focus-group cohorts helped the countries to appraise their status through SWOT analysis and then understand the barriers, and the enabling and mitigation strategies needed to overcome the current and anticipated challenges. Other implications of the study outcomes include:

- One of the most significant outcomes of the focus-group cohorts was the shared collaboration of the countries to develop post-COVID-19 HPV vaccination recovery roadmaps, with specific targets to overcome barriers impeding uptake or introduction.
- The resolve amongst the countries and partners to use the roadmap developed during the focus-group cohort discussions as an updated national strategy for accelerating uptake or introduction.
- The focus groups helped to unravel the problems of vaccine coverage and demand disparities across the Francophone Africa region, in countries such as Senegal, Cameroon, Burkina Faso and Côte d'Ivoire. Also, a challenge to expand HPV vaccine launch to other Francophone African countries, or at least across the remaining seven Francophone West African countries.
- The study discovered a lack of implementation research within all the countries' HPV vaccination programs, in addition to limited research on HPV circulating serotypes and assessment of the clinical, histological and immunological efficacy of a single-dose.
- The study brought to the fore the prevalence of the declining HPV2 dose vaccination across countries in the region, thereby necessitating brainstorming on how to address it, e.g., using new knowledge acquired from the cohorts and lessons from peers that are doing well, such as Rwanda and Ethiopia. Also, the idea of using single-dose as a remedy to the negative trend.
- The use of wives of political figures such as first ladies and female elected leaders as the faces of the HPV vaccination campaign seems a positive strategy. The study outcome showed that countries that adopted this strategy had better uptake than others that did not.
- It was insightful to understand that critical barriers or challenges to HPV vaccination uptake common to all the countries, besides Rwanda, were budget constraints (funding), data quality issues (DHIS 2 versus administrative data) and misconceptions about HPV vaccine or vaccine hesitancy. Myths and misconceptions around the HPV vaccine seem to be recurrent impediments to HPV vaccination uptake among the 14 countries. These were primary ingredients for inflaming vaccine hesitancy.
- Any national HPV vaccination strategy using a school-based approach must integrate the school calendar into its implementation plans, otherwise it will be ineffective, i.e., full involvement from the Ministries of Education in HPV vaccination produced better coverage, based on coverage data from countries who had done so compared to others in the cohorts that had not.
- Across the countries, the outcomes showed there was a problem of inaccurate data reporting which led to disparities between administrative and DHIS 2 data. This data problem needs to be reconciled and systematically aligned across the SSA region for effective decision-making. The COVID-19 pandemic data system could be a useful resource that could be exploited.
- The study approach and methods were very novel, because besides being an empirical study, they facilitated peer mentorship and learning among African countries, especially sharing lessons on strategies that have worked and those that have not. This was inspirational for countries who have just introduced HPV vaccination or are about to do so, e.g., Eswatini, Burkina Faso, Cameroun and Nigeria.
- The study discussion led to clarification of the discordance in the dosage regimen adopted by various countries, from three doses to two doses and a single-dose. There was unanimity across the cohorts that all countries should make a decision on the

- dosage based on the peculiarities of their own country's situation. While some countries such as Nigeria, Kenya, Cameroon are ready for the single dose, others such as Ethiopia, Rwanda, Uganda are not there yet. However, the feelings of the majority of the participants were that the single dose is much better for the particular situation in Africa.
- The poor or stagnant coverage in Côte d'Ivoire and some other countries is largely attributable to vaccine hesitancy and further complicated by other factors such as ineffective communication, low appropriation of vaccination by health workers, poor micro-planning and inadequate awareness. Although Senegal's experience of a drastic decline in coverage from 94% in 2019 to 22% in 2022 was attributed primarily to the uncurbed impacts of misinformation and inadequate community engagement, both situations must be considered independent of each other, despite both being in the Francophone African cluster.
- Broad acknowledgement of Senegal and Cameroon's struggles which were found to be particularly linked to opposition from religious leaders, weak implementation strategies and a lack of commitment in some districts due to poor engagement was significant. The roadmap developed during the study has incorporated these inputs.
- Strategies to optimize coverage were uniquely maximized in Rwanda, Ethiopia, Nigeria, Kenya and a few other countries by leveraging a blend of school-based strategies, community outreach, and health facility delivery. The blend was particularly aimed at reaching in-school and out-of-school girls. This provides template for replication in the region.
- A significant outcome of the study demonstrated that, despite consensus on common strategies for improving HPV vaccination uptake, the success of each country's approach is intricately linked to maximization of their unique local circumstances, opportunities, and how they are able to mitigate obstacles.
- Unique challenges were highlighted for some countries: local political unrest and unreliable administrative data (Ethiopia); sustainability of financing existing school-based initiatives (Kenya); limited experience with adolescent vaccination (Nigeria); the polarity in a country's capacity to reach ambitious targets (Burkina Faso); inadequate HPV vaccine information and communication strategies (Côte d'Ivoire); lack of support from political and religious leaders (Cameroon); insufficient community mobilization to dispel rumors and misinformation (Senegal); discordance between parents and school authorities (Eswatini); poor multi-sectoral collaboration between the Ministries of Education and Health (Malawi and Tanzania); inadequate human resources to deliver on school outreach needs (Uganda); supply chain issues (Zambia); high turnover of HCWs (South Africa), among others.

The limitation of this study was the inability to include more SSA countries in the sample. However, based on the cohort design and the eligibility, 14 countries and the representation of the most important or key actors in each country's immunization program were adequate for any scientific conclusion. Second, the tendency of FGD participants to free-ride (i.e., give socially desirable answers) in group settings is common compared to individual interviews, which are better at mediating such effect. However, it is an effective method for this particular study, because it allows participants who share similar or different experiences to feed off each other's responses, and this generates new ideas which might not have been raised in an individual interview.

5. Conclusions

The study was fully optimized in many respects, principally because participants from 14 countries shared ideas and opinions on the mutual challenges associated with HPV vaccination uptake, the reasons for such outcomes and the approaches suggested to address them. The primary outcome was achieved, because the country-specific challenges driving low HPV vaccination uptake were reported and recovery roadmaps for improving HPV vaccine demand were developed on a country-by-country basis. The participants, most of whom are the coordinators of EPI in their respective countries and senior government representatives, were nudged to adapt the study outcomes (e.g., the roadmaps) and work together to achieve the common goal of reducing the burden of cervical cancer in the SSA region. It is essential that there is continued support for these countries in their efforts to overcome the challenges identified and ensure equitable access to HPV vaccination, in addition to fighting against the misconceptions and misinformation that breed vaccine hesitancy. Collaboration between SSA countries, partners, public health actors and the scientific community is crucial if the region's cervical cancer burden is to be reduced and for collectively working on the identified themes below (as shown in Figure 5) to achieve HPV vaccine uptake.

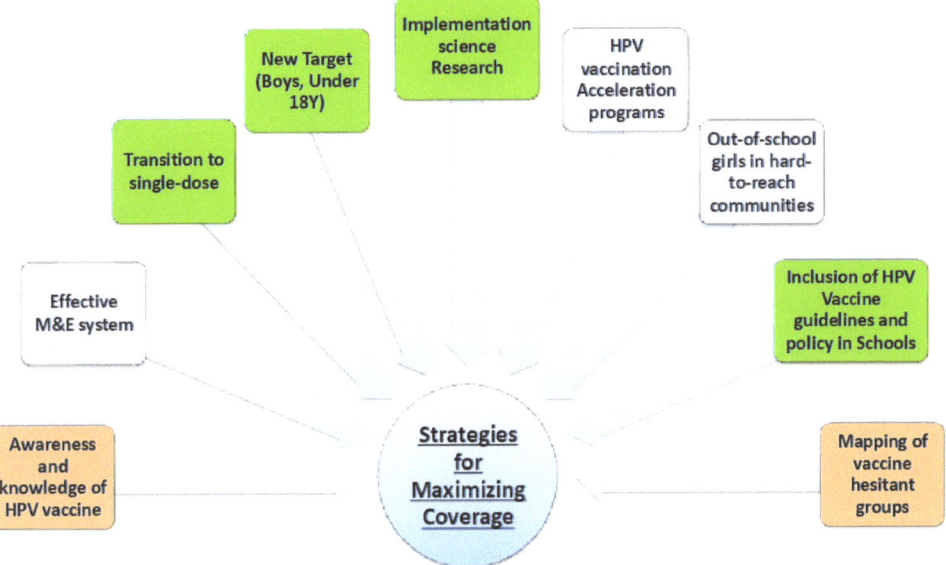

Figure 5. Strategies to foster HPV vaccine uptake.

Vaccine coverage and demand disparities across SSA, especially the Francophone African region underscores the need to strengthen communication, awareness and community engagement efforts in each of the four countries and at least expand the launch of HPV vaccination to the other Francophone African countries. The study brought to bear the significance of scientific approaches that are forward-looking and not just about understanding problems, but are also solution-oriented, one of which was the development of roadmaps with specific targets to overcome country-specific barriers to HPV vaccination uptake. Finally, HPV multi-dose vaccine schedules are expensive and complex to deliver in low-resource settings. Therefore, the SSA countries must evaluate the single-dose HPV vaccine as the best possible option for the obvious reasons discussed in this study.

6. Recommendations

Based on the outcomes of the study, the following recommendations are proffered:

1. A dual anchor system should be initiated to support countries to overcome not only the decline in HPV2 uptake, which the sharing of lessons learnt among peers could help to mitigate, but also to overcome their population's perception issues that contribute to low uptake or vaccine hesitancy.
2. The first anchor should focus on implementation research to support the EPI program with scientific evidence to build resilience and steady uptake. This recommendation is evidence-based owing to a systematic review finding: "To achieve the WHO target

by 2030, we call for studies to understand the barriers and facilitators from the perspectives of stakeholders in order to support the decision-making processes and information required to implement recovery strategies in LMICs" [3].

3. The second anchor, based on the two positive outcomes of this study (sharing opinions/experiences and developing recovery roadmaps), suggest future public health research in low resource settings, such as SSA, should be multifaceted, i.e., understanding the drivers of problems and also finding approaches for solutions.

4. Several countries attributed the decline of HPV vaccination to increased rumors and misinformation as well as to disinformation campaigns. So, concerted efforts using the traditional institutions (religious and cultural) are advised, in addition to the retraining of healthcare workers.

5. NITAGs of various African countries should consider the recommendations for the single-dose option. Multi-dose vaccine schedules are expensive and complex to deliver, and the logistics associated with vast and scattered populations make it less likely that the region will achieve the 2030 target.

6. Strengthening coordination and collaboration. One of the obvious outcomes was the need for close coordination and collaboration because of the similar peculiarities of the challenges surrounding HPV vaccination in the region. There is a need to:

    - Strengthen the intersectoral coordination around HPV vaccination, involving key actors such as the education system, professional associations and community leaders.
    - Promote exchanges and cooperation between SSA countries by creating a research network for sharing information and scientific knowledge.
    - Organize inter-country roadmap appraisal in the form of a bi-annual experience-sharing focus group on HPV vaccination.
    - Revitalize initiatives on the association of first ladies with HPV vaccination. Lessons from peers on how to do so abound.

7. Besides launching a dedicated program of implementation research for HPV vaccination to support the HPV programs, there should also be a strengthening of the diagnosis and monitoring of circulating HPV genotypes in the African region and more inter-country studies to assess the clinical, histological and immunological efficacy of the single-dose HPV vaccine.

Author Contributions: Conceptualization: G.C.A. and T.-A.E. methodology: T.-A.E., G.C.A., A.R.S. and F.K., investigation: G.C.A., A.R.S., F.K. and M.A., results analysis: T.-A.E., G.C.A., A.R.S. and F.K., writing—original draft: G.C.A., writing—review and editing: T.-A.E., G.C.A., A.R.S., F.K. and M.A. All authors have read and agreed to the published version of the manuscript.

Funding: The study was supported by an unconditional educational grant from Merck Sharp & Dohme (MSD) (Ref. No. 60695) through Agence de Médecine Préventive (AMP) Afrique. However, they had no influence on the planning, design, methods, the decision to publish, or the preparation of the manuscript.

Institutional Review Board Statement: Ethical review of protocol was not applicable for this study.

Informed Consent Statement: Informed consent was obtained from all participants.

Data Availability Statement: The datasets used and/or analyzed during the current study are available from the corresponding author on reasonable request.

Acknowledgments: The authors hereby wish to acknowledge the support, contributions and partnership of the following countries' Ministries of Health: Ethiopia, Kenya, Nigeria, Rwanda, Malawi, Tanzania, Zambia, Uganda, Eswatini, South Africa, Côte d'Ivoire, Burkina Faso, Senegal and Cameroon. Similar appreciation goes to the National Immunization Technical Advisory Groups (NITAGs) of Ethiopia, Kenya, Nigeria, Rwanda, Malawi, Tanzania, Zambia, Uganda, Eswatini, South Africa, Côte d'Ivoire, Burkina Faso, Senegal and Cameroon. Finally, we offer big appreciation to the other stakeholders, e.g., WHO country offices, WHO Regional Office for Africa, Solina Centre for International

Development and Research, Gavi, The Vaccine Alliance, Jhpiego, Merck Sharp and Dohme (MSD), University of Erfurt (Germany).

Conflicts of Interest: The authors declare no conflict of interest.

Abbreviations

EPI	Expanded Program on Immunization
HPV	Human papillomavirus
NITAG	National Immunization Technical Advisory Group
SAGE	The Strategic Advisory Group of Experts (SAGE) on Immunization
SSA	Sub-Saharan Africa
CBO	Community-based organizations
MSD	Merck Sharp & Dohme
MCH	Maternal and care health
KENSHE	Kenya Single HPV Vaccine Study
PLWHIV	People living with HIV/AIDS
NCD	Non-communicable diseases
WHO	World Health Organization
MOH	Ministry of Health
DoRIS	A Dose-Reduction Immunobridging and Safety Study
NIP	National Immunization Program
CSOs	Civil Society Organizations
NVI	New vaccines introduction
NPHCDA	National Primary Health Care Development Agency
Q&A	Questions and answers
HF	Health facilities
RI	Routine Immunization
LMIC	Low- and middle-income countries
HIC	High-income countries
SWOT	Strength, weakness, opportunity and threat
HPV1	First dose of HPV vaccine
HVP2	Second dose of HPV vaccine
M&E	Monitoring and evaluation
AUCDC	African Union Centre for Disease Control

References

1. Handler, M.Z.; Handler, N.S.; Majewski, S.; Schwartz, R.A. Human papillomavirus vaccine trials and tribulations: Clinical per-spectives. *J. Am. Acad. Dermatol.* **2015**, *73*, 743–756. [CrossRef] [PubMed]
2. Kutz, J.-M.; Rausche, P.; Gheit, T.; Puradiredja, D.I.; Fusco, D. Barriers and facilitators of HPV vaccination in sub-saharan Africa: A systematic review. *BMC Public Health* **2023**, *23*, 974. [CrossRef] [PubMed]
3. Lee, J.; Ismail-Pratt, I.; Machalek, D.A.; Kumarasamy, S.; Garland, S.M. The recovery strategies to support cervical cancer elimination in lower-and middle-income countries (LMICs) following COVID-19 disruptions. *Prev. Med. Rep.* **2023**, *35*, 102291. [CrossRef] [PubMed]
4. Ba, D.M.; Ssentongo, P.; Musa, J.; Agbese, E.; Diakite, B.; Traore, C.B.; Wang, S.; Maiga, M. Prevalence and determinants of cervical cancer screening in five sub-Saharan African countries: A population-based study. *Cancer Epidemiol.* **2021**, *72*, 101930. [CrossRef]
5. World Health Organization (WHO). Cervical Cancer: Key Facts. 17 November 2023. Available online: https://www.who.int/news-room/fact-sheets/detail/cervical-cancer (accessed on 2 January 2024).
6. World Health Organization (WHO). HPV Vaccination in Africa: A Game-Changer for Women's and Girls' Health, CPHIA 2023. Remarks by WHO Regional Director for Africa, Dr Matshidiso Moeti. Available online: https://www.afro.who.int/regional-director/speeches-messages/hpv-vaccination-africa-game-changer-womens-and-girls-health (accessed on 29 December 2023).
7. Gheit, T. Mucosal and Cutaneous Human Papillomavirus Infections and Cancer Biology. *Front. Oncol.* **2019**, *9*, 355. [CrossRef] [PubMed]
8. Adeyanju, G.C.; Sprengholz, P.; Betsch, C.; Essoh, T.-A. Caregivers' Willingness to Vaccinate Their Children against Childhood Diseases and Human Papillomavirus: A Cross-Sectional Study on Vaccine Hesitancy in Malawi. *Vaccines* **2021**, *9*, 1231. [CrossRef] [PubMed]
9. Adeyanju, G.C.; Betsch, C.; Adamu, A.A.; Gumbi, K.S.; Head, M.G.; Aplogan, A.; Tall, H.; Essoh, T.-A. Examining enablers of vaccine hesitancy toward routine childhood and adolescent vaccination in Malawi. *Glob. Health Res. Policy* **2022**, *7*, 28. [CrossRef]

10. Essoh, T.-A.; Adeyanju, G.C.; Adamu, A.A.; Tall, H.; Aplogan, A.; Tabu, C. Exploring the factors contributing to low vaccination uptake for nationally recommended routine childhood and adolescent vaccines in Kenya. *BMC Public Health* **2023**, *23*, 912. [CrossRef]
11. Amponsah-Dacosta, E.; Blose, N.; Nkwinika, V.V.; Chepkurui, V. Human Papillomavirus Vaccination in South Africa: Programmatic Challenges and Opportunities for Integration with Other Adolescent Health Services? *Front. Public Health* **2022**, *10*, 799984. [CrossRef]
12. Dickson, K.S.; Boateng, E.N.K.; Acquah, E.; Ayebeng, C.; Addo, I.Y. Screening for cervical cancer among women in five countries in sub-saharan Africa: Analysis of the role played by distance to health facility and socio-demographic factors. *BMC Health Serv. Res.* **2023**, *23*, 61. [CrossRef]
13. Perlman, S.; Wamai, R.G.; Bain, P.A.; Welty, T.; Welty, E.; Ogembo, J.G. Knowledge and awareness of HPV vaccine and acceptability to vaccinate in sub-saharan africa: A systematic review. *PLoS ONE* **2014**, *9*, e90912. [CrossRef] [PubMed]
14. Deignan, C.; Swartz, A.; Cooper, S.; Colvin, C.J. Stakeholders' Understandings of Human Papillomavirus (HPV) Vaccination in Sub-Saharan Africa: A Rapid Qualitative Systematic Review. *Vaccines* **2021**, *9*, 496. [CrossRef] [PubMed]
15. Amzat, J.; Kanmodi, K.K.; Aminu, K.; Egbedina, E.A. School-Based Interventions on Human Papillomavirus in Africa: A Systematic Scoping Review. *Venereology* **2023**, *2*, 43–58. [CrossRef]
16. VanBenschoten, H.; Kuganantham, H.; Larsson, E.C.; Endler, M.; Thorson, A.; Gemzell-Danielsson, K.; Hanson, C.; Ganatra, B.; Ali, M.; Cleeve, A. Impact of the COVID-19 pandemic on access to and utilisation of services for sexual and reproductive health: A scoping review. *BMJ Glob. Health* **2022**, *7*, e009594. [CrossRef] [PubMed]
17. Turner, K.; Brownstein, N.C.; Whiting, J.; Arevalo, M.; Vadaparampil, S.; Giuliano, A.R.; Islam, J.Y.; Meade, C.D.; Gwede, C.K.; Kasting, M.L.; et al. Impact of the COVID-19 pandemic on human papillomavirus (HPV) vaccination among a national sample of United States adults ages 18–45: A cross-sectional study. *Prev. Med. Rep.* **2023**, *31*, 102067. [CrossRef] [PubMed]
18. Da Silva, T.M.R.; de Sá, A.C.M.G.N.; Beinner, M.A.; Abreu, M.N.S.; Matozinhos, F.P.; Sato, A.P.S.; Vieira, E.W.R. Impact of the COVID-19 Pandemic on Human Papillomavirus Vaccination in Brazil. *Int. J. Public Health* **2022**, *67*, 1604224. [CrossRef]
19. Olusanya, O.A.; Bednarczyk, R.A.; Davis, R.L.; Shaban-Nejad, A. Addressing Parental Vaccine Hesitancy and Other Barriers to Childhood/Adolescent Vaccination Uptake During the Coronavirus (COVID-19) Pandemic. *Front. Immunol.* **2021**, *12*, 663074.
20. Boucher, J.-C.; Kim, S.Y.; Jessiman-Perreault, G.; Edwards, J.; Smith, H.; Frenette, N.; Badami, A.; Scott, L.A. HPV vaccine narratives on Twitter during the COVID-19 pandemic: A social network, thematic, and sentiment analysis. *BMC Public Health* **2023**, *23*, 694. [CrossRef] [PubMed]
21. Cinelli, M.; Quattrociocchi, W.; Galeazzi, A.; Valensise, C.M.; Brugnoli, E.; Schmidt, A.L.; Zola, P.; Zollo, F.; Scala, A. The COVID-19 social media infodemic. *Sci. Rep.* **2020**, *10*, 16598. [CrossRef]
22. Gisondi, M.A.; Barber, R.; Faust, J.S.; Raja, A.; Strehlow, M.C.; Westafer, L.M.; Gottlieb, M. A Deadly Infodemic: Social Media and the Power of COVID-19 Misinformation. *J. Med. Internet Res.* **2022**, *24*, e35552. [CrossRef]
23. Gountas, I.; Favre-Bulle, A.; Saxena, K.; Wilcock, J.; Collings, H.; Salomonsson, S.; Skroumpelos, A.; Sabale, U. Impact of the COVID-19 Pandemic on HPV Vaccinations in Switzerland and Greece: Road to Recovery. *Vaccines* **2023**, *11*, 258.
24. Schelbar, N.; Ward, C.N.; Phillips, E.; Herr, M.J.; Acevedo, S.; Conner, H.; Greiner, A.; Corriveau, E. Impact of COVID-19 pandemic and vaccine perceptions on HPV vaccine hesitancy. *Am. J. Otolaryngol.* **2023**, *45*, 104172. [CrossRef] [PubMed]
25. SeyedAlinaghi, S.; Karimi, A.; Mojdeganlou, H.; Alilou, S.; Mirghaderi, S.P.; Noori, T.; Shamsabadi, A.; Dadras, O.; Vahedi, F.; Mohammadi, P.; et al. Impact of COVID-19 pandemic on routine vaccination coverage of children and adolescents: A systematic review. *Health Sci. Rep.* **2022**, *5*, e00516. [CrossRef] [PubMed]
26. Daniels, V.; Saxena, K.; Roberts, C.; Kothari, S.; Corman, S.; Yao, L.; Niccolai, L. Impact of reduced human papillomavirus vaccination coverage rates due to COVID-19 in the United States: A model based analysis. *Vaccine* **2021**, *39*, 2731–2735. [PubMed]
27. Global strategy to eliminate cervical cancer as a public health problem: Are we on track? *eClinicalMedicine* **2023**, *55*, 101842. [CrossRef] [PubMed]
28. WHO. Global Strategy to Accelerate the Elimination of Cervical Cancer as a Public Health Problem. 17 November 2020. ISBN 9789240014107. Available online: https://www.who.int/publications/i/item/9789240014107 (accessed on 5 February 2024).
29. Watson-Jones, D.; Changalucha, J.; Whitworth, H.; Pinto, L.; Mutani, P.; Indangasi, J.; Kemp, T.; Hashim, R.; Kamala, B.; Wiggins, R.; et al. Immunogenicity and safety of one-dose human papillomavirus vaccine compared with two or three doses in Tanzanian girls (DoRIS): An open-label, randomised, non-inferiority trial. *Lancet Glob. Health* **2022**, *10*, e1473–e1484. [CrossRef] [PubMed]
30. WHO. Human Papillomavirus Vaccines: WHO Position Paper, December 2022. Weekly Epidemiological Record No 50, 2022; 97, pp. 645–672. Available online: https://iris.who.int/bitstream/handle/10665/365350/WER9750-eng-fre.pdf?sequence=1 (accessed on 4 January 2024).
31. Sharon, K. WHO Global Cervical Cancer Initiative: Key Issues and Priorities for the Africa Region. A Presentation of WHO Office for Africa. Nairobi, 5 July 2023. Available online: https://www.who.int/teams/immunization-vaccines-and-biologicals/diseases/human-papillomavirus-vaccines-(HPV)/hpv-clearing-house/hpv-dashboard (accessed on 4 January 2024).
32. Nhumba, N.; Sunguya, B. Low Uptake of the Second Dose of Human Papillomavirus Vaccine in Dar es Salaam, Tanzania. *Vaccines* **2022**, *10*, 1919. [CrossRef] [PubMed]
33. Bruni, L.; Saura-Lázaro, A.; Montoliu, A.; Brotons, M.; Alemany, L.; Diallo, M.S.; Afsar, O.Z.; LaMontagne, D.S.; Mosina, L.; Contreras, M.; et al. HPV vaccination introduction worldwide and WHO and UNICEF estimates of national HPV immunization coverage 2010–2019. *Prev. Med.* **2021**, *144*, 106399. [CrossRef] [PubMed]

34. Sueyoshi, M.; Huber, K.E. Cohort studies (Chapter 39). In *Handbook for Designing and Conducting Clinical and Translational Research. Translational Radiation Oncology*; Eltorai, A.E.M., Bakal, J.A., Kim, D.W., Wazer, D.E., Eds.; Academic Press: Cambridge, MA, USA, 2023; pp. 231–235.
35. Chido-Amajuoyi, O.G.; Domgue, J.F.; Obi-Jeff, C.; Schmeler, K.; Shete, S. A call for the introduction of gender-neutral HPV vaccination to national immunisation programmes in Africa. *Lancet Glob. Health* **2018**, *7*, E20–E21. [CrossRef]
36. Singh, D.; Vignat, J.; Lorenzoni, V.; Eslahi, M.; Ginsburg, O.; Lauby-Secretan, B.; Arbyn, M.; Basu, P.; Bray, F.; Vaccarella, S. Global estimates of incidence and mortality of cervical cancer in 2020: A baseline analysis of the WHO Global Cervical Cancer Elimination Initiative. *Lancet Glob. Health* **2023**, *11*, e197–e206. [CrossRef]
37. Barnabas, R.V.; Brown, E.R.; Onono, M.A.; Bukusi, E.A.; Njoroge, B.; Winer, R.L.; Galloway, D.A.; Pinder, L.F.; Donnell, D.; Wakhungu, I.; et al. Efficacy of Single-Dose HPV Vaccination among Young African Women. *NEJM Evid.* **2022**, *1*. [CrossRef] [PubMed]
38. Casey, R.M.; Adrien, N.; Badiane, O.; Diallo, A.; Roka, J.L.; Brennan, T.; Doshi, R.; Garon, J.; Loharikar, A. National introduction of HPV vaccination in Senegal—Successes, challenges, and lessons learned. *Vaccine* **2022**, *40* (Suppl. 1), A10–A16. [CrossRef] [PubMed]
39. ICO/IARC HPV Information Centre. Senegal: Human Papillomavirus and Related Cancers, Fact Sheet 2023. 3 October 2023. Available online: https://hpvcentre.net/statistics/reports/SEN_FS.pdf (accessed on 5 November 2023).
40. ICO/IARC HPV Information Centre. Côte d'Ivoire: Human Papillomavirus and Related Cancers, Fact Sheet 2023. 3 October 2023. Available online: https://hpvcentre.net/statistics/reports/CIV_FS.pdf (accessed on 5 November 2023).
41. Ebrahimi, N.; Yousefi, Z.; Khosravi, G.; Malayeri, F.E.; Golabi, M.; Askarzadeh, M.; Shams, M.H.; Ghezelbash, B.; Eskandari, N. Human papillomavirus vaccination in low- and middle-income countries: Progression, barriers, and future prospective. *Front. Immunol.* **2023**, *14*, 1150238. [CrossRef] [PubMed]
42. Haddison, E.; Tambasho, A.; Kouamen, G.; Ngwafor, R. Vaccinators' Perception of HPV Vaccination in the Saa Health District of Cameroon. *Front. Public Health* **2022**, *9*, 748910. [CrossRef] [PubMed]
43. Elit, L.; Ngalla, C.; Afugchwi, G.M.; Tum, E.; Domgue, J.F.; Nouvet, E. Assessing knowledge, attitudes and belief toward HPV vaccination of parents with children aged 9–14 years in rural communities of Northwest Cameroon: A qualitative study. *BMJ Open* **2022**, *12*, e068212. [CrossRef] [PubMed]
44. Kiendrébéogo, J.A.; Sidibe, A.R.O.; Compaoré, G.B.; Nacanabo, R.; Sory, O.; Ouédraogo, I.; Nawaz, S.; Schuind, A.E.; Clark, A. Cost-effectiveness of human papillomavirus (HPV) vaccination in Burkina Faso: A modelling study. *BMC Health Serv. Res.* **2023**, *23*, 1338. [CrossRef] [PubMed]
45. Moucheraud, C.; Whitehead, H.S.; Songo, J.; Szilagyi, P.G.; Hoffman, R.M.; Kaunda-Khangamwa, B.N. Malawian caregivers' experiences with HPV vaccination for preadolescent girls: A qualitative study. *Vaccine X* **2023**, *14*, 100315. [CrossRef] [PubMed]
46. ICO/IARC HPV Information Centre. Malawi: Human Papillomavirus and Related Cancers, Fact Sheet 2023. 3 October 2023. Available online: https://hpvcentre.net/statistics/reports/MWI_FS.pdf (accessed on 27 November 2023).
47. Lubeya, M.K.; Chibwesha, C.J.; Mwanahamuntu, M.; Mukosha, M.; Frank, S.; Kawonga, M. "When you get the HPV vaccine, it will prevent cervical cancer; it will act as a shield": Adolescent girls' knowledge and perceptions regarding the human papillomavirus vaccine in Zambia. *Front. Health Serv.* **2023**, *3*, 1208458. [CrossRef]
48. ICO/IARC HPV Information Centre. Uganda: Human Papillomavirus and Related Cancers, Fact Sheet 2023. 3 October 2023. Available online: https://hpvcentre.net/statistics/reports/UGA_FS.pdf (accessed on 27 November 2023).
49. ICO/IARC HPV Information Centre. South Africa: Human Papillomavirus and Related Cancers, Fact Sheet 2023. 3 October 2023. Available online: https://hpvcentre.net/statistics/reports/ZAF.pdf (accessed on 27 November 2023).
50. Adeyanju, G.C.; Sprengholz, P.; Betsch, C. Understanding drivers of vaccine hesitancy among pregnant women in Nigeria: A longitudinal study. *npj Vaccines* **2022**, *7*, 96.
51. Adeyanju, G.C.; Betsch, C. Vaccination Decision-Making among Mothers of Children Under-5 in Nigeria: A qualitative study. *J. Hum. Vaccine Immunither.* **2023**, *Preprints*, 2023090325. [CrossRef]

Disclaimer/Publisher's Note: The statements, opinions and data contained in all publications are solely those of the individual author(s) and contributor(s) and not of MDPI and/or the editor(s). MDPI and/or the editor(s) disclaim responsibility for any injury to people or property resulting from any ideas, methods, instructions or products referred to in the content.

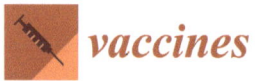

Article

Effect of an HPV Vaccination Multi-Level, Multi-Component Program on HPV Vaccination Initiation and Completion in a Pediatric Clinic Network

Lara S. Savas [1,*], Ross Shegog [1], Erica L. Frost [1], C. Mary Healy [2], Dale S. Mantey [3], Sharon P. Coan [1], L. Aubree Shay [4], Travis A. Teague [1], Juan J. Ferreris [5], Sharice M. Preston [1,†] and Sally W. Vernon [1]

[1] Center for Health Promotion and Prevention Research, UTHealth Houston School of Public Health, Houston, TX 77030, USA; ross.shegog@uth.tmc.edu (R.S.); erica.l.frost@uth.tmc.edu (E.L.F.); sharoncoan@comcast.net (S.P.C.); travis.a.teague@uth.tmc.edu (T.A.T.); sally.w.vernon@uth.tmc.edu (S.W.V.)
[2] Department of Pediatrics, Infectious Diseases Section, Baylor College of Medicine, Houston, TX 77030, USA; chealy@bcm.edu
[3] Michael & Susan Dell Center for Healthy Living, UTHealth Houston School of Public Health in Austin, Austin, TX 78701, USA; dale.s.mantey@uth.tmc.edu
[4] Center for Health Promotion and Prevention Research, UTHealth Houston School of Public Health in San Antonio, San Antonio, TX 78229, USA; laura.aubree.shay@uth.tmc.edu
[5] Christus Health, Children's General Pediatric Clinic, San Antonio, TX 78257, USA; juan.ferreris@christushealth.org
* Correspondence: lara.staub@uth.tmc.edu
† Deceased author.

Abstract: Despite clear evidence of the public health benefits of the human papillomavirus (HPV) vaccine in preventing HPV-related cancers and genital warts, underutilization of HPV vaccination in the United States persists. Interventions targeting multi-level determinants of vaccination behavior are crucial for improving HPV vaccination rates. The study's purpose was to implement and evaluate the adapted Adolescent Vaccination Program (AVP), a clinic-based, multi-level, multi-component intervention aimed at increasing HPV vaccine initiation and completion rates in a five-clinic pediatric network in Bexar County, Texas. The adaptation process was guided by established frameworks and involved formative work with clinic stakeholders. The study utilized a quasi-experimental single group pre- and post- study design, with an external comparison data using the National Immunization Survey-Teen (NIS-Teen) datasets for the same time period to examine the AVP's effect on HPV vaccination initiation and completion. A series of interrupted time series analyses (ITSA) compared the clinic system patient outcomes (HPV vaccination initiation and completion rates) in the post-intervention to the general adolescent population (NIS-Teen). Of the 6438 patients (11–17 years) with clinic visits during the 3-year study period, HPV vaccination initiation rates increased from 64.7% to 80.2% ($p < 0.05$) and completion rates increased from 43.2% to 60.2% ($p < 0.05$). The AVP was effective across various demographic and economic subgroups, demonstrating its generalizability. ITSA findings indicated the AVP improved HPV vaccination initiation and completion rates in clinic settings and that AVP strategies facilitated resilience during the pandemic. The minimal adaptation required for implementation in a new clinic system underscores its feasibility and potential for widespread adoption.

Keywords: human papillomavirus; HPV vaccination; clinic-based multi-level intervention; implementation; quality improvement; adolescents

Citation: Savas, L.S.; Shegog, R.; Frost, E.L.; Healy, C.M.; Mantey, D.S.; Coan, S.P.; Shay, L.A.; Teague, T.A.; Ferreris, J.J.; Preston, S.M.; et al. Effect of an HPV Vaccination Multi-Level, Multi-Component Program on HPV Vaccination Initiation and Completion in a Pediatric Clinic Network. *Vaccines* **2024**, *12*, 510. https://doi.org/10.3390/vaccines12050510

Academic Editors: Li Shi and Yufeng Yao

Received: 26 February 2024
Revised: 13 April 2024
Accepted: 23 April 2024
Published: 8 May 2024

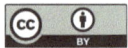

Copyright: © 2024 by the authors. Licensee MDPI, Basel, Switzerland. This article is an open access article distributed under the terms and conditions of the Creative Commons Attribution (CC BY) license (https://creativecommons.org/licenses/by/4.0/).

1. Introduction

The public health benefit of the human papillomavirus (HPV) 9-valent vaccine is clear in its opportunity to prevent infection of 9 HPV types, which cause an estimated 90% of cervical and anal cancers [1–3], 70% of oropharyngeal cancer [4], 75% vaginal cancer [2],

69% of vulvar cancers [2], 63% of penile cancers [2], and 90% of genital warts [2,5]. By preventing nine high-risk HPV infections, the HPV 9-valent vaccine has the potential to prevent approximately 34,400 new cases of HPV-associated cancers in the United States (U.S.) each year [6]. However, each year in the U.S., approximately 196,000 women are diagnosed with high-grade cervical dysplasia [7], 360,000 men and women are affected by genital warts [8], 1.4 million women are diagnosed with low-grade cervical dysplasia [9], and over three million abnormal cervical cancer Pap screenings [9,10]. While the Centers for Disease Control and Prevention (CDC) [11], American Cancer Society [12], and American Academy of Pediatrics [13] recommend completion of the HPV vaccination series by 13 years of age to prevent HPV-related cancers and related morbidity in males and females, HPV vaccine initiation rates fall far below other adolescent vaccines recommended at the same age (i.e., Tdap and meningococcal) [14]. Moreover, after 2018, HPV vaccine series completion, or HPV-up-to-date (HPV-UTD: >3 doses or >2 doses when the first dose was initiated before age 15 years) rates, have stagnated [14] with most states attaining below 50% HPV-UTD rates [15]. In 2022, the national HPV-UTD rate for males 13–17 years (60.6%) [16] and females 13–17 years (64.6%) [16] was far below the Healthy People 2030 goal of 80% [17].

HPV vaccination coverage (with >1 dose) and completion rates differ by ethnicity/race [18]. Minority Hispanic/Latino, Black, and American Indian/Alaskan Native youth have demonstrated greater coverage compared to non-Hispanic (NH) White and NH Asian youth [16,19]. While minority HPV-UTD rates have historically been reported as lower [20], most recent data suggest the NH White HPV-UTD rates now lag behind all minority groups, except for female Hispanics [21].

System-, provider-, and parent-level barriers to HPV vaccination include lack of consistent patient reminders of when vaccination is due, lack of clinician awareness of vaccine-eligible youth and associated missed opportunities, lower parental knowledge about vaccine dosing or scheduling, and inadequate patient-provider communication that alleviates vaccine hesitancy [14]. Evidence for system-, provider- and parent-targeted strategies to mitigate these barriers has been established. Strategies include system-level changes to electronic health records to routinize provider prompts to recommend HPV vaccination and audit and feedback strategies [22], provider-level interventions to promote effective provider communication (including presumptive, bundled, and/or unqualified provider recommendations) [23], and patient reminders [24] and parent education [25] aimed at parent determinants. There is also modest evidence for the implementation of parent- and patient-focused apps to promote HPV education and vaccination [26–28].

Emerging evidence suggests the strength of using multiple intervention strategies through multi-level and multi-component (MLMC) clinic-based intervention approaches to address the complex factors affecting vaccination at the clinic system (organization), provider, and parent levels [29–32]. Recent studies indicate that implementing these evidence-based interventions concurrently has a synergistic impact on HPV vaccination rates [33–35]. The Community Preventive Services Task Force (CPSTF), also known as the 'Community Guide', offers compelling evidence for the effectiveness of these intervention strategies in increasing vaccination rates [36]. Our team developed and evaluated the clinic-based MLMC intervention called the Adolescent Vaccination Program (AVP) to address the need for evidence-based MLMC HPV vaccination interventions designed for clinic organizations to implement to reach diverse patient populations. The AVP comprises six evidence-based strategies that target clinic systems, providers, and parents (Figure 1). AVP development was guided by the Intervention Mapping systematic approach [37], informed by behavioral theory (i.e., Social Cognitive Theory [38], Theory of Reasoned Action [39], Health Belief Model) [40], and guided by formative work with clinic leadership, providers (pediatricians and medical assistants) and parents [41], to increase provider delivery of consistent, bundled (when possible), presumptive and unqualified HPV vaccination recommendations [42].

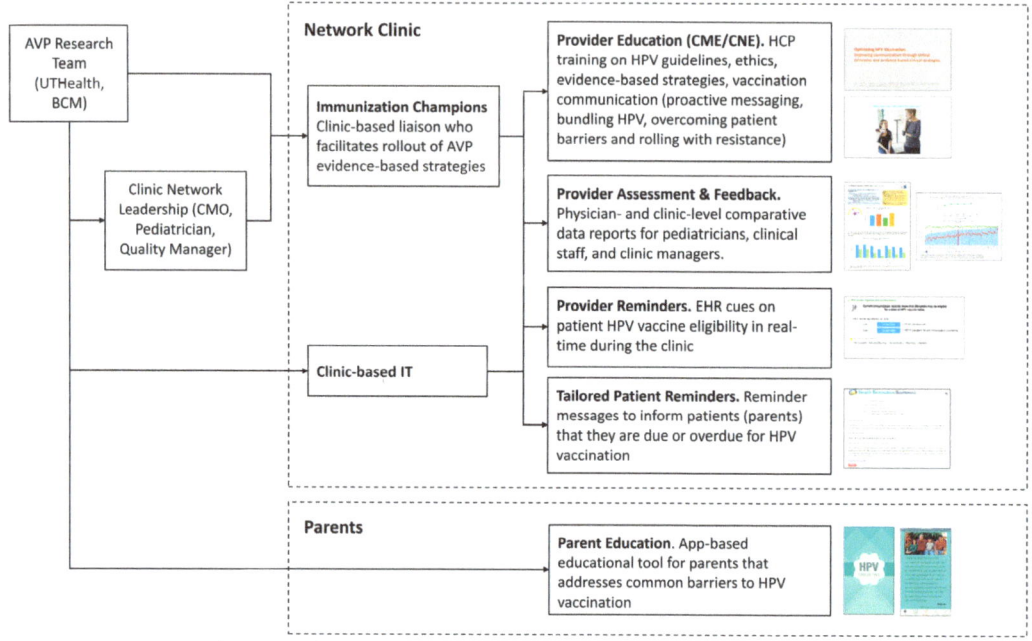

For description of the Adolescent Vaccination Program components see https://avptexas.org

Figure 1. The Adolescent Vaccination Project (AVP) Clinic-Based Multi-level, Multi-Component Evidence-Based Strategies. Note Abbreviations: Information Technology (IT); Health Care Provider (HCP).

We previously demonstrated that the AVP effectively increased HPV vaccination initiation in a 51-clinic pediatric network in Houston, Texas [43]. The patient population in the original study was primarily privately insured (80.3%), identified as English speakers (93.1%), and was demographically diverse (44.4% non-Hispanic White, 24.8% Hispanic and 13.8% Hispanic, and among 17% ethnicity was unknown). The purpose of this study was to adapt, implement, and evaluate the AVP's effect on HPV vaccination initiation and completion in a five-clinic pediatric network. The new clinic setting comprised a primarily insured, English-speaking, and largely diverse patient population, with a slightly larger proportion of Hispanic/Latino patients, reflecting the local population in Bexar County, Texas. This study was designed to increase understanding regarding the generalizability of the AVP and to contribute new evidence regarding its effect on increasing the completion of the HPV vaccination series.

2. Materials and Methods

2.1. The Evidence-Based AVP HPV Vaccination Intervention

The AVP is a pediatric clinic-based intervention that comprises six evidence-based strategies aimed at the clinic organization, providers and parents and designed to synergistically facilitate an increase in HPV vaccination initiation and completion, including (1) HPV immunization champions [44], (2) provider assessment and feedback (A&F) [22,45], (3) continuing medical/nursing education (CME/CNE) [46], (4) electronic health record (EHR)-based provider reminders [47], (5) patient (parent) HPV vaccination reminders [48], and (6) a self-tailored parent education app [49,50].

The champions facilitate the implementation of AVP strategies in their clinic (e.g., by distributing A&F reports, promoting continuing education activity to all clinic staff, training clinic staff on provider and parent reminders, and distributing HPV vaccination education materials for parents in clinic examination and waiting rooms). The provider A&F quarterly reports provide a comparison of each provider's and clinic's HPV vaccination initiation and completion statistics for the previous quarter and HPV vaccination goals for the coming quarter to raise provider awareness of personal and clinic HPV vaccination rates. The online 50 min ethics-accredited CME/CNE HPV vaccination communication education included provider and clinical staff training on HPV vaccine national guidelines, evidence-based strategies to increase HPV vaccination, and communication strategies for providers to deliver strong, presumptive [51], bundled (when concurrent with other vaccines) HPV vaccination recommendations, and to roll with patient resistance [52]. The CME/CNE engaged viewers with real-life case vignettes aimed at enhancing provider communication skills and confidence to deliver strong recommendations. Provider EHR-based real-time HPV vaccination reminders are designed to be delivered during the patient encounter to reduce missed vaccination opportunities. The AVP team worked with the clinic system staff to design reminder messages and coordinate delivery through the EHR system (i.e., Epic software).

The clinic-wide patient registry and HPV vaccination reminder system were developed to notify parents of their child's vaccine initiation due date (triggered by birth date) and to remind parents of completion due dates for the 2nd (or 3rd) HPV vaccination dose. This system was designed for automated delivery through the Epic MyChart patient portal. The parent educational materials promoted positive messaging about the HPV vaccine, as well as provided a QR code for parents to download the AVP *HPVcancerFree* parent education app. Outcome analyses of the original AVP conducted in a 51-pediatric clinic network indicated the AVP MLMC intervention approach effectively increased HPV vaccination initiation 28% from baseline to 3-year follow-up compared with a 20% change for Houston reported by the NIS-Teen data for the same age group and period (2014 through 2018) [43].

2.2. The Adapted AVP Intervention

In the current study, our team, comprising UTHealth behavioral scientists and a Baylor College of Medicine pediatric infectious disease specialist, adapted, implemented, and evaluated the AVP intervention for a new five-clinic pediatric network. Adaptation was guided by the Intervention Mapping approach and CDC Replicating Effective Programs (REP) frameworks [37,53]. The REP framework includes four phases: (1) preconditions (to identify need, target population, and suitability of the intervention); (2) pre-implementation activities (e.g., adapting the program for the new practice setting and patient population with stakeholder input and planning implementation rollout with clinic leadership); (3) implementation (e.g., delivery of the AVP strategies); and (4) maintenance (e.g., preparing the AVP intervention for sustainability).

Focus groups and surveys were conducted with clinic staff and managers to identify psychosocial factors in patients and providers (e.g., social and cultural norms) and clinic structural factors (e.g., EHR capabilities) that affect the implementation of the clinic-based AVP strategies. We did not identify new cultural-related determinants of vaccination that required adaption to parent education. Adaptation included updates to CME and CNE content, including updated HPV vaccination guidelines, new information on HPV vaccine safety, and more evidence for vaccinating at the recommended age (11–12 years). Working with the clinic partners, we identified the need to tailor the A&F preparation strategy to fit with the clinic Athena EHR system capabilities. In addition, the delivery of A&F reports to each provider was designed to align with the clinic organization. Reports were compiled by the AVP team and delivered to champions via email. Champions at each clinic site printed the reports and distributed them to physicians and other clinic staff.

To adapt and integrate the provider reminder strategy into the new clinic system EHR platform, the AVP team worked with the medical director and EHR team. The result was the creation of provider HPV vaccination job aids that outline HPV vaccination best practices and instructions for providers that included the following steps to set up vaccination reminder prompts: (1) use the EHR's (i.e., Athena) quality tab to check whether the patient is due for HPV, (2) subscribe to a customized order set that includes HPV, and (3) manually add HPV immunization alerts to patient's records. These job aids were distributed to all physicians and managers. Champions and managers promoted the job aids and posted them in exam rooms for easy reference by physicians and clinical staff.

Parent reminder delivery methods were also adapted to align with the clinic patient communication infrastructure, changing the delivery method, which was developed with the previous clinic system [43], to sending reminders through an automated email reminder campaign to align with the clinic system's current patient communication methods. The AVP *HPVcancerFree* parent education app adaptation was informed by the formative work with the new system adoptees. In addition, we reviewed the parent survey and app usage data from the original AVP evaluation to improve user engagement and improved relevance to parents. AVP *HPVcancerFree* parent education app adaptations included the addition of (1) an animated, infographic-based video on HPV and the HPV vaccine, and (2) biweekly push notifications containing factual information to serve as reminders to app users and as an additional source of information. The AVP intervention strategies are presented in Figure 1 below and may be viewed at the AVP URL https://avptexas.org (accessed on 29 April 2004).

2.3. Study Setting and Population

Eligible clinics were part of an urban pediatric clinic network in Bexar County, Texas, which serves approximately 7000 children and adolescents aged 11–17 years per year, and served approximately 26,000 11–17-year-olds from 2018 to 2022. No clinics in this system were excluded. At the time of AVP intervention implementation, the system had five clinic sites, 18 pediatricians, and 40 clinical staff (e.g., CMA, RN, LVN). Of those patients, most were privately insured (85%) and identified as Hispanic. (Table 1).

Table 1. Demographics and HPV Vaccine Initiation by Year, Patients Aged 11–17 Years.

Characteristics	Mean Number of Patients per Year	% of Patient Pop.	Baseline N	%	Year 1 N	%	Year 2 N	%	Year 3 N	%	End of Study N	%
Total	6771		6438	64.7	6703	70.5	6715	79.1	7229	80.2	5469	81.6
Ages 11–12	2253	33.3	2430	52.1	2048	57.9	2304	70.5	2228	70.9	1551	70.5
Ages 13–17	4519	66.7	4008	72.3	4655	76.0	4410	83.7	5001	84.3	3918	86.0
Female	3526	52.1	3387	66.6	3498	72.1	3482	79.7	3737	81.6	2756	83.5
Male	3245	47.9	3051	62.6	3205	68.7	3232	78.6	3492	78.6	2713	79.7
Non-Hispanic White	2290	33.8	1540	62.3	3692	70.8	1606	77.6	2322	79.4	1445	79.3
Non-Hispanic Black	292	4.3	231	62.8	319	69.3	267	77.9	350	80.6	256	84.4
Hispanic	2914	43.0	3739	67.8	823	78.7	3846	81.0	3249	82.5	2860	83.5
Other	860	12.7	602	67.8	1339	68.2	620	77.4	878	78.4	589	79.0
Missing or Unknown	415	6.1	326	50.3	530	62.6	375	70.1	430	70.5	319	77.4
Commercial Insurance	5774	85.3	5571	65.0	5723	71.5	5734	79.9	6069	80.6	4486	81.7
Medicare/Medicaid	707	10.4	613	68.8	682	70.2	708	78.8	824	81.7	733	83.8
Other Insurance	120	1.8	88	45.5	96	56.3	123	59.4	172	72.1	154	75.3
None	170	2.5	166	49.4	202	51.0	149	66.4	164	65.9	96	71.9
English Language	6488	95.8	6265	65.1	6514	71.0	6504	79.4	6669	80.7	5264	81.7
Spanish Language	141	2.1	116	59.5	137	59.1	150	76.0	159	78.6	157	81.5
Other Language	3	0.0	1	100.0	0	-	7	14.3	4	100.0	1	100.0
Unknown Language	140	2.1	56	32.1	52	44.2	53	60.4	397	72.0	47	74.5

Baseline = 1 September 2017–31 August 2018; Year 1 = 1 September 2018–31 August 2019; Year 2 = 1 September 2019–31 August 2020; Year 3 = 1 September 2020–31 August 2021; End = 1 September 2021–31 May 2022.

2.4. Study Design

We conducted a quasi-experimental single group, pre- and post-study design with an external comparison group to examine the effect of the adapted AVP intervention on HPV vaccination initiation and completion rates and compare the HPV vaccination initiation rates to the original AVP study. This research was approved by the Institutional Review Board at the University of Texas Health Sciences Center at Houston (HSC-SPH-18-0733).

2.5. Measures

The primary outcomes include HPV vaccination initiation among 11–12-year-olds and HPV vaccination completion, or up-to-date (UTD), by age 13. UTD status is defined as having ≥3 doses, or 2 doses when the first HPV vaccine dose was initiated before age 15 years of age and there were at least 5 months between the first and second dose. We also examined HPV vaccination among 13–17-year-olds to examine the effect of the intervention on the catch-up age groups. We ascertained HPV vaccination outcomes from EHR data at baseline and follow-up. Patient sociodemographic characteristics were also obtained through EHR data, including age (11–12 and 13–17), sex, race/ethnicity (NH Black, Hispanic/Latino, NH White), and health insurance status (public or private).

2.6. Comparison Data

Comparison data are from the National Immunization Survey-Teen (NIS-Teen) datasets for the years 2017–2021, which provides vaccination surveillance data based on a representative sample of adolescents 13–17 years of age, collected among U.S. parents (mailed questionnaires) and providers (by telephone) [54]. The NIS-Teen dataset includes HPV vaccination uptake (≥1 dose) and vaccination UTD rates (≥3 doses, or 2 doses when the first HPV vaccine dose was initiated before age 15 years of age and there were at least 5 or more months minus 4 days, between the first and second dose). The age group reported by NIS-Teen was 13–17 years so we used that age group as our comparison to examine secular trends. The NIS-Teen database presents coverage rates (≥1 dose of HPV vaccine) based on a representative sample of males and females nationally (sample sizes in the years 2017–2021 range from 990–2256 in Texas and 296–336 in Bexar County, Texas.

2.7. Statistical Methods

Before testing the study hypotheses, we calculated patient-level mean and prevalence figures (i.e., descriptive statistics) for study variables among all patients presenting for care during the study period. To test the study hypotheses, we conducted a series of interrupted time series analyses (ITSA) [55,56]. First, we used an ITSA to compare trends in HPV vaccine initiation before delivery of the intervention (1 September 2017 to August 2018) and relative to after delivery of the intervention (1 September 2018 to 31 May 2022). Second, we conducted a similar ITSA to compare trends in HPV vaccine competition before delivery of the intervention, relative to after delivery of the intervention. This method is used to compare the outcome (HPV vaccination initiation) in the post-intervention among the clinic system patient population period to the counterfactual [57]. Each ITSA controlled for age, sex, race/ethnicity, and health insurance status. We also conducted an interaction between interruption and race/ethnicity to test for any possible differences in treatment effect. In addition, we conducted a comparison of clinic HPV initiation and completion (UTD) trends with trends in the general adolescent population provided by NIS-Teen data (2017–2021). All analyses were conducted in Stata 17.2 (College Station, TX, USA).

3. Results

During this three-year intervention study, an average of 6771 patients, aged 11 through 17 years, completed a clinical appointment (52.1% female and 47.9% male). Patients' sociodemographic characteristics, as ascertained from EHRs, indicate that 43% of patients were identified as Hispanic, 33.8% NH White, and 4.3% NH Black. Patients were primarily covered by private insurance, with 10.4% covered by Medicaid, and the majority spoke English (Table 1).

AVP Intervention Effect on HPV Initiation and Completion Rates

We examined HPV vaccination initiation and completion trends from the baseline period (1 September 2017–31 August 2018) to year 1, before rolling out the AVP intervention strategies, and annually through year 3 (1 September 2020–31 August 2021), as well as at a 9-month post-intervention follow-up period. Results indicate a significant increase in initiation rates among 11–17-year-olds from baseline to 3-year follow-up (64.7% to 80.2%; *p*-value < 0.001) (Table 1). Similarly, initiation rates increased from baseline to the 3-year follow-up among both younger adolescents (11–12-year-olds: 52.1% to 70.9%) and older adolescents (13–17-year-olds: 72.3% to 84.3%) (Figure 2). Initiation rates also increased for patients across all races/ethnicities and insurance coverage types, including those with commercial insurance, Medicare/Medicaid, and those with no insurance (Table 1 and Figures 3 and 4).

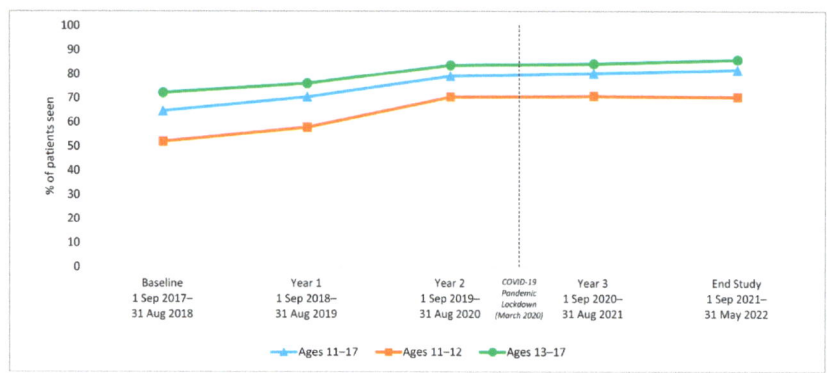

Figure 2. HPV Vaccine Initiation for Clinic System Patients by Age Group, 2017–2022.

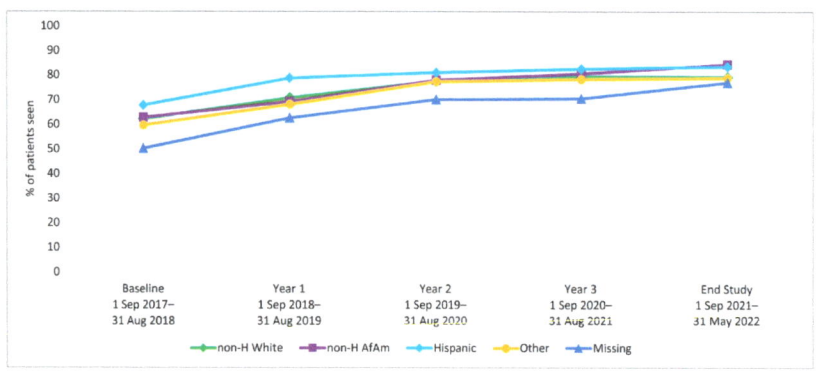

Figure 3. HPV Vaccine Initiation by Race/Ethnicity for Clinic System Patients Aged 11–17.

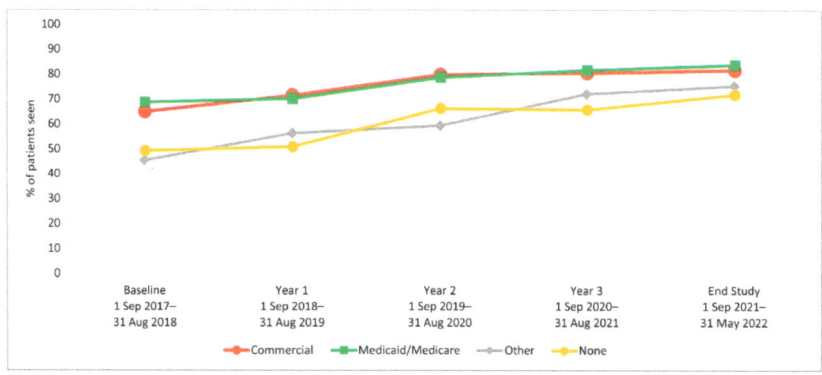

Figure 4. HPV Vaccine Initiation by Patients' Insurance Type Aged 11–17.

HPV vaccination completion rates also increased significantly among 11–17-year-olds from baseline to the 3-year follow-up (43.2% to 60.2%; p-value < 0.001) (Table 2). The increase was observed among both younger adolescents (11–12-year-olds: 20.9% to 28.6%) and older adolescents (13–17-year-olds: 56.7% to 74.2%) (Figure 5). In addition to age, the increase over time was observed across all race/ethnicity and insurance groups (Table 2 and Figures 6 and 7).

Table 2. Sample Demographics and HPV Vaccine Series Completion * by Year, Patients Aged 11–17 Years.

Characteristics	Mean Number of Patients per Year	% of Patient Pop.	Baseline N	%	Year 1 N	%	Year 2 N	%	Year 3 N	%	End of Study N	%
Total	6771		6438	43.2	6703	45.7	6715	53.9	7229	60.2	5469	61.3
Ages 11–12	2253	33.3	2430	20.9	2048	17.5	2304	24.8	2228	28.6	1551	27.0
Ages 13–17	4519	66.7	4008	56.7	4655	58.1	4410	69.1	5001	74.2	3918	74.9
Female	3526	52.1	3387	45.7	3498	47.7	3482	55.2	3737	61.6	2756	62.9
Male	3245	47.9	3051	40.4	3205	43.5	3232	52.5	3492	58.6	2713	59.7
Non-Hispanic White	2290	33.8	1540	40.1	3692	46.6	1606	51.7	2322	60.6	1445	60.4
Non-Hispanic Black	292	4.3	231	38.1	319	43.3	267	50.6	350	61.1	256	62.9
Hispanic	2914	43.0	3739	46.5	823	53.3	3846	56.8	3249	62.9	2860	63.4
Other	860	12.7	602	38.7	1339	41.7	620	51.1	878	55.0	589	57.7
Missing or Unknown	415	6.1	326	31.0	530	39.4	375	41.1	430	46.7	319	52.0
Commercial Insurance	5774	85.3	5571	43.2	5723	46.6	5734	55.0	6069	61.0	4486	62.1
Medicare/Medicaid	707	10.4	613	48.6	682	44.0	708	50.7	824	60.2	733	61.3
Other Insurance	120	1.8	88	30.7	96	34.4	123	39.0	172	48.8	154	50.7
None	170	2.5	166	30.1	202	32.7	149	41.6	164	42.1	96	41.7
English Language	6488	95.8	6265	43.4	6514	46.1	6504	54.5	6669	60.7	5264	61.5
Spanish Language	141	2.1	116	38.8	137	38.0	150	41.3	159	54.7	157	58.0
Other Language	3	0.0	1	100.0	0	-	7	0.0	4	25.0	1	100.0
Unknown Language	140	2.1	56	23.2	52	23.1	53	28.3	397	52.9	47	51.1

* Completion was defined as completing 2 doses by age 15 and 3 doses from 15–17 years of age. Baseline = 1 September 2017–31 August 2018; Year 1 = 1 September 2018–31 August 2019; Year 2 = 1 September 2019–31 August 2020; Year 3 = 1 September 2020–31 August 2021; End = 1 September 2021–31 May 2022.

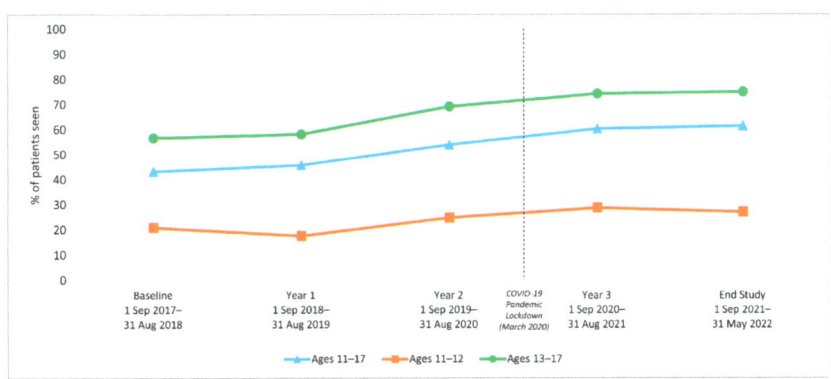

Figure 5. HPV Vaccine Completion for Clinic System Patients by Age Group, 2017–2022.

Overall, a greater increase in initiation and completion rates occurred from year 1 to year 2, following the rollout of A&F, patient reminders, provider CME/CNE, and the parent education app (Figure 8).

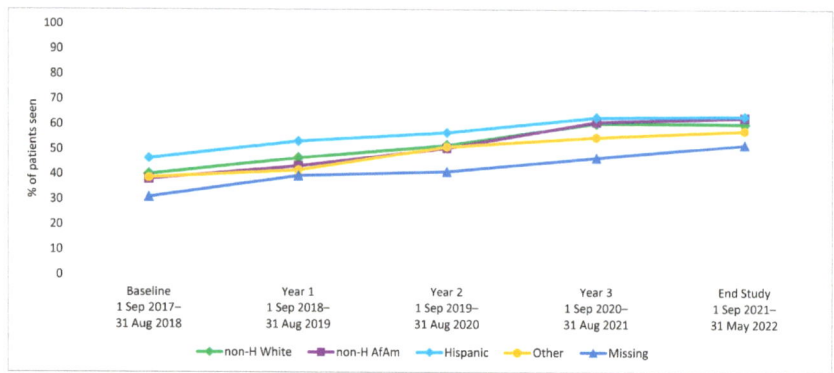

Figure 6. HPV Vaccine Completion by Race/Ethnicity for Clinic System Patients Aged 11–17.

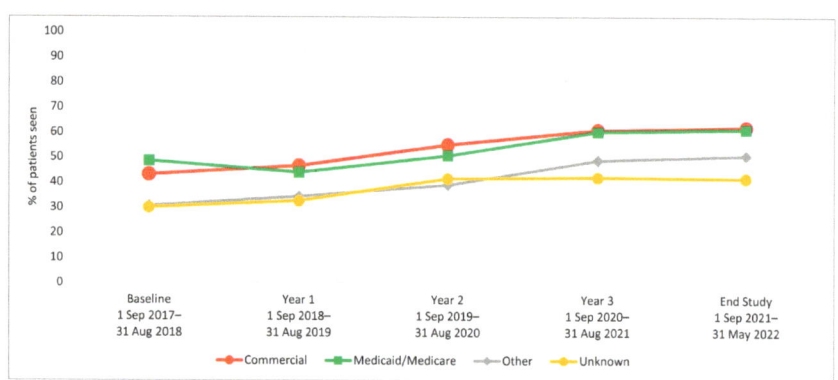

Figure 7. HPV Vaccine Completion by Patients' Insurance Type Aged 11–17.

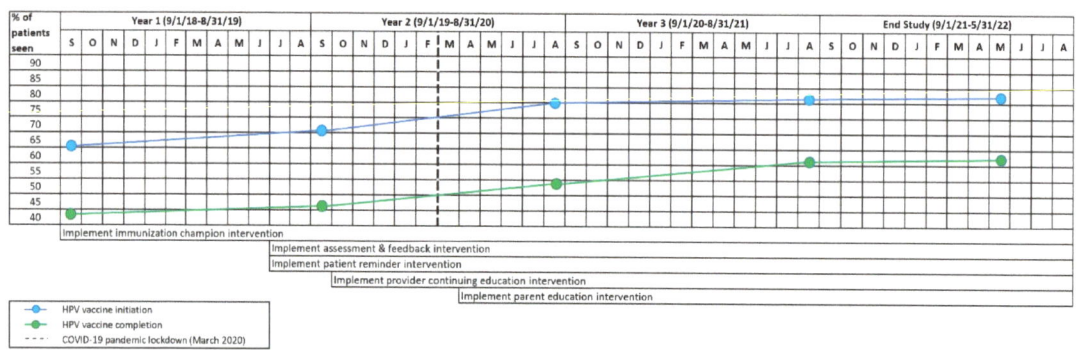

Figure 8. Increase HPV Initiation and Completion Among Patients Aged 11–17 Years, by Year and Adolescent Vaccination Project (AVP) Intervention Strategy Roll-Out.

Figures 9 and 10 present HPV vaccination rates comparing the intervention clinic network patient population initiation and series completion rates to adolescents in the same age groups residing in Bexar County (where the clinic system is located) and Texas. The external comparison was based on NIS-Teen data provided for 13–17-year-olds in the same period (January 2017–February 2022) [58–60].

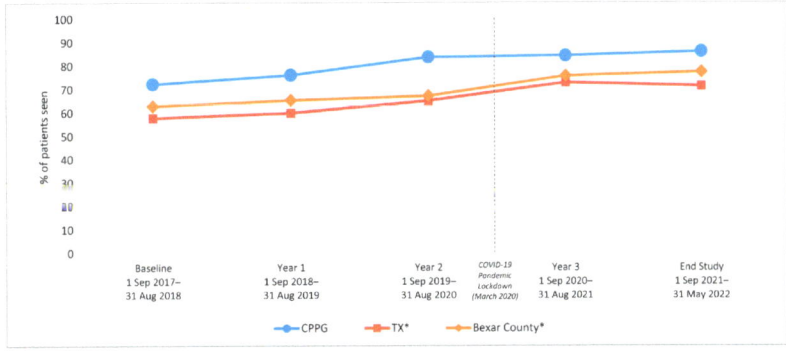

Figure 9. HPV Vaccine Initiation Comparing Intervention Clinics, Texas, and Bexar County Rates, Ages 13–17 *.

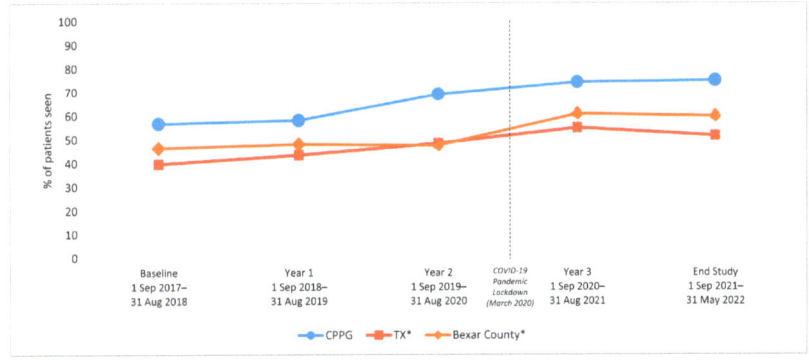

Figure 10. HPV Vaccine Series Completion Comparing Intervention Clinics, Texas, and Bexar County Rates, Ages 13–17 *.

Figure 11 presents the ITSA of the network HPV vaccination initiation data results, which indicate that prior to the intervention, HPV vaccine initiation prevalence was significantly increasing at ~0.34% per month ($p = 0.002$), relative to ~0.18% after the intervention. These trends were not statistically different ($p = 0.173$); however, the onset of the intervention (i.e., the "interruption") was associated with a significant increase in HPV vaccine initiation (+3.0%; $p = 0.002$). No statistical differences were observed between race/ethnicity categories with Hispanic as the referent group or NH White as the referent group.

Figure 12 presents HPV vaccination completion ITSA results, which indicate that prior to the intervention, HPV vaccination completion was unchanged (~0.04% per month; $p = 0.812$) and then increased to 0.43% per month following the intervention ($p < 0.001$). These trends were significantly different, indicating that HPV vaccine competition increased significantly following the intervention ($p = 0.033$). There was no immediate change in the prevalence of HPV vaccination completion ($p = 0.077$) at the onset of the intervention (i.e., interruption).

Because the COVID-19 pandemic lockdown was initiated on 15 March 2020 [61], we assessed the potential effect of the pandemic on HPV vaccination rates during the 3-year intervention period. We found no decrease in HPV vaccination when comparing HPV vaccination rates pre-COVID with post-COVID within the five-clinic network.

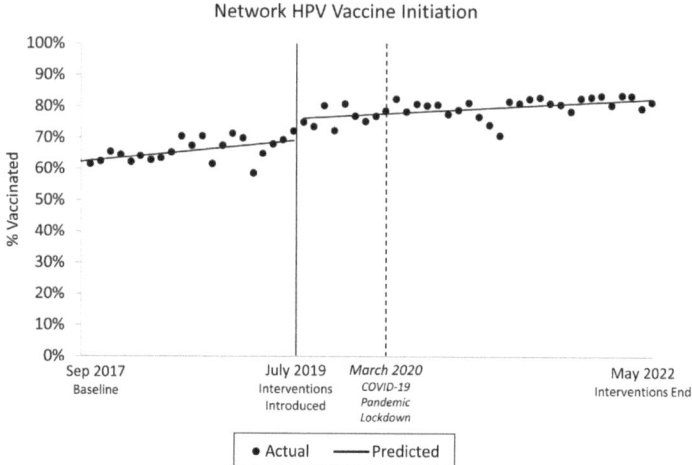

Figure 11. Interrupted Time Series for the Five-Clinic Network, 2017–2022.

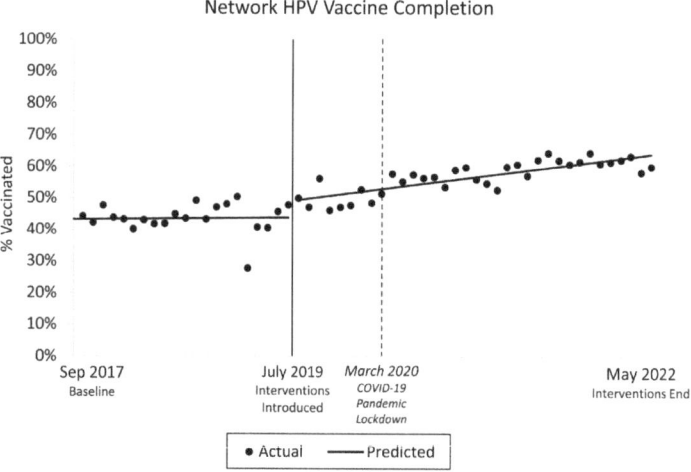

Figure 12. Interrupted Time Series for the Five-Clinic Network, 2017–2022.

4. Discussion

To improve vaccination efforts, we developed the AVP, comprised of evidence-based strategies [48,62–64] to address clinic system-, provider- and patient-related factors influencing HPV vaccination in clinic settings (Figure 1). In our first evaluation of the MLMC intervention (2015–2017), in a 51-clinic network with 44.4% NH White, 24.8% Hispanics, and 13.8% NH Black patients, and predominately English speakers (93.1%), we found the AVP effectively increased HPV initiation rates among 11–17-year-olds by 36% from baseline to 3-year follow-up across all clinic sites [43]. In this current study (2018–2022), in the five-clinic network with fewer NH White (33.8%) and NH Black patients (4.3%), a larger proportion of Hispanic patients (43%), and a slightly higher proportion of English speakers (95.8%), we found the adapted AVP again effectively increased HPV vaccination initiation rates by 24% from baseline to 3-year follow-up, to an overall 80% initiation among 11–17-year-olds. However, we observed the rates began to plateau once clinic site initiation rates approached 80%, indicating there could be a threshold effect. Additionally, this current study establishes the effectiveness of the AVP on increasing HPV vaccination completion rates from 43.2% at baseline to 60.2% at 3-year follow-up (while varying, an increase was observed across each subgroup) (Table 2). Comparing clinic initiation and completion ITSA rates with those among adolescents in the same age groups residing in Bexar County during the same period, we observed that the onset of the intervention was associated with a significant increase in initiation prevalence (+3.0%; $p = 0.002$). In addition, we observed a 0.43% per month increase in completion rates following the intervention ($p < 0.001$). No differences in treatment effect were found by race/ethnic subgroups, indicating that the positive effect of the AVP intervention was observed across race/ethnicity groups. This replicates the findings of our original AVP effectiveness study focused on increasing HPV vaccination initiation [43] and adds new findings regarding effectively increasing completion rates.

The success of the AVP also indicates that minimal adaptation of the MLMC AVP program for the new clinic system was needed to retain its effectiveness on initiation, as well as to positively affect HPV vaccination completion rates. This study thus provides strong evidence of feasibility regarding the minimal burden on AVP program clinic adopters to adapt the AVP strategies for new clinic settings and implement them with fidelity. Thus, the results from this study indicate promise regarding the generalizability of the strategies and scalability of the AVP approach. Moreover, this study adds to the evidence in the literature regarding using MLMC clinic-based intervention strategies [65], including training HPV vaccination champions to implement provider reminder job aids and assessment and feedback (A&F), encouraging providers to complete the CME/CNE to obtain HPV vaccination-specific communication training focused on increasing providers' consistent and effective HPV vaccination recommendation style with adolescent patients/parents and delivering parent education via an HPV vaccination self-tailored app [66].

Importantly, during this study, the COVID-19 pandemic shutdown in the U.S. began in mid-March 2020. During the early pandemic period that coincided with this study, the vaccination initiation and completion rates in the AVP clinic sites continued to rise, albeit with slightly depressed increases (Figures 2, 5, 8 and 9). This increase occurred despite a marked decline in pediatric vaccine administration during the COVID-19 pandemic [67,68]. Moreover, while the NIS-Teen data indicate a significant decrease in HPV vaccination initiation rates among Medicaid and uninsured adolescents during the pandemic period [16], in the present study, these groups continued to experience a slight increase in both initiation and completion rates, suggesting the AVP strategies mitigated the COVID-19-related decline in HPV vaccination rates. Findings of AVP effectiveness during the pandemic were supported by a smaller HPV vaccination quality improvement project conducted in two clinics during the pandemic, which also found the HPV vaccination strategies helped to sustain both HPV initiation and completion rates during the pandemic [69].

This study also has several limitations, particularly related to study design. We used a one-group pre- and post-study design, and the analysis methods did not control for time-varying confounders [57]. We also cannot control for secular trends; however, during the pandemic, secular vaccination trends would not have supported an increase in vaccination rates, and rather, our examination of the vulnerable subgroups most affected by the pandemic (uninsured and Medicaid-covered adolescents) suggests the AVP mitigated negative effects on these vulnerable patient groups receiving care at the AVP clinics. Finally, implementation of the AVP was partially supported by the UTHealth research team, particularly in facilitating the adaptation of the AVP strategies to fit with the capacity and EHR infrastructure of the adopting clinic system. This study also has several strengths. First, this study replicates the original AVP's effect on increasing HPV vaccination initiation, as well as provides new evidence that the AVP had a significant effect on increasing HPV completion rates during the COVID-19 pandemic. By replicating the AVP in a smaller clinic network in a different city, with different patient population demographic profiles, EHR systems, and organizational factors, the results provide insight into the generalizability of the AVP approach across clinic systems. The HPV vaccination outcome data were also ascertained using EHR data.

Findings from this intervention study further establish the AVP as an EBI that supports an increase in HPV vaccination initiation and completion in a pediatric clinic network. This study also serves as an example of the minimal adaptation required to prepare the AVP for new clinic systems. Finally, our findings suggest that the AVP vaccination strategies facilitated resilience during the pandemic, helping to support best practices to promote HPV vaccination initiation and completion. To promote scale-up and sustainment of the evidence-based AVP, research is underway to design implementation support strategies to guide clinic leaders and staff in safety-net clinic systems in the adoption, implementation planning, and delivery of the AVP [70].

Author Contributions: The authors contributing to the study and manuscript development were as follows: Conceptualization, L.S.S., S.W.V., E.L.F., R.S. and C.M.H.; methodology, L.S.S., S.P.C., E.L.F., R.S., S.W.V. and D.S.M.; software, D.S.M.; validation, L.S.S., D.S.M. and E.L.F.; formal analysis, S.P.C. and D.S.M.; investigation L.S.S., E.L.F., R.S., S.W.V., J.J.F. and S.M.P.; resources, L.S.S., R.S., S.W.V., C.M.H., J.J.F., L.A.S., S.M.P. and E.L.F.; data curation, S.P.C. and D.S.M.; writing—original draft preparation, L.S.S. and E.L.F.; writing—review and editing, L.S.S., E.L.F., T.A.T., R.S., L.A.S. and C.M.H.; visualization, E.L.F., D.S.M. and S.P.C.; supervision, L.S.S.; project administration, E.L.F.; funding acquisition, L.S.S., S.W.V., R.S. and E.L.F. All authors have read and agreed to the published version of the manuscript.

Funding: This research was funded by The Cancer Prevention and Research Institute of Texas (CPRIT), grant number PP180089.

Institutional Review Board Statement: This study was approved by the University of Texas Health Science Center at Houston Institutional Review Board (HSC-SPH-18-0733).

Informed Consent Statement: Not applicable.

Data Availability Statement: The data presented in this study are available on request from the corresponding author. The data are not publicly available due to security restrictions.

Conflicts of Interest: The authors declare no conflicts of interest.

Abbreviations

AVP	Adolescent Vaccination Program
A&F	Assessment and feedback
CDC	Centers for Disease Control and Prevention
CME/CNE	Continuing medical/nursing education
HER	Electronic health record
HCP	Health Care Provider
HPV	Human papillomavirus
IT	Information Technology
ITSA	Interrupted time series analyses
MLMC	Multi-level and multi-component
NIS-Teen	National Immunization Survey-Teen
REP	Replicating Effective Programs
U.S.	United States
UTD	Up-to-date

References

1. Senkomago, V.; Henley, S.J.; Thomas, C.C.; Mix, J.M.; Markowitz, L.E.; Saraiya, M. Human Papillomavirus-Attributable Cancers—United States, 2012–2016. *MMWR Morb. Mortal Wkly. Rep.* **2019**, *68*, 724–728. [CrossRef] [PubMed]
2. Saraiya, M.; Unger, E.R.; Thompson, T.D.; Lynch, C.F.; Hernandez, B.Y.; Lyu, C.W.; Steinau, M.; Watson, M.; Wilkinson, E.J.; Hopenhayn, C.; et al. US assessment of HPV types in cancers: Implications for current and 9-valent HPV vaccines. *J. Natl. Cancer Inst.* **2015**, *107*, djv086. [CrossRef] [PubMed]
3. de Martel, C.; Georges, D.; Bray, F.; Ferlay, J.; Clifford, G.M. Global burden of cancer attributable to infections in 2018: A worldwide incidence analysis. *Lancet Glob. Health* **2020**, *8*, e180–e190. [CrossRef] [PubMed]

4. Mahal, B.A.; Catalano, P.J.; Haddad, R.I.; Hanna, G.J.; Kass, J.I.; Schoenfeld, J.D.; Tishler, R.B.; Margalit, D.N. Incidence and Demographic Burden of HPV-Associated Oropharyngeal Head and Neck Cancers in the United States. *Cancer Epidemiol. Biomark. Prev.* **2019**, *28*, 1660–1667. [CrossRef] [PubMed]
5. Garland, S.M.; Steben, M.; Sings, H.L.; James, M.; Lu, S.; Railkar, R.; Barr, E.; Haupt, R.M.; Joura, E.A. Natural history of genital warts: Analysis of the placebo arm of 2 randomized phase III trials of a quadrivalent human papillomavirus (types 6, 11, 16, and 18) vaccine. *J. Infect. Dis.* **2009**, *199*, 805–814. [CrossRef]
6. Centers for Disease Control and Prevention. *Cancers Associated with Human Papillomavirus, United States—2015–2019*; Centers for Disease Control and Prevention, US Department of Health and Human Services: Atlanta, GA, USA, October 2022. Available online: https://www.cdc.gov/cancer/uscs/about/data-briefs/no31-hpv-assoc-cancers-unitedstates-2015-2019.htm (accessed on 2 April 2024).
7. McClung, N.M.; Gargano, J.W.; Park, I.U.; Whitney, E.; Abdullah, N.; Ehlers, S.; Bennett, N.M.; Scahill, M.; Niccolai, L.M.; Brackney, M.; et al. Estimated Number of Cases of High-Grade Cervical Lesions Diagnosed Among Women—United States, 2008 and 2016. *MMWR Morb. Mortal Wkly. Rep.* **2019**, *68*, 337–343. [CrossRef]
8. Centers for Disease Control and Prevention. *Genital HPV Infection—Basic Fact Sheet*; Centers for Disease Control and Prevention, US Department of Health and Human Services: Atlanta, GA, USA, 2023. Available online: https://www.cdc.gov/std/hpv/hpv-Fs-July-2017.pdf (accessed on 2 April 2024).
9. Centers for Disease Control and Prevention. *Priority: Cervical Cancer Statistics*; Centers for Disease Control and Prevention, US Department of Health and Human Services: Atlanta, GA, USA, 2023. Available online: https://www.cdc.gov/cancer/cervical/statistics/index.htm (accessed on 4 April 2024).
10. Sirovich, B.E.; Welch, H.G. The frequency of Pap smear screening in the United States. *J. Gen. Intern. Med.* **2004**, *19*, 243–250. [CrossRef]
11. Centers for Disease Control and Prevention. HPV Vaccination Recommendations. 2021. Available online: https://www.cdc.gov/vaccines/vpd/hpv/hcp/recommendations.html (accessed on 2 April 2024).
12. American Cancer Society. Guideline for Human Papillomavirus (HPV) Vaccine Use. 2023. Available online: https://www.cancer.org/health-care-professionals/american-cancer-society-prevention-early-detection-guidelines/hpv-guidelines.html (accessed on 2 April 2024).
13. O'Leary, S.C.; Frost, H.M. Does HPV vaccination initiation at age 9, improve HPV initiation and vaccine series completion rates by age 13? *Hum. Vaccin. Immunother.* **2023**, *19*, 2180971. [CrossRef]
14. Chido-Amajuoyi, O.G.; Talluri, R.; Wonodi, C.; Shete, S. Trends in HPV Vaccination Initiation and Completion Within Ages 9-12 Years: 2008–2018. *Pediatrics* **2021**, *147*, e2020012765. [CrossRef]
15. Centers for Disease Control and Prevention. *Vaccination Coverage among Adolescents (13–17 Years)*; Centers for Disease Control and Prevention, US Department of Health and Human Services: Atlanta, GA, USA, 2021. Available online: https://www.cdc.gov/mmwr/volumes/71/wr/mm7135a1.htm (accessed on 2 April 2024).
16. Pingali, C.; Yankey, D.; Elam-Evans, L.D.; Markowitz, L.E.; Valier, M.R.; Fredua, B.; Crowe, S.J.; DeSisto, C.L.; Stokley, S.; Singleton, J.A. Vaccination Coverage Among Adolescents Aged 13–17 Years—National Immunization Survey-Teen, United States, 2022. *MMWR Morb. Mortal Wkly. Rep.* **2023**, *72*, 912–919. [CrossRef]
17. Department of Health and Human Services: Office of Disease Prevention and Health Promotion. Increase the Proportion of Adolescents Who Get Recommended Doses of the HPV Vaccine—IID-08 Healthy People 2030. Available online: https://health.gov/healthypeople/objectives-and-data/browse-objectives/vaccination/increase-proportion-adolescents-who-get-recommended-doses-hpv-vaccine-iid-08 (accessed on 2 April 2024).
18. Chao, C.R.; Xu, L.; Cannizzaro, N.; Bronstein, D.; Choi, Y.; Riewerts, R.; Mittman, B.; Zimmerman, R.K.; Gilkey, M.; Glenn, B.; et al. Trends in HPV vaccine administration and HPV vaccine coverage in children by race/ethnicity and socioeconomic status during the COVID-19 pandemic in an integrated health care system in California. *Vaccine* **2022**, *40*, 6575–6580. [CrossRef] [PubMed]
19. National Center for Immunization and Respiratory Diseases Supplemental Table 1: Estimated vaccination coverage with selected vaccines and doses among adolescents aged 13–17* years, by Race and Ethnicity—National Immunization Survey–Teen (NIS-Teen), United States. 2021. Available online: https://www.cdc.gov/ncird/surveillance/hpvimpact/overview.html (accessed on 5 February 2024).
20. Spencer, J.C.; Calo, W.A.; Brewer, N.T. Disparities and reverse disparities in HPV vaccination: A systematic review and meta-analysis. *Prev. Med.* **2019**, *123*, 197–203. [CrossRef] [PubMed]
21. National Center for Immunization and Respiratory Diseases. Supplemental Table 1. Estimated Vaccination Coverage with Selected Vaccines and Doses among Adolescents Aged 13–17* Years, by Race and Ethnicity—National Immunization Survey–Teen (NIS-Teen), United States, 2021; Centers for Disease Control and Prevention. National Center for Immunization and Respiratory Diseases. 24 August 2022. Available online: https://www.cdc.gov/vaccines/imz-managers/coverage/teenvaxview/pubs-presentations/NIS-teen-vac-coverage-estimates-2021-tables.html (accessed on 5 February 2024).
22. Groom, H.C.; Irving, S.A.; Caldwell, J.; Larsen, R.; Beaudrault, S.; Luther, L.M.; Naleway, A.L. Implementing a Multipartner HPV Vaccination Assessment and Feedback Intervention in an Integrated Health System. *J. Public Health Manag. Pract.* **2017**, *23*, 589–592. [CrossRef] [PubMed]

23. Bright, T.J.; Wong, A.; Dhurjati, R.; Bristow, E.; Bastian, L.; Coeytaux, R.R.; Samsa, G.; Hasselblad, V.; Williams, J.W.; Musty, M.D.; et al. Effect of clinical decision-support systems: A systematic review. *Ann. Intern. Med.* **2012**, *157*, 29–43. [CrossRef]
24. Hanley, K.; Chung, T.H.; Nguyen, L.K.; Amadi, T.; Stansberry, S.; Yetman, R.J.; Foxhall, L.E.; Bello, R.; Diallo, T.; Le, Y.L. Using Electronic Reminders to Improve Human Papillomavirus (HPV) Vaccinations among Primary Care Patients. *Vaccines* **2023**, *11*, 872. [CrossRef] [PubMed]
25. Potts, J.; Southard, E. Teaching It Forward: Educating Parents About HPV/HPV Vaccine. *J. Dr. Nurs. Pract.* **2019**, *12*, 46–58. [CrossRef] [PubMed]
26. Gockley, A.A.; Pena, N.; Vitonis, A.; Welch, K.; Duffey-Lind, E.C.; Feldman, S. Tablet-Based Patient Education Regarding Human Papillomavirus Vaccination in Colposcopy Clinic. *J. Low. Genit. Tract Dis.* **2019**, *23*, 188–192. [CrossRef] [PubMed]
27. Ruiz-Lopez, T.; Sen, S.; Jakobsen, E.; Trope, A.; Castle, P.E.; Hansen, B.T.; Nygard, M. FightHPV: Design and Evaluation of a Mobile Game to Raise Awareness About Human Papillomavirus and Nudge People to Take Action Against Cervical Cancer. *JMIR Serious Games* **2019**, *7*, e8540. [CrossRef] [PubMed]
28. Savas, L.S.; Loomba, P.; Shegog, R.; Alaniz, A.; Costa, C.; Adlparvar, E.; Allicock, M.A.; Chenier, R.; Goetz, M.; Markham, C.M.; et al. Using Implementation Mapping to Increase the Implementation of Salud en Mis Manos: A Breast and Cervical Cancer Screening and HPV Vaccination Intervention for Latinas. *Front. Public Health* **2022**, *11*, 966553. [CrossRef]
29. Walling, E.B.; Dodd, S.; Bobenhouse, N.; Reis, E.C.; Sterkel, R.; Garbutt, J. Implementation of Strategies to Improve Human Papillomavirus Vaccine Coverage: A Provider Survey. *Am. J. Prev. Med.* **2019**, *56*, 74–83. [CrossRef]
30. Rodriguez, A.M.; Do, T.Q.N.; Goodman, M.; Schmeler, K.M.; Kaul, S.; Kuo, Y.F. Human Papillomavirus Vaccine Interventions in the U.S.: A Systematic Review and Meta-analysis. *Am. J. Prev. Med.* **2019**, *56*, 591–602. [CrossRef] [PubMed]
31. Khalid, K.; Lee, K.Y.; Mukhtar, N.F.; Warijo, O. Recommended Interventions to Improve Human Papillomavirus Vaccination Uptake among Adolescents: A Review of Quality Improvement Methodologies. *Vaccines* **2023**, *11*, 1390. [CrossRef] [PubMed]
32. Kelly, M.K.; Katzenellenbogen, R.A.; Fiks, A.G. What Health Systems Can Do Now to Improve Human Papillomavirus Vaccination. *JAMA Pediatr.* **2024**, *178*, 13–14. [CrossRef] [PubMed]
33. Siddiqui, F.A.; Padhani, Z.A.; Salam, R.A.; Aliani, R.; Lassi, Z.S.; Das, J.K.; Bhutta, Z.A. Interventions to Improve Immunization Coverage Among Children and Adolescents: A Meta-analysis. *Pediatrics* **2022**, *149*, e2021053852D. [CrossRef] [PubMed]
34. Finney Rutten, L.J.; Griffin, J.M.; St Sauver, J.L.; MacLaughlin, K.; Austin, J.D.; Jenkins, G.; Herrin, J.; Jacobson, R.M. Multilevel Implementation Strategies for Adolescent Human Papillomavirus Vaccine Uptake: A Cluster Randomized Clinical Trial. *JAMA Pediatr.* **2024**, *178*, 29–36. [CrossRef] [PubMed]
35. Fiks, A.G.; Grundmeier, R.W.; Mayne, S.; Song, L.; Feemster, K.; Karavite, D.; Hughes, C.C.; Massey, J.; Keren, R.; Bell, L.M.; et al. Effectiveness of decision support for families, clinicians, or both on HPV vaccine receipt. *Pediatrics* **2013**, *131*, 1114–1124. [CrossRef] [PubMed]
36. Guide to Community Preventive Services. CPSTF Findings for Increasing Vaccination. 16 April 2019. Available online: https://www.thecommunityguide.org/pages/task-force-findings-increasing-vaccination.html (accessed on 10 January 2022).
37. Bartholomew, L.K.; Parcel, G.S.; Kok, G.; Gottlieb, N.; Fernandez, M.E. *Planning Health Promotion Programs: An Intervention Mapping Approach*, 3rd ed.; Jossey-Bass: San Francisco, CA, USA, 2011.
38. Bandura, A. Human agency in social cognitive theory. *Am. Psychol.* **1989**, *44*, 1175–1184. [CrossRef]
39. Fishbein, M. A reasoned action approach to health promotion. *Med. Decis. Mak.* **2008**, *28*, 834–844. [CrossRef] [PubMed]
40. Glanz, K.; Rimer, B.K.; Viswanath, K. *Health Behavior and Health Education: Theory, Research, and Practice*; Jossey-Bass: San Franciso, CA, USA, 2008; Volume 4.
41. Becker, E.R.; Shegog, R.; Savas, L.S.; Frost, E.L.; Healy, C.M.; Spinner, S.W.; Vernon, S.W. Informing Content and Feature Design of a Parent-Focused Human Papillomavirus Vaccination Digital Behavior Change Intervention: Synchronous Text-Based Focus Group Study. *JMIR Form. Res.* **2021**, *5*, e28846. [CrossRef]
42. Crawford, C.A.; Shegog, R.; Savas, L.S.; Frost, E.L.; Healy, C.M.; Coan, S.P.; Gabay, E.K.; Spinner, S.W.; Vernon, S.W. Using Intervention Mapping to Develop an Efficacious Multicomponent Systems-Based Intervention to Increase Human Papillomavirus (HPV) Vaccination in a Large Urban Pediatric Clinic Network. *J. Appl. Res. Child.* **2019**, *10*, 9. [CrossRef]
43. Vernon, S.W.; Savas, L.S.; Shegog, R.; Healy, C.M.; Frost, E.L.; Coan, S.P.; Gabay, E.K.; Preston, S.M.; Crawford, C.A.; Spinner, S.W.; et al. Increasing HPV Vaccination in a Network of Pediatric Clinics using a Multi-component Approach. *J. Appl. Res. Child.* **2019**, *10*, 11. Available online: https://www.ncbi.nlm.nih.gov/pubmed/34231977 (accessed on 5 February 2024). [CrossRef] [PubMed]
44. Santos, W.J.; Graham, I.D.; Lalonde, M.; Demery Varin, M.; Squires, J.E. The effectiveness of champions in implementing innovations in health care: A systematic review. *Implement. Sci. Commun.* **2022**, *3*, 80. [CrossRef] [PubMed]
45. Centers for Disease Control and Prevention. Vaccination Programs: Provider Assessment and Feedback. Available online: https://www.thecommunityguide.org/findings/vaccination-programs-provider-assessment-and-feedback (accessed on 10 January 2022).
46. Perkins, R.B.; Zisblatt, L.; Legler, A.; Trucks, E.; Hanchate, A.; Gorin, S.S. Effectiveness of a provider-focused intervention to improve HPV vaccination rates in boys and girls. *Vaccine* **2015**, *33*, 1223–1229. [CrossRef]

47. Centers for Disease Control and Prevention. Vaccination Programs: Provider Reminders. Available online: https://www.thecommunityguide.org/findings/vaccination-programs-provider-reminders (accessed on 10 January 2022).
48. Centers for Disease Control and Prevention. Vaccination Programs: Client Reminder and Recall Systems. Available online: https://www.thecommunityguide.org/findings/vaccination-programs-client-reminder-and-recall-systems (accessed on 10 January 2022).
49. The Community Preventive Services Task Force. Vaccination Programs: Community-Wide Education When Used Alone. 2020. Available online: https://www.thecommunityguide.org/findings/vaccination-programs-community-wide-education-when-used-alone.html (accessed on 10 January 2022).
50. Henrikson, N.B.; Zhu, W.; Baba, L.; Nguyen, M.; Berthoud, H.; Gundersen, G.; Hofstetter, A.M. Outreach and Reminders to Improve Human Papillomavirus Vaccination in an Integrated Primary Care System. *Clin. Pediatr.* **2018**, *57*, 1523–1531. [CrossRef] [PubMed]
51. Constable, C.; Ferguson, K.; Nicholson, J.; Quinn, G.P. Clinician communication strategies associated with increased uptake of the human papillomavirus (HPV) vaccine: A systematic review. *CA Cancer J. Clin.* **2022**, *72*, 561–569. [CrossRef] [PubMed]
52. Gilkey, M.B.; McRee, A.L. Provider communication about HPV vaccination: A systematic review. *Hum. Vaccin. Immunother.* **2016**, *12*, 1454–1468. [CrossRef] [PubMed]
53. Kilbourne, A.M.; Neumann, M.S.; Pincus, H.A.; Bauer, M.S.; Stall, R. Implementing evidence-based interventions in health care: Application of the replicating effective programs framework. *Implement. Sci.* **2007**, *2*, 42. [CrossRef] [PubMed]
54. Centers for Disease Control and Prevention. About the National Immunization Surveys (NIS). 2018. Available online: https://www.cdc.gov/nchs/hus/sources-definitions/nis.htm (accessed on 2 April 2024).
55. Linden, A. Conducting interrupted time-series analysis for single-and multiple-group comparisons. *Stata J.* **2015**, *15*, 480–500. [CrossRef]
56. Linden, A. A comprehensive set of postestimation measures to enrich interrupted time-series analysis. *Stata J.* **2017**, *17*, 73–88. [CrossRef]
57. Bernal, J.L.; Cummins, S.; Gasparrini, A. Interrupted time series regression for the evaluation of public health interventions: A tutorial. *Int. J. Epidemiol.* **2017**, *46*, 348–355. [CrossRef]
58. Centers for Disease Control and Prevention. *NIS-Teen Data and Documentation for 2015 to Present*; CDC: Atlanta, GA, USA, 2023. Available online: https://www.cdc.gov/vaccines/imz-managers/nis/datasets-teen.html (accessed on 5 February 2024).
59. Bavley, R.; Skalland, B.; Tao, X.; Wolter, K.; Elam-Evans, L.D.; Singleton, J.A.; Walker, T.Y. *A User's Guide for the 2017 Public-Use Data File*; Centers for Disease Control and Prevention: Atlanta, GA, USA, October 2018. Available online: https://www.cdc.gov/vaccines/imz-managers/nis/downloads/NIS-TEEN-PUF17-DUG.pdf (accessed on 10 January 2022).
60. Elam-Evans, L.D.; Mu, Y.; Pingali, C.; Singleton, J.A.; Francis, R.; Skalland, B.; Wolter, K.; Yarbrough, M. *A User's Guide for the 2021 Public-Use Data File*; Centers for Disease Control and Prevention: Atlanta, GA, USA, November 2022. Available online: https://www.cdc.gov/vaccines/imz-managers/nis/downloads/nis-teen-puf21-dug.pdf (accessed on 5 February 2024).
61. Ochani, R.; Asad, A.; Yasmin, F.; Shaikh, S.; Khalid, H.; Batra, S.; Sohail, M.R.; Mahmood, S.F.; Ochani, R.; Hussham Arshad, M.; et al. COVID-19 pandemic: From origins to outcomes. A comprehensive review of viral pathogenesis, clinical manifestations, diagnostic evaluation, and management. *Infez. Med.* **2021**, *29*, 20–36. [PubMed]
62. The Community Preventive Services Task Force. Increasing Appropriate Vaccination: Provider Assessment and Feedback; 1/4/2016. Available online: https://www.thecommunityguide.org/findings/vaccination-programs-provider-assessment-and-feedback.html (accessed on 5 February 2024).
63. The Community Preventive Services Task Force. Increasing Appropriate Vaccination: Provider Reminders; 1/4/2016. Available online: https://www.thecommunityguide.org/findings/vaccination-programs-provider-reminders.html (accessed on 10 January 2022).
64. Centers for Disease Control and Prevention. Vaccination Programs: Health Care System-Based Interventions Implemented in Combination. Available online: https://www.thecommunityguide.org/findings/vaccination-programs-health-care-system-based-interventions-implemented-combination (accessed on 10 January 2022).
65. Smulian, E.A.; Mitchell, K.R.; Stokley, S. Interventions to increase HPV vaccination coverage: A systematic review. *Hum. Vaccin. Immunother.* **2016**, *12*, 1566–1588. [CrossRef] [PubMed]
66. Escoffery, C.; Petagna, C.; Agnone, C.; Perez, S.; Saber, L.B.; Ryan, G.; Dhir, M.; Sekar, S.; Yeager, K.A.; Biddell, C.B.; et al. A systematic review of interventions to promote HPV vaccination globally. *BMC Public Health* **2023**, *23*, 1262. [CrossRef] [PubMed]
67. Patel Murthy, B.; Zell, E.; Kirtland, K.; Jones-Jack, N.; Harris, L.; Sprague, C.; Schultz, J.; Le, Q.; Bramer, C.A.; Kuramoto, S.; et al. Impact of the COVID-19 Pandemic on Administration of Selected Routine Childhood and Adolescent Vaccinations—10 U.S. Jurisdictions, March-September 2020. *MMWR Morb. Mortal Wkly. Rep.* **2021**, *70*, 840–845. [CrossRef] [PubMed]
68. Ryan, G.; Gilbert, P.A.; Ashida, S.; Charlton, M.E.; Scherer, A.; Askelson, N.M. Challenges to Adolescent HPV Vaccination and Implementation of Evidence-Based Interventions to Promote Vaccine Uptake During the COVID-19 Pandemic: "HPV Is Probably Not at the Top of Our List". *Prev. Chronic Dis.* **2022**, *19*, E15. [CrossRef] [PubMed]

69. Zorn, S.; Darville-Sanders, G.; Vu, T.; Carter, A.; Treend, K.; Raunio, C.; Vasavada, A. Multi-level quality improvement strategies to optimize HPV vaccination starting at the 9-year well child visit: Success stories from two private pediatric clinics. *Hum. Vaccin. Immunother.* **2023**, *19*, 2163807. [CrossRef] [PubMed]
70. Shegog, R.; Savas, L.S.; Frost, E.L.; Thormaehlen, L.C.; Teague, T.; Steffy, J.; Healy, C.M.; Shay, L.A.; Preston, S.; Vernon, S.W. Adaptation and Formative Evaluation of Online Decision Support to Implement Evidence-Based Strategies to Increase HPV Vaccination Rates in Pediatric Clinics. *Vaccines* **2023**, *11*, 1270. [CrossRef]

Disclaimer/Publisher's Note: The statements, opinions and data contained in all publications are solely those of the individual author(s) and contributor(s) and not of MDPI and/or the editor(s). MDPI and/or the editor(s) disclaim responsibility for any injury to people or property resulting from any ideas, methods, instructions or products referred to in the content.

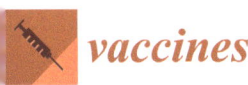

Article

Overview of the Implementation of the First Year of Immunization against Human Papillomavirus across Different Administrative Units in Serbia and Montenegro

Mirjana Štrbac [1,*], Milko Joksimović [2], Vladimir Vuković [1,2,†], Mioljub Ristić [1,3], Goranka Lončarević [4], Milena Kanazir [4], Nataša Nikolić [1,3], Tatjana Pustahija [1,3], Smiljana Rajčević [1,3], Stefan Ljubičić [1], Marko Koprivica [1], Dragan Laušević [2] and Vladimir Petrović [1,3]

1. Institute of Public Health of Vojvodina, Futoška 121, 21000 Novi Sad, Serbia; mioljub.ristic@izjzv.org.rs (M.R.)
2. Institute of Public Health of Montenegro, Džona Džeksona bb, 81110 Podgorica, Montenegro
3. Faculty of Medicine, University of Novi Sad, Hajduk Veljkova 3, 21000 Novi Sad, Serbia
4. Institute of Public Health of Serbia "Dr Milan Jovanović Batut", 11000 Belgrade, Serbia
* Correspondence: mirjana.strbac@izjzv.org.rs (M.Š.); vladimir.vukovic@mf.uns.ac.rs (V.V.); Tel.: +381-21-4897-800 (M.Š.)

Citation: Štrbac, M.; Joksimović, M.; Vuković, V.; Ristić, M.; Lončarević, G.; Kanazir, M.; Nikolić, N.; Pustahija, T.; Rajčević, S.; Ljubičić, S.; et al. Overview of the Implementation of the First Year of Immunization against Human Papillomavirus across Different Administrative Units in Serbia and Montenegro. *Vaccines* **2024**, *12*, 803. https://doi.org/10.3390/vaccines12070803

Academic Editors: Yufeng Yao and Li Shi

Received: 11 June 2024
Revised: 12 July 2024
Accepted: 15 July 2024
Published: 19 July 2024

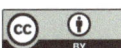

Copyright: © 2024 by the authors. Licensee MDPI, Basel, Switzerland. This article is an open access article distributed under the terms and conditions of the Creative Commons Attribution (CC BY) license (https:// creativecommons.org/licenses/by/ 4.0/).

Abstract: Despite the availability of a safe and effective vaccination, uptake of human papillomavirus (HPV) vaccination remains low worldwide. We aimed to analyze the coverage of HPV immunization during the first year of the immunization program and the sociodemographic characteristics across different administrative units in Serbia and Montenegro. Coverage of HPV vaccination in Serbia for females aged 9–14 and 15–19 years was 5.5% and 5.9%, respectively. The coverage rate of immunization against HPV in Montenegro for girls aged 9–14 years was 22.1%. Within Serbia, only one administrative region (Moravica) had HPV immunization coverage in girls 9–19 years old above 10%, 11 districts had coverage from 5 to 10%, while 13 districts had coverage below 5%. As per Montenegro, two administrative units, Cetinje and Berane, reported the highest coverage, with 39% and 36.4% of vaccinated eligible girls, respectively. When we explored the coverage of HPV immunization among girls aged 9–19 years across different regions in Serbia, we observed that the level of coverage did not correlate with the number of pediatricians or with the population density. In Montenegro, we observed a similar situation. On the other hand, we noticed a statistically significant moderate negative correlation ($r = -0.446$; $p = 0.026$) between HPV immunization coverage and the percentage of illiterate women in the administrative units. Comparing the coverage between the two countries we found that the higher coverage in Montenegro corresponded with a smaller number of female populations aged 9–14 years, with higher average net monthly income, with smaller population density and smaller number of pediatricians, among divorced persons, and among those without formal education or incompletely primary education. Taking into account the experiences in Montenegro, increasing immunization coverage in Serbia could be achieved through a more vigorous educational campaign targeting schools, the general population, and healthcare workers as well as by additionally incentivizing those engaged in these activities.

Keywords: human papillomavirus; HPV vaccine; prevention; oncology; Serbia; Montenegro

1. Introduction

Cervical cancer is the 10th leading cause of female cancer and the third most common cancer in women aged 15 to 44 years in Europe, but in Serbia, it is the fifth most common female cancer overall and the second most common in the age group of 15–44 years [1]. Montenegro, on the other hand, has the highest rate of cervical cancer in Europe, according to WHO's estimates from 2020 the age-standardized incidence rate is 26.2/100,000 women and 10.5 women died from the disease for every 100,000 women in the country [2]. Regarding the geographical world regions, the incidence and mortality of cervical cancer vary. They are higher in underdeveloped areas (e.g., Sub-Saharan African and Southeastern Asian countries), which can be explained by limited healthcare infrastructure, lack of screening programs, and minimal access to HPV vaccination, contributing to very high incidence rates of cervical cancer (ASRI > 26.26/100,000). Contrary to that, economically developed countries (e.g., Western Europe) have a low burden of cervical cancer. These countries typically have robust healthcare systems with widespread access to screening programs (such as Pap smears) and HPV vaccination. Early detection and treatment options are advanced, leading to lower incidence rates and improved survival rates among cervical cancer patients (ASRI < 7.56/100,000). Somewhere in between, developing countries, such as Serbia and Montenegro, have a moderate to high burden of incidence and mortality of cervical cancer (ASRI 17.10–26.26/100,000). In these countries, healthcare resources may be limited, leading to challenges in implementing comprehensive cervical cancer prevention and control measures. Screening programs may be sporadic, and access to HPV vaccination could be limited, especially in rural or underserved areas [3].

Persistent infection with an oncogenic strain of the human papillomavirus (HPV) is considered a necessary factor for the formation of precancerous lesions and the occurrence of cervical cancer. In fact, oncogenic strains of the HPV, of which type 16 and type 18 are most common, cause almost 100% of cases of cervical cancer, along with 90% of anal, 70% of vaginal, 40% of vulvar, 50% of penile and 13% to 72% of oropharyngeal cancers [4]. Considering that HPV prevalence and genotype distribution of normal and abnormal cervical lesions are missing in the updated IARC Human Papillomavirus and Related Diseases Report for Serbia and Montenegro, only recent publications can provide insight into data on the prevalence of HPV-infected women. According to them, the HPV infection rate in Serbian and Montenegrin women is nearly the same (43% vs. 41%) [5,6] emphasizing the importance and need for vaccination. The WHO Cervical Cancer Elimination strategy includes coverage targets for scale-up by 2030 of HPV vaccination to 90% of all adolescent girls, twice-lifetime cervical screening to 70%, and treatment of pre-invasive lesions and invasive cancer to 90% [7].

Currently, there are six licensed HPV vaccines available to the population: three bivalent, two quadrivalent, and one nonavalent vaccine. All of these have proven their effectiveness in preventing infection with HPV types 16 and 18, which together cause about 70% of global cervical cancer cases [8,9]. The nonavalent vaccine has the widest prophylactic spectrum, offering additional protection against HPV types 31, 33, 45, 52, and 58, which are responsible for a smaller number of HPV-related cancers. The most common genotypes in Serbian women are HPV 16, 31, 33, and 51 [10]. With this in mind, the prophylactic value of HPV vaccines that target these high-risk strains is evident, and in many countries with implemented HPV vaccination programs and high vaccine coverage, a reduction in the number of HPV infections, genital warts, and cervical precancerous lesions is seen, and reduction in cervical cancer and other HPV related cancers is expected [11,12]. In Serbia, since 2008, the HPV vaccination has been recommended for young adults before their first sexual experience, although the cost of the vaccine was not covered by the national health care insurance. Since June 2022, the nonavalent HPV vaccine was introduced in the National Immunization Program in Serbia and started to be implemented nationwide, targeting persons aged 9–19 years [13]. The vaccine is applied free of charge in two doses for children aged 9–15 and in three doses for young adults aged 15–19 years. In Montenegro, the HPV vaccination campaign started on 26 September 2022, with a one-dose schedule for 9-year-old girls (cohort 2013) as part of the National Immunization Program using the nonavalent HPV vaccine. From 15 February 2023, the catch-up vaccination for all girls aged 9–14 years started (cohorts 2008–2013). Before the start of vaccination, education activities were conducted, especially for healthcare workers at the primary health level (pediatric specialists, pediatric nurses, and gynecologists) and partially among the parents. The program is facility-based and is implemented nationwide. Vaccines are administered by teams that consist of pediatric specialists and pediatric nurses. In Serbia, as well as in

Montenegro, immunization against HPV is recommended. During the observed period, the vaccines against HPV were continuously available in both countries.

Lack of parent awareness about vaccination, low level of parental education, gender inequality, and poverty contribute to lower vaccination coverage of children. Similarly, lower education, maternal knowledge, and social prejudices were demonstrated to significantly impact vaccination coverage. Also, various socioeconomic and demographic factors demonstrate a significant relationship with high vaccine coverage, as evidenced by numerous studies conducted at the local and regional levels [14–17]. The objective of our study was to analyze the coverage of immunization against HPV taking into account available sociodemographic characteristics of different administrative units (districts and municipalities) in Serbia and Montenegro.

2. Materials and Methods

2.1. Country Characteristics

Both Serbia and Montenegro are divided into administrative units. Observed characteristics of administrative units in our study were: average monthly income, number of pediatricians per 10,000 children, educational attainment of women aged 15 and up (without formal education or incompletely primary education, primary, secondary, and tertiary level of education, or unknown), marital status of women over 15 years old, population density and area (in km^2) of the district/municipality [18,19]. For the territory of Serbia, the average age of the women aged 15 and over, the degree of urbanization, and the percentage of illiteracy in the population over 10 years old were also observed. In Montenegro, healthcare on the primary health level for 25 administrative units is covered by 18 primary healthcare centers (PHCCs) and seven Health Stations (HSs). HSs are located in small municipalities and administrative parts of some primary healthcare centers.

2.2. HPV Vaccine Coverage

We used depersonalized coverage data from the National Immunization Registries of the Public Health Institute of Serbia and Institute of Public Health of Montenegro, which contain data on vaccinated girls with the HPV vaccine. Data were collected for one year from the time of the introduction of nine-valent HPV vaccine at the national level, i.e., from June 2022 in Serbia, and from February 2023 in Montenegro. Additionally, Serbia initiated HPV vaccination, adopting a gender-neutral strategy and targeting ages 9–19 without prior campaign or promotion. In contrast, Montenegro focused initially on 9-year-olds with extensive promotional efforts. It was not until February 2023 that Montenegro expanded its vaccination program to include ages 9–14. We analyzed coverage in cohorts of girls aged 9 to 14 years, 15 to 19, and 9 to 19 years in Serbia, and of girls aged 9–14 years in Montenegro for the mentioned period. The analysis of vaccine coverage was based on the initiated HPV immunization, i.e., every child who received at least one dose of the vaccine was considered vaccinated, in both countries. The coverage by administrative units was calculated by dividing the number of vaccinated female persons by the number of female persons in the observed cohorts according to the population census [20,21].

2.3. Data Analyses

Comparisons of categorical data between groups were made by Fisher's exact test (two-tailed) or chi-square test, where appropriate, while the analysis of variance (ANOVA) was used for continuous data. Tests of proportion were performed in order to compare sociodemographic characteristics and coverage of immunization against HPV between two countries. For the purpose of statistical analyses, different administrative units per country were distributed into tertiles based on the values of the evaluated sociodemographic characteristics, where the first tertile contained the lowest and the third represented the highest values. Pearson's correlation was used to explore potential correlations between values of different sociodemographic characteristics of the administrative units and the corresponding level of HPV coverage. Data analysis was performed using the SPSS version 22 software and $p < 0.05$ was considered statistically significant across the analyses.

3. Results

According to the latest available census data, the total female population aged 9 to 14 is about 188,000 in Serbia and around 25,000 in Montenegro. The average monthly net wage in Montenegro at the beginning of the HPV vaccination program (2022) was USD 776, while in Serbia was USD 670.8. Population density was 79 inhabitants per km^2 in Serbia and 46 in Montenegro, while the number of pediatricians in primary healthcare was 28.7 per 10,000 children in Serbia and 6.4 in Montenegro. Marital status of females $\geq$15 years old was represented with the highest percent of married females in both countries, around 53%, while the education of the same population was mostly of secondary level, 48.1% in Serbia and 47% in Montenegro, followed by tertiary (24%) and primary (19.1%) level in Serbia, and primary (22.4%) and tertiary (16.1%) in Montenegro. The average HPV vaccination uptake rate ($\geq$1 dose) of females aged 9–19 years after the first year of immunization in Serbia was 5.72%, (county range across the administrative units 0.92–11.07%, median = 4.80%). On the other hand, in the cohort of females 9–14 years old in Serbia was 5.53%, while in Montenegro was 22.10% for the same age cohort, as presented in Table 1.

Table 1. Selected sociodemographic characteristics of Serbia and Montenegro.

	Serbia		Montenegro		p Value
Female population, aged 9 to 14 (n)	188,043		24,929		<0.0001 *
Average net monthly income (2022, in USD)	670.8		776		<0.0001 *
Population density (per km^2)	79		46		0.0054 *
No of pediatrician in primary health care	1012		76		<0.0001 *
No of pediatrician in primary health care (per 10,000 children)	28.67		6.4		NA
Marital status of females aged 15 and up, n (%)					
Unmarried	731,559	22.90%	70,107	27.30%	
Married	1,702,581	53.40%	13,702	53.40%	
Widow	562,384	17.60%	10,328	4.00%	**<0.0001 ****
Divorced	181,351	5.70%	38,666	15.10%	
Unknown	11,841	0.40%	687	0.30%	
Educational attainment of females aged 15 and up, n (%)					
Without formal education or incomplete primary education	247,375	8.40%	35,993	14.0%	
Primary education	562,523	19.10%	57,442	22.40%	
Secondary education	1,420,971	48.10%	120,888	47.0%	**<0.0001 ****
Tertiary education	709,436	24.0%	41,278	16.10%	
Unknown	11,507	0.40%	1207	0.50%	
HPV vaccine coverage in the age group 9–14 years (%)	5.53		22.10		NA
HPV vaccine coverage in the age group 15–19 years (%)	5.94		-		NA
HPV vaccine coverage in the age group 9–19 years (%)	5.72		-		NA

* Test of proportion; ** chi-square test. NA—not applicable. In bold are significant results at $p < 0.05$.

Within Serbia, only one administrative region (Moravica) reported HPV immunization coverage in girls 9–19 years old above 10%, 11 districts had coverage from 5 to 10%, while 13 districts of Serbia had coverage below 5%, as presented in Figure 1. On the other hand, the HPV vaccination uptake in Serbia was almost equal between younger females

(9–14 years of age) and females aged 15–19 years (5.53% and 5.94%). As per Montenegro, two administrative units, Cetinje and Berane, had the highest coverage, with 39% and 36.4% of vaccinated girls 9–14 years old, respectively. The other four units had coverage between 25 and 30%, another five from 20 to 25%, and the majority was in the range between 15% and 20% of vaccinated eligible girls. Finally, two administrative units, Žabljak and Šavnik administered just a few vaccines and were in the lowest coverage category.

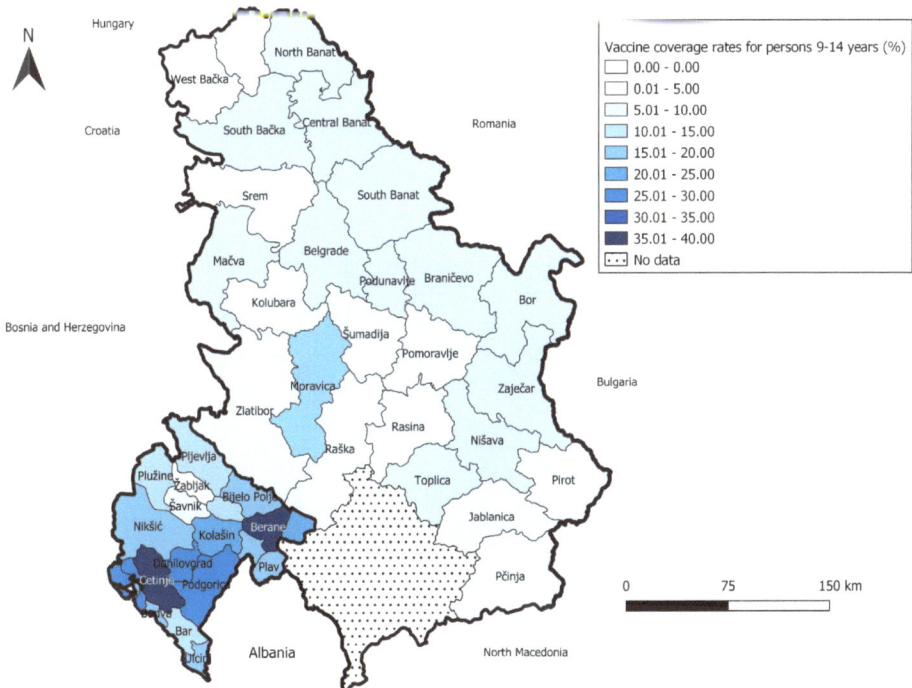

Figure 1. HPV vaccine coverage in girls 9–14 years after first year of immunization across administrative units in Serbia and Montenegro.

When we explored the coverage of HPV immunization among girls aged 9–19 years across different regions in Serbia, ordering coverage from the highest to the lowest, we observed that the level of coverage did not correlate with the number of pediatricians (Figure 2A) or with the population density (Figure 2B). Likewise, the Pčinja region with the lowest vaccination coverage has more pediatricians than the Moravica region, where vaccination coverage is the highest. Also, it can be observed that units with a higher percentage of population density have lower vaccination coverage as we can see in Belgrade and South Bačka, which are more urban than the Moravica region. In the Moravica district, the coverage rate is 11.0%, and in the Pčinja region, 0.9%, while the observed indicator population density is almost equal.

Vaccine coverage by administrative units in Montenegro (girls 9–14 years), from the highest to the lowest administrative unit is presented in Figure 3. We observed a similar situation as per Serbia's administrative units, the level of coverage did not correlate with the number of pediatricians or population density. In fact, the administrative units that do not have pediatricians employed in primary healthcare centers (Zeta, Gusinje, Petnjica, Tuzi, Plužine, Šavnik, and Žabljak) have immunization coverage, from 0% in Žabljak to 25% in Zeta region. The administrative unit Cetinje, which has the highest HPV immunization coverage (nearly 40%), counts four employed pediatricians, on the contrary administrative unit Kolašin with 15 employed pediatricians has 20% HPV immunization coverage (Figure 3A). The level of population density (Figure 3B) also did not correlate with the percentage of immunization coverage (Tivat population density 350.0 per km^2 and coverage below 20%).

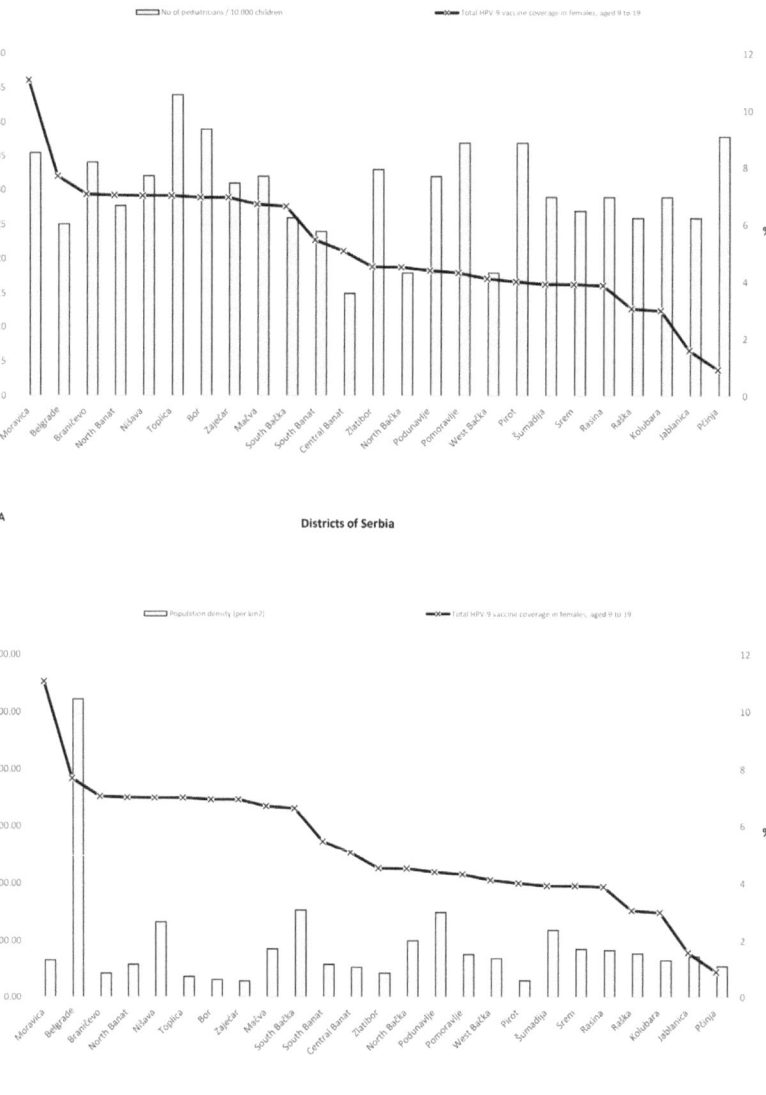

Figure 2. Relation between HPV vaccine coverage in girls 9–19 years old and (**A**) the number of pediatricians in administrative units; (**B**) the district's population density, across administrative units in Serbia.

When dividing Serbia's administrative units into tertiles by the distribution of the values of selected sociodemographic variables, we noticed that those units that are in the first tercile (the lowest percentage) by the variable "Illiterate female population aged 10 and up" have the highest mean values of the vaccine coverage (mean = 6.14%, SD = 2.14), although not at the statistically significant level. Administrative units in the third tertile (highest percentage) of the explored variables, "Educational attainment of females aged 15 and up" and "Illiterate female population aged 10 and up", had the lowest mean values of HPV vaccine coverage (mean 4.33, SD = 2.45 and 4.63, SD = 2.49, respectively). On the other hand, in the administrative units with the highest percentage of married females aged 15 and up (third tertile), the lowest mean value of HPV vaccine coverage has been recorded (mean = 4.00, SD = 2.22) (Table 2).

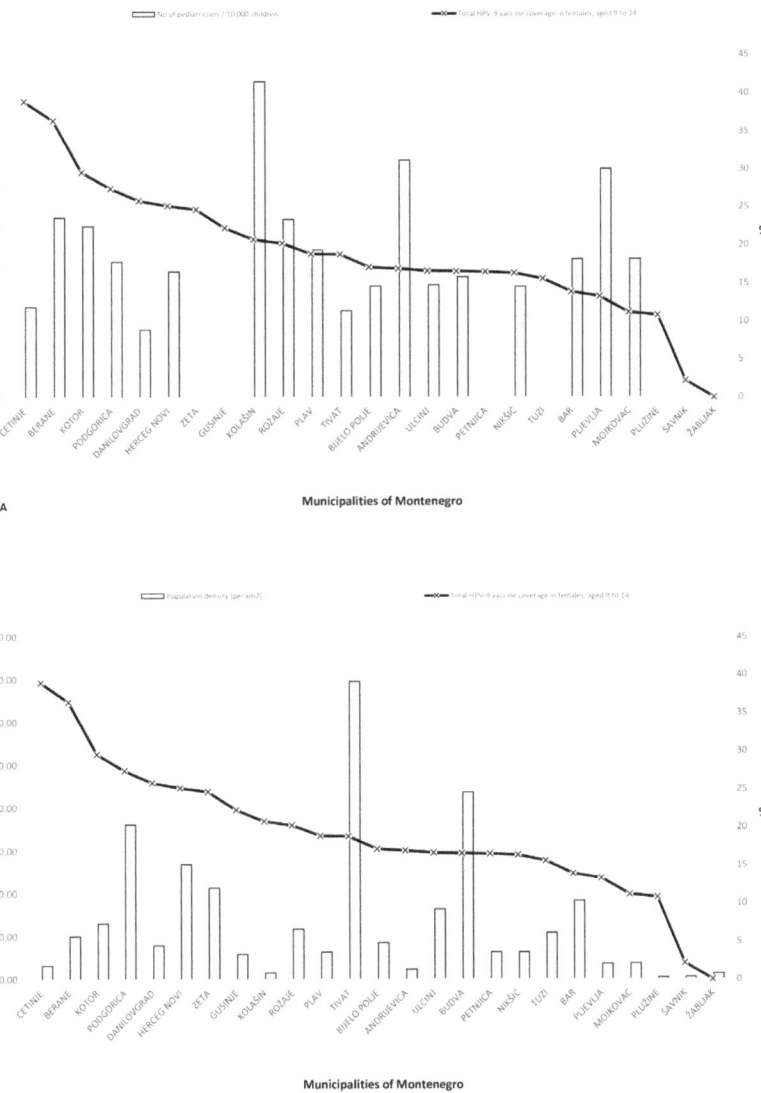

Figure 3. Relation between HPV vaccine coverage in girls 9–14 years old and (**A**) number of pediatricians in administrative units; (**B**) population density, across administrative units in Montenegro.

Table 2. Mean value of HPV-9 vaccine coverage in girls 9–19 years old across administrative units of Serbia by terciles of selected sociodemographic variables.

Administrative Units of Serbia		HPV Vaccine Coverage in Girls 9–19 Years Old		p-Value *
		Mean	(SD)	
Degree of Urbanization (2018 Estimate)	1st tertile	4.05	2.07	
	2nd tertile	5.83	2.53	0.456
	3rd tertile	5.96	1.54	
Average net monthly income (2022, in USD)	1st tertile	4.28	2.25	
	2nd tertile	5.62	2.64	0.248
	3rd tertile	5.91	1.35	
	Without or incomplete primary education			
	1st tertile	5.77	2.56	
	2nd tertile	5.53	1.23	0.157
	3rd tertile	4.33	2.45	
	Primary education			
	1st tertile	5.85	2.78	
	2nd tertile	4.68	1.21	0.116
	3rd tertile	5.08	2.3	
	Secondary education			
	1st tertile	4.9	2.21	
	2nd tertile	5.69	1.62	0.386
	3rd tertile	5.15	2.8	
	Tertiary education			
	1st tertile	5.75	1.95	
	2nd tertile	3.59	1.29	0.302
	3rd tertile	6.29	2.39	
Illiterate female population aged 10 and up (2022 census)	1st tertile	6.14	2.42	
	2nd tertile	4.8	1.36	0.271
	3rd tertile	4.63	2.49	
	Unmarried			
	1st tertile	5.39	2.84	
	2nd tertile	5.19	2.22	0.261
	3rd tertile	5.09	1.49	
	Married			
	1st tertile	5.89	1.32	
	2nd tertile	5.69	2.8	0.138
	3rd tertile	4	2.22	
	Widow			
	1st tertile	4.36	2.37	
	2nd tertile	5.89	2.4	0.56
	3rd tertile	5.56	1.63	
	Divorced			
	1st tertile	3.85	2.05	
	2nd tertile	5.84	2.47	0.281
	3rd tertile	6.16	1.3	
Average age of females aged 15 and up (2022 census)	1st tertile	4.74	2.12	
	2nd tertile	5.48	2.91	0.284
	3rd tertile	5.53	1.56	
Population density (per km^2) by district	1st tertile	5.5	2.11	
	2nd tertile	4.56	2.87	0.299
	3rd tertile	5.6	1.55	
Area (in km^2), by district	1st tertile	4.68	1.39	
	2nd tertile	5.88	2.89	0.168
	3rd tertile	5.19	2.24	
No of pediatrician/10,000 children	1st tertile	4.67	1.83	
	2nd tertile	5.36	1.72	0.257
	3rd tertile	5.73	3	
Number of girls 9–19 yrs old	1st tertile	5.68	1.64	
	2nd tertile	4.4	3.04	0.173
	3rd tertile	5.55	1.72	

* Using Analysis of variance (ANOVA).

Further on, when analyzing a potential correlation between HPV immunization coverage and different sociodemographic characteristics of administrative units in Serbia, we noticed a statistically significant moderate negative correlation (r = −0.446; p = 0.026) with the percentage of illiterate women in the administrative units (Figure 4).

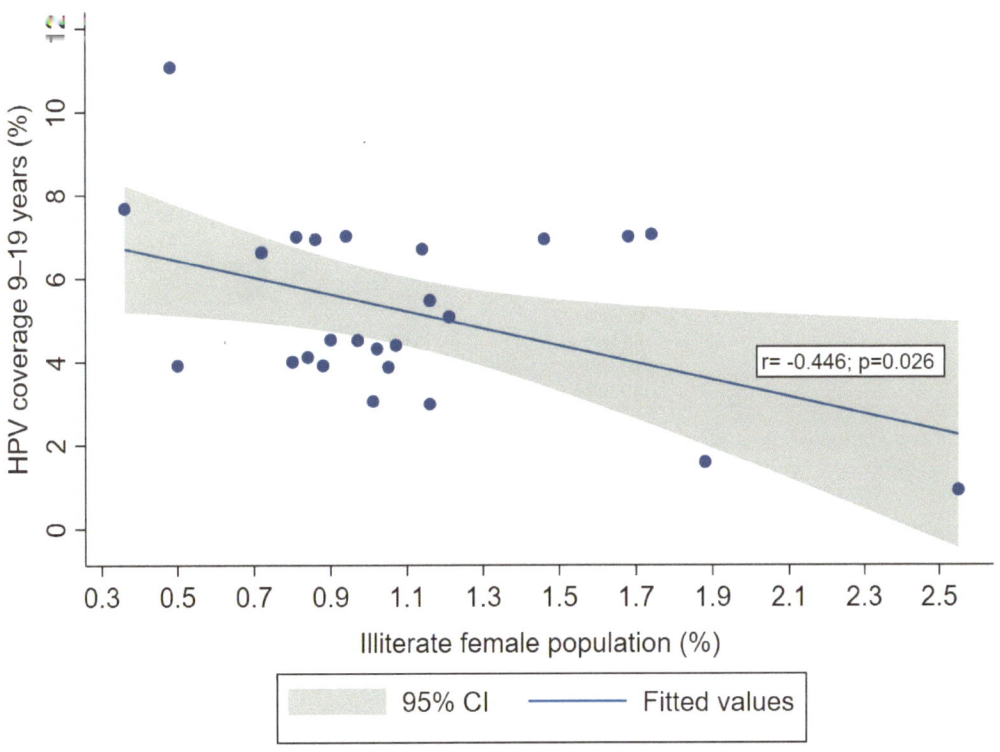

Figure 4. Correlation between administrative units' percent of illiterate females and the HPV coverage in girls 9–19 yrs old, across districts in Serbia.

In Table 3, we explored the level of vaccine coverage in girls aged 9–14 years across administrative units of Montenegro by terciles of selected sociodemographic variables and observed that the municipalities that are in the level of the second tercile of the observed variable "Married, marital status of females aged 15 and up" reported the highest mean values of coverage (mean 22.77, SD = 8.47) with a statistically significant difference in the level of coverage compared to the first and third tercile ($p = 0.003$). There is also a statistically significant difference in the mean value of the vaccine coverage ($p = 0.013$) across the units from the first tercile (lowest values) of the "Area (in km^2)" compared to the coverage values in the municipalities that are in the other two terciles (Table 3).

Table 3. Mean value of HPV-9 vaccine coverage in girls 9–14 years old across administrative units of Montenegro by terciles of selected sociodemographic variables.

Administrative Units of Montenegro		HPV Vaccine Coverage in Girls 9–14 Years Old		p-Value *
		Mean	(SD)	
Marital status of females aged 15 and up (2011 census)	Unmarried			
	1st tertile	20.15	8.18	
	2nd tertile	20.49	5.94	0.136
	3rd tertile	16.03	13.73	
	Married			
	1st tertile	16.93	14.15	
	2nd tertile	22.77	8.47	**0.003**
	3rd tertile	16.96	2.61	
	Widow			
	1st tertile	13.81	6.89	
	2nd tertile	18.54	10.85	0.567
	3rd tertile	24.33	8.68	
	Divorced			
	1st tertile	18.65	4.33	
	2nd tertile	23.33	8.53	0.054
	3rd tertile	14.69	13.04	
Population density (per km^2) by district	1st tertile	15.13	11.66	
	2nd tertile	20.85	7.1	0.155
	3rd tertile	21.58	5.81	
Area (in km^2), by district	1st tertile	19.43	3.68	
	2nd tertile	19.25	11.44	**0.013**
	3rd tertile	18.35	11.1	
No of pediatrician/10,000 children	1st tertile	22.27	8.91	
	2nd tertile	18.83	6.35	0.748
	3rd tertile	22.86	8.57	
Number of girls 9–14 yrs old	1st tertile	13.26	7.91	
	2nd tertile	22.9	8.59	0.947
	3rd tertile	21.64	7.57	

* Using ANOVA. In bold = significant p-values at <0.05.

4. Discussion

HPV is the most common viral infection in the human reproductive tract, capable of causing cervical cancer in women, other types of cancer, and genital warts in both men and women. By the end of 2022, 130 Member States had incorporated the HPV vaccine into their national immunization programs, including 14 new introductions [11,22]. Despite this progress on the global level, many countries are facing suboptimal vaccine coverage. In 2022, only 21% of girls received the first dose of the HPV vaccine [22]. Challenges in achieving adequate HPV immunization coverage have been observed in various regions. A recent systematic review and meta-analysis, which included 18,611 females from 27 European countries, concluded that personalized interventions targeting population- and country-specific characteristics are necessary to enhance HPV vaccination coverage [23]. However, there exists a dearth of quantitative studies examining the correlation between the socioeconomic characteristics of Eastern and Central European regions, perceptions regarding the severity of specific diseases, and attitudes towards vaccination, particularly in high-income countries within the region, where vaccine hesitancy is most prevalent [22]. Vaccination hesitancy stands as one of the foremost global health threats and has emerged as a critical public health concern worldwide [14].

Although our study only analyzed the first year of vaccination program implementation, we found that the HPV immunization coverage in Serbia was 5.5% for girls aged 9–14 years and 5.9% for those aged 15–19 years. In contrast, Montenegro achieved HPV immunization coverage of 22.1% for girls aged 9–14 years. Despite both countries having high rates of HPV-related cancers, the first-year immunization coverage differed significantly between them [2,8]. Several factors contributed to the differences in immunization coverage between Serbia and Montenegro. The process of introducing the HPV vaccine at the national level differed significantly between the two countries. In Serbia, the HPV vaccine was introduced abruptly, without prior national promotional campaigns, as a gender-neutral vaccination for individuals aged 9–19 and was offered free of charge to those eligible by age [20]. Montenegro had established a structured approach to prepare the target population for the vaccine's introduction. Conversely, extensive educational campaigns, expert media coverage, school visits, and communication with parents preceded the vaccine's introduction. This included involving epidemiologists and healthcare workers in promoting and emphasizing the vaccine's importance to the public. Additionally, financial incentives were provided to those involved in administering the HPV vaccine. These factors, rather than the number of pediatricians, population density, level of education, and other sociodemographic variables investigated in our study, appear to have had a more significant influence on the level of HPV immunization coverage [24].

In Serbia, the national immunization program with the nonavalent HPV vaccine, free of charge for all interested girls and boys aged 9–19, started in June 2022. By the end of June 2023, about 5% of eligible young people had been vaccinated. Although there were no clear reasons for this, the immunization coverage with the nonavalent HPV vaccine in the Moravica District was significantly higher compared to other districts in Serbia. One possible reason could be that epidemiologists from the local Public Health Department had a more prominent presence in local media and communication with schools and healthcare workers in their district compared to other districts. Additionally, immunization coverage against HPV was higher in Montenegro, where there was a smaller population of girls in the appropriate age group for vaccination, making it potentially easier to achieve higher coverage. Furthermore, at the administrative unit's level, the monthly incomes are higher and population density is lower in Montenegro compared to Serbia, even though the number of pediatricians is inversely proportional to the level of coverage in these two countries. Our research found that the coverage of HPV immunization in Serbia by district was not correlated with the number of pediatricians. The coverage for girls aged 9–14 years was 5.5% in Serbia and 22.1% in Montenegro, indicating that effective organization within the pediatric health service plays a more significant role in implementing HPV immunization than the number of employed pediatricians.

It is noteworthy that in the administrative units in Serbia that fall into the third tertile for the variables "Educational attainment of females aged 15 and up: Without or incomplete primary education" and "Illiterate female population aged 10 and up", the mean values of average immunization coverage are lower compared to the other tertiles. This suggests that those sociodemographic variables might be relevant to the success of immunization programs. Although the overall HPV coverage is low (5.72%), our study found a correlation between the percentage of illiterate females and the HPV immunization coverage across administrative units in Serbia. This indicates that illiterate individuals might be harder to reach and inform about vaccination.

Considering these findings, along with previously published common reasons for rejecting the HPV vaccine—such as fear of side effects, perception of the vaccine as being too new or experimental, belief that the chances of being infected are low, and concerns regarding safety and inadequate information—it is important to emphasize the significant impact that highly motivated healthcare workers can have on vaccination uptake. Additionally, support from friends or family members, or encouragement from acquaintances, can positively influence vaccination rates against HPV [23]. Considering the prediction that HPV immunization coverage achieved in the first few years tends to be sustained, it is crucial to address these sociodemographic challenges early on. This includes focusing on areas with lower educational attainment and higher illiteracy rates among females, as these factors are significant in achieving successful immunization. Our findings highlight the need for targeted interventions, such as comprehensive educational campaigns and community engagement efforts, particularly in regions with higher illiteracy rates. Additionally, addressing common concerns about the vaccine—like fear of side effects, perceptions of it being new or experimental, and doubts about safety and necessity—can further improve vaccination rates. The most effective preventive measure against human papillomavirus remains vaccination. In Serbia, there is a growing initiative to professionalize educational campaigns involving highly motivated professionals. These campaigns aim to raise awareness among parents and children in schools across every district of the country. Additionally, there is a concerted effort to engage more healthcare workers in educational campaigns tailored for schools in every county. The goal is to ensure that every parent receives crucial information about HPV vaccination directly through the school system. Epidemiologists responsible for each district should have digital information on the number of vaccinated persons, gender, and place of residence, and then analyze vaccination rates more frequently to identify districts with low vaccination coverage. This analysis guides the strengthening of targeted promotional campaigns in those specific areas.

With the advent of the internet, while it brought significant benefits, it also introduced challenges such as the rise of vaccine opponents and their theories. These opposing views have had a considerable impact on public perception regarding vaccination as a crucial preventive measure. It is essential to address these challenges effectively in future national strategies, leveraging media, especially electronic platforms, to counter misinformation and promote evidence-based information about the HPV vaccine. By doing so, we can reinforce the understanding of the vaccine's importance and encourage higher vaccination rates across communities [25]. These platforms play a pivotal role in disseminating accurate information and effectively reaching a wide audience. In Serbia, utilizing electronic media channels enhances the visibility and understanding of HPV vaccination among the public. This approach ensures that key messages about the vaccine's benefits and availability are widely accessible, thereby fostering increased vaccination rates nationwide.

Highly motivated healthcare workers play a key role in this process, as do supportive networks involving friends, family, and acquaintances. By leveraging these influences and addressing the specific barriers identified, we can enhance the overall success and sustainability of the HPV immunization programs [26], there is an urgent need to utilize all available resources to increase the uptake of the HPV vaccine in our territory. Considering that the HPV vaccine is proven safe, effective, and provided free of charge for children aged 9–19 years in Serbia, one potential solution could be the implementation of mandatory instead of recommended HPV immunization in our country.

5. Conclusions

Despite the fact that the vaccines against HPV were continuously available in both countries, vaccination coverage against HPV in Serbia was low during the first year of the immunization program. One potentially influencing factor might be the literacy levels among the female population at the administrative unit's level. Drawing on the experiences and successes of HPV immunization in Montenegro, Serbia could improve its vaccination coverage through a robust educational campaign. This campaign should target schools, the general population, and healthcare workers, and include incentives for those involved in these efforts.

Author Contributions: Conceptualization, M.Š., V.V., M.R. and V.P.; methodology, M.Š., V.V. and M.R.; software, V.V. and M.R.; validation, N.N., T.P., S.R. and M.K. (Marko Koprivica); formal analysis, V.V. and M.R.; investigation, M.Š., M.J., G.L., M.K. (Milena Kanazir). and S.L.; resources, M.Š., M.J., G.L., M.K. (Milena Kanazir), D.L. and V.P.; data curation, M.Š., M.J., V.V. and M.R.; writing—original draft preparation, M.Š., M.J., V.V. and M.R.; writing—review and editing, M.Š., V.V., M.R. and V.P.; visualization, V.V., M.R., S.L., S.R., M.K. (Marko Koprivica) and T.P.; supervision, D.L. and V.P.; project administration, M.Š. All authors have read and agreed to the published version of the manuscript.

Funding: This research received no external funding.

Institutional Review Board Statement: Ethical review and approval were waived for this study due to the study design and the analysis of secondary data collected as part of routine public health surveillance.

Informed Consent Statement: No consent was required since the study consisted of the analysis of secondary data collected as part of a routine surveillance of vaccine administration.

Data Availability Statement: The data that support the findings of this study are available from the corresponding author upon reasonable request.

Conflicts of Interest: The authors declare no conflicts of interest.

References

1. World Health Organization Cancer Today. Available online: https://gco.iarc.fr/today/en/dataviz/tables?mode=population (accessed on 14 May 2024).
2. World Health Organization. Introducing HPV Vaccines for a Cervical Cancer-Free Generation in Montenegro. 2020. Available online: https://www.who.int/about/accountability/results/who-results-report-2020-mtr/country-story/2022/introducing-hpv-vaccines-for-a-cervical-cancer-free-generation-in-montenegro (accessed on 16 March 2024).
3. Bruni, L.; Albero, G.; Serrano, B.; Mena, M.; Collado, J.J.; Gómez, D.; Muñoz, M.; Bosch, F.X.; de Sanjosé, S. *Human Papillomavirus and Related Diseases Report WORLD*; 2023.
4. Elrefaey , S.; Massaro , M.A.; Chiocca , S.; Chiesa , F.; Ansarin , M. HPV in oropharyngeal cancer: The basics to know in clinical practice. *Acta. Otorhinolaryngol.* **2014**, *34*, 299–309. [PubMed] [PubMed Central]
5. Nikolic, N.; Basica, B.; Strbac, M.; Terzic, L.; Patic, A.; Kovacevic, G.; Velicki, R.; Petrovic, D.; Mandic, A.; Petrovic, V. Prevalence of Carcinogenic Genotypes of HPV-Infected Women in a Ten-Year Period (2014–2023) in Vojvodina, Serbia. *Medicina* **2024**, *60*, 922. [CrossRef] [PubMed]
6. Lopicic, M.; Raonic, J.; Antunovic, M.; Milicic, B.; Mijovic, G. Distribution of Vaccine-Related High-Risk Human Papillomaviruses and Their Impact on the Development of Cervical Dysplasia in Women in Montenegro. *Acta Microbiol. Immunol. Hung.* **2021**, *68*, 297–303. [CrossRef] [PubMed]
7. WHO. *Director-General Calls for All Countries to Take Action to Help End the Suffering Caused by Cervical Cancer*; WHO: Geneva, Switzerland, 2018.
8. World Health Organization. Immunization, Vaccines and Biologicals. Available online: https://www.who.int/teams/immunization-vaccines-and-biologicals/diseases/human-papillomavirus-vaccines-(HPV) (accessed on 12 May 2024).
9. World Health Organization. *Global Strategy to Accelerate the Elimination of Cervical Cancer As a Public Health Problem*; WHO: Geneva, Switzerland, 2020.
10. Nikolic, N.; Basica, B.; Mandic, A.; Surla, N.; Gusman, V.; Medic, D.; Petrovic, T.; Strbac, M.; Petrovic, V. E6/E7 mRNA Expression of the Most Prevalent High-Risk HPV Genotypes in Cervical Samples from Serbian Women. *Diagnostics* **2023**, *13*, 917. [CrossRef] [PubMed]
11. World Health Organization. *Immunization Coverage*; World Health Organization: Geneva, Switzerland, 2023.
12. Lee, L.-Y.; Garland, S.M. Human Papillomavirus Vaccination: The Population Impact. *F1000Research* **2017**, *6*, 866. [CrossRef] [PubMed]
13. Štrbac, M.; Vuković, V.; Pustahija, T.; Nikolić, N.; Rajčević, S.; Ilić, S.; Dugandžija, T.; Patić, A.; Ristić, M.; Petrović, V. Motives and Attitudes of Parents toward HPV Vaccination: Results from the Initial Period of HPV Vaccine Rollout in Serbia. *PLoS ONE* **2023**, *18*, e0287295. [CrossRef] [PubMed]
14. Kirbiš, A. The Impact of Socioeconomic Status, Perceived Threat and Healthism on Vaccine Hesitancy. *Sustainability* **2023**, *15*, 6107. [CrossRef]
15. Dong, L.; Nygård, M.; Hansen, B.T. Sociodemographic Correlates of Human Papillomavirus Vaccine Uptake: Opportunistic and Catch-Up Vaccination in Norway. *Cancers* **2021**, *13*, 3483. [CrossRef] [PubMed]
16. Vickers, M.; Green, C.L.; Lee, H.Y.; Pierce, J.Y.; Daniel, C.L. Factors Associated with HPV Vaccination Uptake and HPV-Associated Cancers: A County-Level Analysis in the State of Alabama. *J. Community Health* **2019**, *44*, 1214–1223. [CrossRef] [PubMed]
17. Sacre, A.; Bambra, C.; Wildman, J.M.; Thomson, K.; Bennett, N.; Sowden, S.; Todd, A. Socioeconomic Inequalities in Vaccine Uptake: A Global Umbrella Review. *PLoS ONE* **2023**, *18*, e0294688. [CrossRef] [PubMed]
18. International Monetary Fund. *Report on Government Finance Statistics Technical Assistance: Republic of Serbia*; International Monetary Fund: Washington, DC, USA, 2024.
19. Statistical Office Republic of Serbia. *Census Data 2022*; Statistical Office Republic of Serbia: Belgrade, Serbia, 2023.
20. Ministry of Health. Pravilnik o Imunizaciji i Načinu Zaštite Lekovima. Available online: https://www.paragraf.rs/propisi/pravilnik_o_imunizaciji_i_nacinu_zastite_lekovima.html (accessed on 12 May 2023).
21. Ministry of Health of the Republic Serbia. Zakon o Zaštiti Stanovništva Od Zaraznih Bolesti: 15/2016-31, 68/2020-4, 136/2020-3. Available online: https://www.pravno-informacioni-sistem.rs/SlGlasnikPortal/eli/rep/sgrs/skupstina/zakon/2016/15/8/reg (accessed on 16 January 2023).
22. European Centre for Disease Prevention and Control. *Let's Talk about Hesitancy*; ECDC: Stockholm, Sweden, 2016.

23. Jiboc, N.-M.; Paşca, A.; Tăut, D.; Băban, A.-S. Factors Influencing Human Papillomavirus Vaccination Uptake in European Women and Adolescents: A Systematic Review and Meta-Analysis. *Psychooncology* **2024**, *33*, e6242. [CrossRef] [PubMed]
24. Institute of Public Health of Montenegro. *Program HPV Vakcinacije u Crnoj Gori*; Institute of Public Health of Montenegro: Podgorica, Montenegro, 2022.
25. Galagali, P.M.; Kinikar, A.A.; Kumar, V.S. Vaccine Hesitancy: Obstacles and Challenges. *Curr. Pediatr. Rep.* **2022**, *10*, 241–248. [CrossRef] [PubMed]
26. Bruni, L.; Saura-Lázaro, A.; Montoliu, A.; Brotons, M.; Alemany, L.; Diallo, M.S.; Afsar, O.Z.; LaMontagne, D.S.; Mosina, L.; Contreras, M.; et al. HPV Vaccination Introduction Worldwide and WHO and UNICEF Estimates of National HPV Immunization Coverage 2010–2019. *Prev. Med.* **2021**, *144*, 106399. [CrossRef] [PubMed]

Disclaimer/Publisher's Note: The statements, opinions and data contained in all publications are solely those of the individual author(s) and contributor(s) and not of MDPI and/or the editor(s). MDPI and/or the editor(s) disclaim responsibility for any injury to people or property resulting from any ideas, methods, instructions or products referred to in the content.

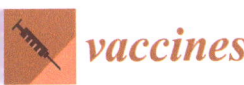

Article

Longitudinal Screening for Oral High-Risk Non-HPV16 and Non-HPV18 Strains of Human Papillomavirus Reveals Increasing Prevalence among Adult and Pediatric Biorepository Samples: A Pilot Study

Jordan Jacobs [1], Eugene Chon [1] and Karl Kingsley [2],*

[1] Department of Clinical Sciences, School of Dental Medicine, University of Nevada-Las Vegas, 1700 W. Charleston Boulevard, Las Vegas, NV 89106, USA
[2] Department of Biomedical Sciences, School of Dental Medicine, University of Nevada-Las Vegas, 1001 Shadow Lane, Las Vegas, NV 89106, USA
* Correspondence: karl.kingsley@unlv.edu; Tel.: +1-702-774-2623

Abstract: Most high-risk oral human papillomavirus research has focused on prevalent HPV16 and HPV18, with fewer studies focused on other high-risk strains incorporated into the nine-valent HPV vaccine. Therefore, the objective of this study was to determine the oral prevalence of non-HPV16 and non-HPV18 high-risk strains. A total of $n = 251$ existing biorepository saliva samples were screened using validated primers and qPCR. A total of $n = 72$ samples tested positive for HPV, including HPV31, HPV33, HPV35, HPV52, and HPV58. In addition, there were also significant increases in the prevalence of these high-risk strains (2011–2014, 21.3%) following the nine-valent HPV vaccine's introduction (2015–2019, 36.2%). However, the distribution of HPV-positive samples was nearly equal among males and females (52.8%, 47.2%, respectively, $p = 0.5485$), although the majority (66.7%) of the HPV-positive samples were within the HPV vaccination age (11 to 26 years) or catch-up range (27 to 45 years). These data demonstrated that the prevalence of high-risk oral HPV may be higher than anticipated, highly concentrated among patients within the recommended vaccination age range, and may be increasing over time—providing new evidence and support for the nine-valent HPV vaccine that covers these additional high-risk HPV strains.

Keywords: clinical sampling; human papillomavirus (HPV); biorepository saliva screening; high-risk oral HPV; nine-valent HPV vaccine

1. Introduction

High-risk oncogenic strains of human papillomavirus (HPV) have been demonstrated to be involved with many oral and head and neck tumors [1,2]. Recent evidence has demonstrated that high-risk HPV strains are capable of mediating and modulating the progression of oropharyngeal and other types of head and neck cancers, thereby influencing patient outcomes and reducing patient survival [3,4]. Moreover, many of these high-risk HPV strains have also been associated with the initiation and development of oral and other head and neck cancers, which presents many potential opportunities for prevention [5,6].

The vast majority of the research into the prevalence of high-risk oral strains has focused on HPV16 and HPV18, which are known to comprise the largest proportion of known infections to date [7,8]. These high-risk strains may also be associated with the vast majority of cervical cancers and other HPV-related diseases, exerting their effects through HPV early proteins E6 and E7 that downregulate tumor suppressors Retinoblastoma (Rb) and TP53 [9,10]. However, a growing number of studies now demonstrate that additional non-HPV16 and non-HPV18 high-risk strains that were not originally included in the initial studies of oral and head and neck cancers may not only be present but also functional in the initiation, development, and progression of these tumors [11,12].

Although HPV16 and HPV18 are very important high-risk HPV strains, many additional strains including HPV31, HPV33, HPV45, HPV52, and HPV58 are also associated with many types of cancer development and progression in a variety of tissues and organs, including oropharyngeal and head and neck cancers [13,14]. The recognition that the prevention of infection by these additional high-risk strains may significantly reduce morbidity and mortality has led to the incorporation of these additional high-risk strains into the modified nine-valent HPV vaccine, covering high-risk HPV16, HPV18, HPV31, HPV33, HPV45, HPV52, and HPV58, as well as the low-risk strains HPV6 and HPV11 associated with the majority of anogenital warts [15–17]. Although these additional high-risk strains are well studied among other cancers, fewer studies have focused on these high-risk strains among oral or head and neck cancers [18–20].

In addition, most of the research in these areas has been focused on obtaining the one-time, cross-sectional prevalence of high-risk HPV16 and HPV18, although some researchers have started to perform longitudinal studies to track changes in prevalence over time [21–23]. These studies have demonstrated increases in both the prevalence and incidence of HPV16 and HPV18 over time, although much less is known about high-risk non-HPV16 and non-HPV18 strains [24–26]. For example, although a recent systematic review and meta-analysis of oral HPV strains confirmed the high prevalence of HPV16 and HPV18 among oropharyngeal cancer patients, HPV33 and HPV58 (included in the nine-valent HPV vaccine), as well as the additional strain HPV35, were also among the most prevalent in the oral cavity [27]. This report of high oral HPV35 prevalence has been demonstrated in numerous other screening studies of oropharyngeal cancer, which suggest that this strain may be much more common among oral cancer patients than the high-risk cervical cancer-associated strain HPV45 that is covered by the nine-valent vaccine [20,28–30]. Some evidence now suggests that the oral prevalence of HPV35 may not only be high but may also be increasing over time, suggesting that the screening of this strain may be of particular relevance for screening studies of high-risk oral HPV strains [31–33]. In fact, despite the high prevalence of the high-risk strain HPV45 in cervical cancers, the few studies screening for this strain have revealed a strikingly low prevalence among oral and oropharyngeal cancers [34,35].

Due to the recent nature of these discoveries and the limited information available regarding non-HPV16 and non-HPV18 high-risk HPV strains, the primary goal within the current study involved the analysis and screening of saliva samples within an existing biorepository to reveal a more complete understanding of oral HPV infections, as well as any temporal trends or associations over time.

2. Materials and Methods

2.1. Study Approval

This study involved a retrospective analysis of previously collected samples stored within a biorepository. As a retrospective study with no clinical sample collection or patient interactions, this study was reviewed and approved by the Institutional Review Board (IRB) as Research Exempt for studies that do not require informed consent according to the United States (US) Department of Health and Human Services (HHS) code of federal regulations (CFR) 45 CFR 46, which states that research using previously collected data or specimens that cannot be linked with patient-identifying information or personal private information. The protocol titled "Retrospective analysis of microbial prevalence from DNA isolated from saliva samples originally obtained from the University of Nevada, Las Vegas (UNLV) School of Dental Medicine (SDM) pediatric and clinical population" was filed and approved by the UNLV Office for the Protection of Research Subjects (OPRS) and IRB under Protocol 1717625-1.

2.2. Biorepository Sample Collection

The biorepository consisted of clinical saliva samples derived under the original sample collection Protocol 1305-4466M titled "The Prevalence of Oral Microbes in Saliva from the University of Nevada, Las Vegas School of Dental Medicine (UNLV-SDM) Pediatric Adult Clinical Population". The original study inclusion criteria required that samples be collected from UNLV-SDM patients of record and that participation be strictly voluntary. Exclusion criteria included any patients that did not wish to participate. Briefly, unstimulated saliva was collected using sterile collection tubes and stored for processing at −80 °C. Labels with randomly generated identifiers were used to prevent any personal or private patient information from being associated with any particular sample. Only basic demographic information was noted, such as patient age, sex, and race or ethnicity. No chart numbers, patient birth dates, or other specific information was collected or available to the study authors. Samples were collected on randomly selected days on alternating months over the time period between 2011 and 2019.

2.3. DNA Isolation

DNA was previously isolated from all saliva samples within the biorepository using the TRIzol (phenol–chloroform) extraction procedure from Invitrogen (Waltham, MA, USA), as detailed in previous studies [19,20]. The quantification and assessment of the sample-derived DNA were performed using a NanoDrop 2000 spectrophotometer obtained from Fisher Scientific (Fair Lawn, NJ, USA). The quantity and quality of sample-derived DNA were evaluated utilizing the A260 and A280 nm absorbance readings and ratio, as outlined previously [19,20].

2.4. qPCR Screening

This study involved n = 251 DNA biorepository samples isolated from patient saliva. Screening for high-risk non-HPV16 and non-HPV18 was performed using validated primers for each specific HPV strain (HPV31, −33, −35, −52, −58). The screening protocol involved the use of the SYBR Green Universal qPCR Master Mix obtained from Applied Biosystems (Waltham, MA, USA) and the manufacturer's recommended protocol, as previously described [19,20]. Previously validated primer sequences were obtained from Eurofins Scientific (Louisville, KY, USA), as outlined in Table 1 below [19,20]:

Table 1. Screening primer sequences.

Primer	Primer Sequence	Length (nt)	GC%	Tm
GAPDH forward	5'-ATCTTCCAGGAGCGAGATCC-3'	20 nt	55%	66 °C
GAPDH reverse	5'-ACCACTGACACGTTGGCAGT-3'	20 nt	55%	70 °C
HPV31 forward	5'-ATTCCACAACATAGGAGGAAGGTG-3'	24 nt	46%	66 °C
HPV31 reverse	5'-CACTTGGGTTTCAGTACGAGGTCT-3'	24 nt	50%	68 °C
HPV33 forward	5'-ATATTTCGGGGTCGTTGGGCA-3'	21 nt	52%	69 °C
HPV33 reverse	5'-ACGTCACAGTGCAGTTTCTCTACGT-3'	25 nt	48%	70 °C
HPV35 forward	5'-TCGGTGTATGTCTGTTGGAAAC-3'	22 nt	45%	65 °C
HPV35 reverse	5'-CATAGTCTTGCAATGTAGTTATTTCTCCA-3'	29 nt	34%	64 °C
HPV52 forward	5'-AAAGCAAAAATTGGTGGACGA-3'	21 nt	38%	63 °C
HPV52 reverse	5'-TGCCAGCAATTAGCGCATT-3'	19 nt	47%	66 °C
HPV52 forward	5'-GGCATGTGGATTTAAACAAAAGGT-3'	24 nt	38%	64 °C
HPV52 reverse	5'-TCTCATGGCGTTGTTACAGGTTAC-3'	24 nt	46%	67 °C

Key: nucleotide = nt; melting temperature = Tm.

2.5. Statistical Analysis

Data regarding the demographic characteristics of the study sample were compiled for analysis using Chi Square, the recommended method for statistical comparisons of non-parametric, categorical data. In addition, the qPCR results were also categorized (HPV-positive, HPV-negative) and analyzed using Chi Square statistics. Descriptive statistics and Pearson's correlations (R) were generated using Microsoft Excel 2021, Office 365 Version (Redmond, WA, USA), and Chi Square analysis was performed using GraphPad Prism software, Version 8 (San Diego, CA, USA), as previously described [19,20,36].

3. Results

3.1. Demographic Analysis of Study Sample

This study screened $n = 251$ biorepository samples (Table 2). An analysis of the demographics demonstrated that these samples were nearly equal with respect to the proportion of males (50.6%) and females (49.4%) which closely matched the overall proportion within the clinical population, $p = 0.8414$. Most samples had some demographic characteristics regarding race or ethnicity (95.6% or $n = 240/251$). This analysis revealed that most samples were derived from non-White or minority patients (74.2%), similar to the percentage within the overall patient clinic population (70.6%), $p = 0.5085$. More detailed analysis revealed that these samples were derived from minority patients that self-identified as Hispanic or Latino (30.4%), Black or African American (20.4%), and Asian or Pacific Islander (20.0%). In addition, the average age for all study samples was 25.2 years, which was similar to the overall clinical population of 26.4 years, $p = 0.1806$.

Table 2. Demographic characteristics of study sample.

	Study Sample	Clinic Population	Statistical Analysis
Sex			
Female	49.4% ($n = 124/251$)	49.1%	$X^2 = 0.040$, d.f. = 1 $p = 0.8414$
Male	50.6% ($n = 127/251$)	50.9%	
Race or ethnicity			
White or Caucasian	25.8% ($n = 62/240$)	29.4%	$X^2 = 0.4027$, d.f. = 1 $p = 0.5085$
Minority	74.2% ($n = 178/240$)	70.6%	
Hispanic or Latino	30.4% ($n = 73/240$)	49.3%	
Black or African American	20.4% ($n = 49/240$)	10.7%	
Asian or Pacific Islander	20.0% ($n = 48/240$)	8.1%	
Other/Mixed race	3.3% ($n = 8/240$)	2.5%	
Age			
Average	25.19 years	26.35	Two-tailed t-test
Range	7–51 years	0–89 years	$p = 0.1806$

3.2. High-Risk Oral HPV Screening Results

To determine if the samples identified met the standards for qPCR screening, an analysis of DNA quality and quantity was performed (Table 3). These data demonstrated that the average DNA concentration for pediatric samples was 312.4 ng/uL with a range of 221 to 452 ng/uL, which was well above the recommended minimum concentration of 10 ng/uL for optimal qPCR screening. Adult samples had a higher average DNA concentration of 431.2 ng/uL with a range of 347 to 558 ng/uL, which also met the minimum recommended DNA concentration standard for qPCR processing. The purity of pediatric and adult samples was calculated using the ratio of absorbance readings measured at absorbances of A260 and A280 nm. These data demonstrated that the quality of DNA from pediatric (A260:A280 ratio of 1.76) and adult (A260:A280 ratio of 1.79) samples met the minimum qPCR standard of an A260:A280 ratio of 1.70.

All samples met the minimum standard for qPCR quantity and were then confirmed as having human DNA using the positive control primer for glyceraldehyde 3-phosphate dehydrogenase (GAPDH) prior to screening for high-risk HPV using qPCR (Figure 1). The screening results demonstrated that 28.7% ($n = 72/251$) of samples were found to harbor at least one of these high-risk HPV strains. In addition, an increasing trend in prevalence was observed between 2011 (23.1%) and 2019 (40.0%). Although there was one year with an unusually high number of HPV-positive samples (2015), the overall average of the four years 2011 to 2014 prior to the introduction of the nine-valent vaccine (21.3%) was significantly lower than the average of the five years following the modified HPV vaccine rollout and introduction from 2015 to 2019 (36.2%), $p = 0.019$. This revealed a moderate, positive correlation between the year the sample was taken and the potential for HPV positivity, $R = 0.584$.

Table 3. Qualitative and quantitative analysis of study sample DNA.

Study Sample	DNA Concentration [ng/uL]	DNA Purity Ratio [A260:A280]
Pediatric samples ($n = 110$)	312.4 ng/uL +/− 63 range: 221–452 ng/uL	1.76 range: 1.71–1.82
Adult samples ($n = 141$)	431.2 ng/uL +/− 71 range: 347–558 ng/uL	1.79 range: 1.73–1.88

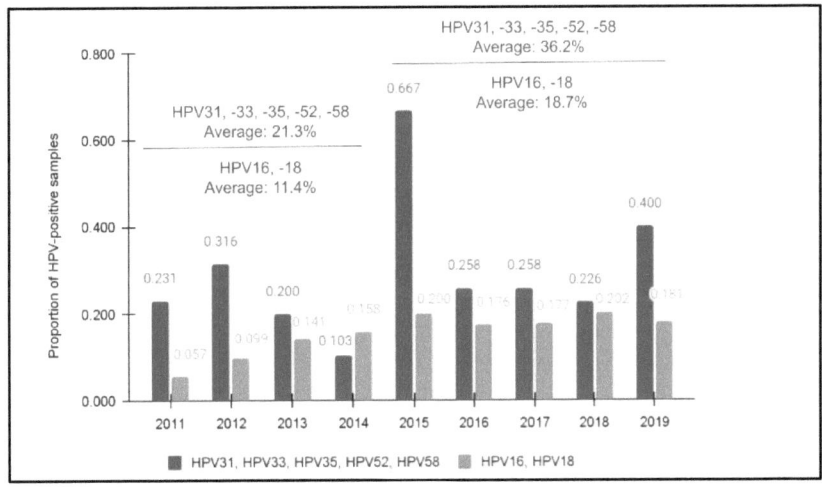

Figure 1. The results of qPCR screening for HPV31, HPV33, HPV35, HPV52, and HPV58. Screening demonstrated that 28.7% ($n = 72/251$) were HPV-positive for one or more of the high-risk strains with an increase observed between 2011 (23.1%) and 2019 (40.0%). The overall average of 2011 to 2014 (21.3%) was significantly lower than following the nine-valent vaccine introduction from 2015 to 2019 (36.2%), $p = 0.019$. In addition, previous data from this clinic population for HPV16 and HPV18 data also revealed increasing trends between 2011 (5.7%) and 2019 (18.1%).

Comparative data from a previous study of this clinic population revealed that HPV positivity for HPV16 and HPV18 data also demonstrated an increasing trend in prevalence between 2011 (5.7%) and 2019 (18.1%) that also had an increased average for the latter five years following the nine-valent HPV vaccine's introduction from 2015 to 2019 (18.7%) compared with the first four years of the analysis from 2011 to 2014 (11.4%) [27]. Overall, a higher percentage of samples tested positive for one of the five high-risk HPV strains in each year compared with the percentage of samples previously testing positive for either HPV16 or HPV18.

A more detailed analysis of the HPV-positive and HPV-negative results was performed (Table 4). This analysis revealed that no significant differences were found between females and males in the HPV-positive (47.2% and 52.8%, respectively) or HPV-negative (50.3% and 49.7%, respectively) categories, $p = 0.5485$. Moreover, the percentage of samples from

White and minority patients was also similar between the HPV-positive (20.8% and 72.3%, respectively) and HPV-negative (26.3% and 70.4%, respectively) groups, $p = 0.1951$. The proportion of HPV-positive and HPV-negative minority subgroups was also similar, such as the percentages of Hispanics or Latinos (29.2% and 29.1%, respectively), Black or African Americans (20.8% and 18.9%, respectively), and Asian or Pacific Islanders (18.1% and 19.6%, respectively). Furthermore, two-thirds (66.7%) of the HPV-positive samples were within the HPV vaccination age (11 to 26 years) or catch-up range (27 to 45 years), which was similar to the percentage of HPV-negative samples within the same age ranges (64.8%), $p = 0.4443$.

Table 4. Demographic analysis of HPV screening samples.

	HPV-Positive	HPV-Negative	Statistical Analysis
Sex			
Female	47.2% ($n = 34/72$)	50.3% ($n = 90/179$)	$X^2 = 0.360$, d.f. = 1 $p = 0.5485$
Male	52.8% ($n = 38/72$)	49.7% ($n = 89/179$)	
Race or ethnicity			
White or Caucasian	20.8% ($n = 15/72$)	26.3% ($n = 47/179$)	$X^2 = 3.269$, d.f. = 2 $p = 0.1951$
Minority	72.3% ($n = 52/72$)	70.4% ($n = 126/179$)	
Hispanic or Latino	29.2% ($n = 21/72$)	29.1% ($n = 52/179$)	
Black or African American	20.8% ($n = 15/72$)	18.9% ($n = 34/179$)	
Asian or Pacific Islander	18.1% ($n = 13/72$)	19.6% ($n = 35/179$)	
Not declared	11.1% ($n = 8/72$)	6.1% ($n = 11/179$)	
Age			
Average	22.8 years	27.7 years	
7–10 years (ORVA) *	8.3% ($n = 6/72$)	10.1% ($n = 18/179$)	$X^2 = 2.676$ d.f. = 3 $p = 0.4443$
11–26 years (RVA)	50.0% ($n = 36/72$)	43.0% ($n = 77/179$)	
26–45 years (VCA)	16.7% ($n = 12/72$)	21.8% ($n = 39/179$)	
45 and older (ORVA) *	25.0% ($n = 18/72$)	25.1% ($n = 45/179$)	

Key: ORVA = outside recommended vaccination age, RVA = recommended vaccination age, VCA = vaccination catch-up age, * denotes outside recommended vaccination age (ORVA).

3.3. Comparison of HPV Screening Results with Recommended Vaccination Age

A graphical analysis of the vaccination ages for the HPV-positive and HPV-negative samples was performed (Figure 2). This analysis demonstrated that the proportion of samples outside the recommended vaccination age between seven and ten years of age was similar between the HPV-positive (8.3%) and HPV-negative (10.1%) samples. Similarly, those within the recommended vaccination age between 11 and 26 years of age were also similar among the HPV-positive and -negative samples (50.0% and 42.0%, respectively), as were those within the vaccination catch-up age range of 27 to 45 years (16.7% and 21.8%, respectively). Finally, nearly identical proportions of samples above the recommended vaccination age (45 years and over) were found between the HPV-positive and -negative samples (25.0% and 25.1%, respectively).

To more closely evaluate the relationship between age and HPV screening results, the HPV-positive and HPV-negative results were then sorted into pediatric and adult groups (Figure 3). These data demonstrated that slightly less than half of the HPV-positive (44.4%) and HPV-negative (43.6%) samples were derived from pediatric patients under the age of 18 years old. The proportion of HPV-positive (55.6%) and HPV-negative (56.4%) samples derived from adults over the age of 18 years old was also similar, which was not statistically significant, $p = 0.8399$.

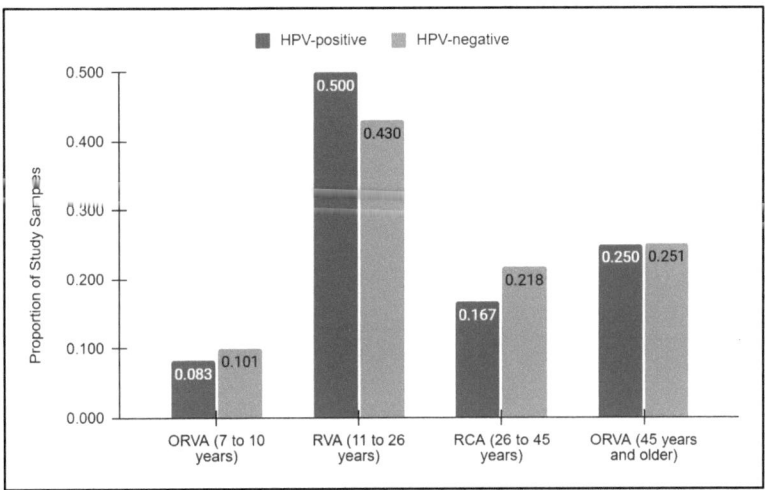

Figure 2. Vaccination grouped ages for the HPV-positive and HPV-negative samples. Samples below or outside the recommended vaccination age (ORVA) of 7 to 10 years were similar between the HPV-positive and -negative (8.3%, 10.1%) samples, as were those above the recommended vaccination age of 45 and older (25.0%, 25.1%, respectively). Similar proportions of HPV-positive and -negative samples within the recommended vaccination age (RVA) were observed (50.0% and 42.0%, respectively), as were those within the vaccination catch-up age range of 27 to 45 years (16.7% and 21.8%, respectively).

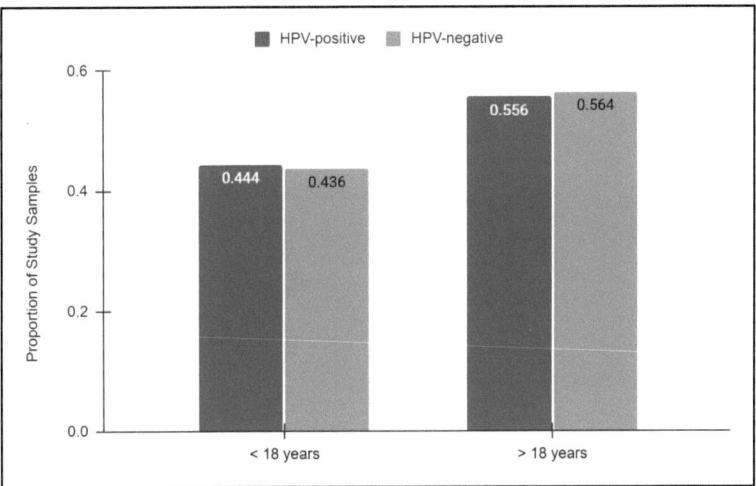

Figure 3. Pediatric and adult HPV screening results. Pediatric samples represented less than half of the HPV-positive (44.4%) and HPV-negative (43.6%) samples, while similar proportions of HPV-positive (55.6%) and HPV-negative (56.4%) samples were derived from adults, which was not statistically significant, $p = 0.8399$.

3.4. Analysis of High-Risk Oral HPV Strains

The HPV-positive samples were further analyzed to determine the overall prevalence of each high-risk strain detected (Figure 4). These data revealed striking differences in prevalence among each of the high-risk strains analyzed, with the highest proportion observed among HPV33-positive samples (34.7%) followed by HPV58 (27.8%), HPV31

(19.4%), and HPV52 (13.9%). However, HPV35 was only observed among a very small proportion of the overall HPV-positive samples (4.2%).

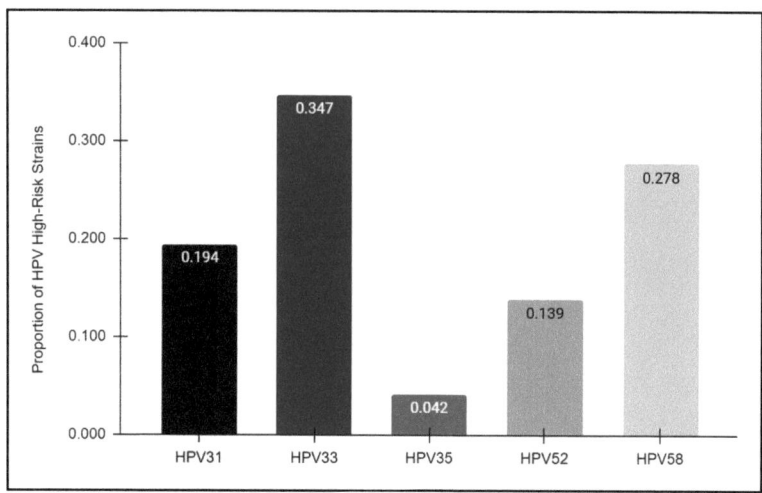

Figure 4. The prevalence of high-risk HPV strains. The highest proportion of HPV-positive samples was observed among HPV33 (34.7%), followed by HPV58 (27.8%), HPV31 (19.4%), HPV52 (13.9%), and HPV35 (4.2%).

3.5. Analysis of Pediatric HPV Vaccination Status

Finally, vaccination status for the pediatric clinic population was evaluated (Figure 5). These data demonstrated that approximately half (48.0%) of pediatric patients within the clinic population self-reported that no HPV vaccine doses had been received. In addition, only 22.1% reported having received one or more doses of the HPV vaccine, although the clinic charting does not automatically separate and categorize the number of vaccinations (one, two, or three dosages). It is worth noting that 30.9% of patients (or their parents and guardians) declined to offer this information, which may suggest that HPV vaccination may be less likely among this subgroup.

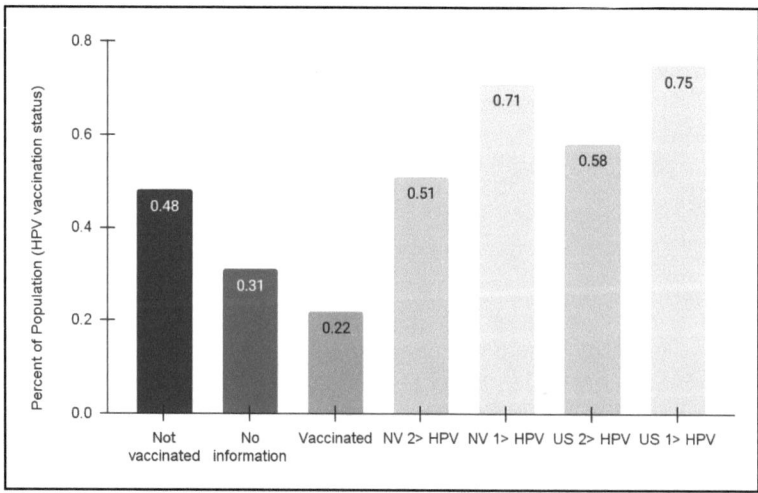

Figure 5. HPV vaccination status for pediatric patients. An analysis of data from pediatric patients aged 11–17 years revealed nearly half (48.0%) had not received any HPV vaccination. Less than one-

quarter (22.1%) reported having received one or more doses of the HPV vaccine, while 30.9% of patients (or their parents and guardians) declined to offer this information. No data regarding HPV vaccination for the adult patient population were available at this time of this analysis. State and national HPV vaccination data revealed NV vaccination rates for HPV adolescents (13–17 years) were 51% (one dose) and 71% (two or more dosages), respectively, which were lower than the national averages of 58% and 75%, respectively.

Regional and national HPV vaccination status data from the Centers for Disease Control and Prevention (CDC) were also compiled and graphed for this analysis. These data demonstrated that state-level population statistics for at least one HPV vaccination dosage for adolescents (13–17 years) were approximately 71%, which was lower but similar to the national average of 75%. For the full dosage series of two or three HPV vaccinations, the percentages for Nevada and the US were lower (51% and 58%, respectively)—although both were much higher than the percentage of clinic patients within this same age range (13–17 years). Unfortunately, no data regarding HPV vaccination for adult patients were available at this time of this analysis.

4. Discussion

This study sought to determine the oral prevalence of high-risk HPV strains from within an existing salivary biorepository. These data revealed that several high-risk HPV strains, including most of those contained within the nine-valent HPV vaccine, were present. These data demonstrated that the oral prevalence for these high-risk HPV strains may be two-fold greater (40%) than another recent study of HPV16 and HPV18 prevalence (18.1%) from the same biorepository [36]. Moreover, these results correspond with other recent studies and reviews of oral HPV prevalence that screened for the additional non-HPV16 and non-HPV18 high-risk strains of HPV covered by the nine-valent HPV vaccine [37,38].

In addition, the longitudinal and temporal analysis incorporated into the study design demonstrated that these strains may be becoming more prevalent within this patient population over time—increasing from 23.1% to 40.0% between 2011 and 2019 [24,25,36]. These data reflect similar reviews and reports of increasing oral HPV prevalence that demonstrated marked increases in these high-risk HPV strains within the most recent ten to fifteen years among various patient populations [39–41]. An analysis of these data also revealed that the average prevalence of HPV over the first four years of this analysis (2011 to 2014) prior to the approval and introduction of the nine-valent vaccine in December 2014 was actually lower than the prevalence of these high-risk strains following this approval and vaccine rollout (2015 to 2019). It is important to note that these data also revealed that oral HPV positivity was equally distributed among both males and females, which has been a topic of increasing public health interest as HPV vaccination rates for young males within the recommended vaccination age continue to lag significantly behind those of young females [42–44].

These data revealed the overwhelming majority of samples with high-risk HPV came from patient samples within the recommended HPV vaccination age (11 to 26 years) or the recommended catch-up vaccination age range (27 to 45 years). These data correspond to other systematic reviews and meta-analyses that suggested oral HPV16 and HPV18 prevalence may also be found among patients within similar age ranges [45–47]. Despite numerous studies confirming the safety and efficacy of the nine-valent HPV vaccine, rising levels of vaccine hesitancy fueled by vaccine myths and misinformation spread on social media have created significant barriers and challenges to this straightforward and effective HPV-related prevention method [48–51]. Among the most effective strategies to increase provider willingness to engage and counter these misconceptions are data demonstrating the increasing trends and prevalence of HPV among vaccine-eligible adolescents and young adults, which may help to highlight the importance of these findings and the risks associated with failure to use evidence-based decisions among parents and caregivers [52–55].

This study also presents significant findings as the overwhelming majorities of both clinical biorepository samples and the clinical patient population are under-represented minorities [19,20,36]. These data are increasingly important as more and more studies have demonstrated that multiple challenges and barriers to vaccination in general, and HPV vaccination in particular, may be faced by ethnic and racial minorities within the United States, which have often led to lower rates of health prevention in general and HPV vaccination in particular that have been demonstrated by the rising prevalence of HPV among this patient population even after the introduction of the nine-valent HPV vaccine [56–58]. Despite the advances made in language proficiency and cultural competency, additional issues surrounding communication practices and long-standing trust issues between minority parents and physicians further complicate the landscape regarding HPV vaccination hesitancy [59–62].

These findings are also important considerations as more and more data now suggest that oral healthcare providers, including dentists and hygienists, may be able to engage more patients in a wide range of discussions that help to increase HPV awareness and HPV vaccination uptake [63,64]. For example, research from this group has demonstrated that vaccine myths, misconceptions, and hesitancy among dental students and post-graduate residents were mediated, in part, by up-to-date evidence-based knowledge regarding HPV vaccine safety and efficacy, as well as data and evidence regarding oral HPV prevalence and vaccine hesitancy within the clinical patient population [65,66]. This study adds to the growing body of evidence that may help to increase community awareness and engagement with HPV prevalence and the importance of HPV vaccination among vaccine-eligible adolescents and youth [67,68].

This study has several implicit limitations that should be considered. For example, this study does not provide the most up-to-date information on oral HPV prevalence due to the retrospective nature of this study. Therefore, any data regarding oral HPV prevalence between 2020 and 2024 were not available for analysis [19,20]. Another limitation is the nature of the convenience sample, which was drawn from a low minority-serving, low-income open clinic within a public dental school that may not accurately reflect the local or regional community at large [59,65,66]. Moreover, some limitations of this study included both the number and availability of previously collected samples, as well as any additional limitations and biases that could have been associated with the original sample collection that could not be controlled for within the parameters of the current study.

Despite these limitations, this study presented significant findings that may be important for public and oral health researchers for several reasons. First, these data revealed that the prevalence of high-risk oral HPV may be much higher than in other recent studies of healthy adult populations (4.5% to 6.6%) but within the range of oral HPV prevalence found by some oral health researchers (0.67% to 35%), which may be due to the extremely low vaccination rates among this low-income, minority patient population as well as the many challenges and barriers faced by these subgroups [41,69,70]. Next, these data demonstrated that despite the increase in vaccination rates among adolescents and teenagers in other industrialized countries following the nine-valent vaccine release, high oral HPV prevalence rates combined with low vaccination rates were observed within this patient population and may suggest that these phenomena could be present among other low-income, minority populations where prevention messages and implementation measures remain comparatively low and could be the basis for future studies in this area [71,72]. Finally, a more detailed analysis of these research studies also demonstrated nearly the same proportion of oral HPV-16 among males and females, which was similar to the result of this current study that showed no significant difference between high-risk oral HPV among females and males (47.2% and 52.8%, respectively) [71,72].

5. Conclusions

This study provides new evidence regarding the oral prevalence of the additional high-risk HPV strains covered by the nine-valent HPV vaccine evaluated over time. These data demonstrated that the oral HPV prevalence of these additional strains may be higher than that of HPV16 and HPV18 within this low-income and mostly minority patient population, which was found mainly among patients within the recommended or catch-up HPV vaccination age. Moreover, oral HPV prevalence also appears to be increasing over time, providing new evidence and support for the importance of the nine-valent HPV vaccine that covers these additional high-risk HPV strains, such as HPV31, HPV33, HPV52, and HPV58, and the public health measures that must be employed to increase knowledge, awareness, and acceptance.

Author Contributions: Conceptualization, K.K.; methodology, K.K.; formal analysis, J.J., E.C., and K.K.; investigation, J.J. and E.C.; resources, K.K.; data curation, K.K.; writing—original draft preparation, J.J., E.C., and K.K.; writing—review and editing, J.J., E.C., and K.K.; supervision, K.K. All authors have read and agreed to the published version of the manuscript.

Funding: This research received no external funding.

Institutional Review Board Statement: This study was conducted in accordance with the Declaration of Helsinki and approved by the Institutional Review Board of The University of Nevada, Las Vegas (UNLV) as Exempt under Protocol #171612-1, "Retrospective analysis of microbial prevalence from DNA isolated from saliva samples originally obtained from the University of Nevada, Las Vegas (UNLV) School of Dental Medicine (SDM) pediatric and clinical population", on 3 March 2021.

Informed Consent Statement: The samples analyzed in this retrospective study were originally collected for the biorepository under approved protocol OPRS#1305-4466M, "The Prevalence of Oral Microbes in Saliva from the UNLV School of Dental Medicine Pediatric and Adult Clinical Population". The patients of record voluntarily provided informed consent, and pediatric patients provided pediatric assent in addition to informed consent from the parent or designated guardian.

Data Availability Statement: The primary data may be available upon request from the corresponding author. These data are not publicly available according to the protection parameters for the study protocol, which were required by the IRB and OPRS for the study approval.

Conflicts of Interest: The authors declare no conflicts of interest.

References

1. Rahman, R.; Shaikh, M.H.; Gopinath, D.; Idris, A.; Johnson, N.W. Human papillomavirus and Epstein-Barr virus co-infection in oral and oropharyngeal squamous cell carcinomas: A systematic review and meta-analysis. *Mol. Oral Microbiol.* **2023**, *38*, 259–274. [CrossRef] [PubMed]
2. Katirachi, S.K.; Grønlund, M.P.; Jakobsen, K.K.; Grønhøj, C.; von Buchwald, C. The Prevalence of HPV in Oral Cavity Squamous Cell Carcinoma. *Viruses* **2023**, *15*, 451. [CrossRef] [PubMed]
3. Santacroce, L.; Di Cosola, M.; Bottalico, L.; Topi, S.; Charitos, I.A.; Ballini, A.; Inchingolo, F.; Cazzolla, A.P.; Dipalma, G. Focus on HPV Infection and the Molecular Mechanisms of Oral Carcinogenesis. *Viruses* **2021**, *13*, 559. [CrossRef] [PubMed]
4. Fiorillo, L.; Cervino, G.; Surace, G.; De Stefano, R.; Laino, L.; D'Amico, C.; Fiorillo, M.T.; Meto, A.; Herford, A.S.; Arzukanyan, A.V.; et al. Human Papilloma Virus: Current Knowledge and Focus on Oral Health. *BioMed Res. Int.* **2021**, *2021*, 6631757. [CrossRef] [PubMed]
5. Saikia, P.J.; Pathak, L.; Mitra, S.; Das, B. The emerging role of oral microbiota in oral cancer initiation, progression and stemness. *Front. Immunol.* **2023**, *14*, 1198269. [CrossRef] [PubMed]
6. Das, T.; Zhong, R.; Spiotto, M.T. Notch Signaling and Human Papillomavirus-Associated Oral Tumorigenesis. *Adv. Exp. Med. Biol.* **2021**, *1287*, 105–122; Erratum in *Adv. Exp. Med. Biol.* **2021**, *1287*, C1. [CrossRef] [PubMed]
7. Yete, S.; D'Souza, W.; Saranath, D. High-Risk Human Papillomavirus in Oral Cancer: Clinical Implications. *Oncology* **2018**, *94*, 133–141. [CrossRef] [PubMed]
8. Zhao, M.; Zhou, D.; Zhang, M.; Kang, P.; Cui, M.; Zhu, L.; Luo, L. Characteristic of persistent human papillomavirus infection in women worldwide: A meta-analysis. *PeerJ* **2023**, *11*, e16247. [CrossRef] [PubMed] [PubMed Central]
9. Wolf, J.; Kist, L.F.; Pereira, S.B.; Quessada, M.A.; Petek, H.; Pille, A.; Maccari, J.G.; Mutlaq, M.P.; Nasi, L.A. Human papillomavirus infection: Epidemiology, biology, host interactions, cancer development, prevention, and therapeutics. *Rev. Med. Virol.* **2024**, *34*, e2537. [CrossRef]
10. Plotzker, R.E.; Vaidya, A.; Pokharel, U.; Stier, E.A. Sexually Transmitted Human Papillomavirus: Update in Epidemiology, Prevention, and Management. *Infect. Dis. Clin. N. Am.* **2023**, *37*, 289–310. [CrossRef]
11. Yousefi, Z.; Aria, H.; Ghaedrahmati, F.; Bakhtiari, T.; Azizi, M.; Bastan, R.; Hosseini, R.; Eskandari, N. An Update on Human Papilloma Virus Vaccines: History, Types, Protection, and Efficacy. *Front. Immunol.* **2022**, *12*, 805695. [CrossRef] [PubMed]

12. Wakabayashi, R.; Nakahama, Y.; Nguyen, V.; Espinoza, J.L. The Host-Microbe Interplay in Human Papillomavirus-Induced Carcinogenesis. *Microorganisms* **2019**, *7*, 199. [CrossRef] [PubMed]
13. McNamara, M.; Batur, P.; Walsh, J.M.E.; Johnson, K.M. HPV Update: Vaccination, Screening, and Associated Disease. *J. Gen. Intern. Med.* **2016**, *31*, 1360–1366. [CrossRef] [PubMed]
14. Zou, K.; Huang, Y.; Li, Z. Prevention and treatment of human papillomavirus in men benefits both men and women. *Front. Cell. Infect. Microbiol.* **2022**, *12*, 1077651. [CrossRef] [PubMed]
15. Bhattacharjee, R.; Kumar, L.; Dhasmana, A.; Mitra, T.; Dey, A.; Malik, S.; Kim, B.; Gundamaraju, R. Governing HPV-related carcinoma using vaccines: Bottlenecks and breakthroughs. *Front. Oncol.* **2022**, *12*, 977933. [CrossRef] [PubMed]
16. Charde, S.H.; Warbhe, R.A. Human Papillomavirus Prevention by Vaccination: A Review Article. *Cureus* **2022**, *14*, e30037. [CrossRef] [PubMed]
17. Zhang, Z.; Zhang, J.; Xia, N.; Zhao, Q. Expanded strain coverage for a highly successful public health tool: Prophylactic 9-valent human papillomavirus vaccine. *Hum. Vaccines Immunother.* **2017**, *13*, 2280–2291. [CrossRef] [PubMed]
18. Okerosi, S.; Mokoh, L.W.; Rubagumya, F.; Niyibizi, B.A.; Nkya, A.; Van Loon, K.; Buckle, G.; Bent, S.; Ha, P.; Fagan, J.J.; et al. Human Papillomavirus-Associated Head and Neck Malignancies in Sub-Saharan Africa: A Systematic Review. *JCO Glob. Oncol.* **2023**, *9*, e2200259. [CrossRef] [PubMed]
19. Hinton, H.; Herrera, L.; Valenzuela, S.; Howard, K.M.; Kingsley, K. Screening for High-Risk Human Papillomavirus Reveals HPV52 and HPV58 among Pediatric and Adult Patient Saliva Samples. *Dent. J.* **2024**, *12*, 56. [CrossRef]
20. Hinton, H.; Coleman, S.; Salem, J.R.; Kingsley, K. Screening for High-Risk Oral Human Papillomavirus (HPV31, HPV33, HPV35) in a Multi-Racial Pediatric and Adult Clinic Patient Population. *Cancers* **2023**, *15*, 4501. [CrossRef]
21. Hedges, J.; Sethi, S.; Garvey, G.; Whop, L.J.; Canfell, K.; Dodd, Z.; Larkins, P.; Antonsson, A.; Smith, M.A.; Mittinty, M.; et al. The Indigenous Australian Human Papillomavirus (HPV) Cohort Study 2, Continuation for 5 to 10 Years: Protocol for a Longitudinal Study. *JMIR Res. Protoc.* **2023**, *12*, e44593. [CrossRef] [PubMed]
22. Wei, F.; Goodman, M.T.; Xia, N.; Zhang, J.; Giuliano, A.R.; D'Souza, G.; Hessol, N.A.; Schim van der Loeff, M.F.; Dai, J.; Neukam, K.; et al. Incidence and Clearance of Anal Human Papillomavirus Infection in 16 164 Individuals, According to Human Immunodeficiency Virus Status, Sex, and Male Sexuality: An International Pooled Analysis of 34 Longitudinal Studies. *Clin. Infect. Dis.* **2023**, *76*, e692–e701. [CrossRef] [PubMed]
23. Brouwer, A.F.; Campredon, L.P.; Walline, H.M.; Marinelli, B.M.; Goudsmit, C.M.; Thomas, T.B.; Delinger, R.L.; Lau, Y.K.; Andrus, E.C.; Nair, T.; et al. Incidence and clearance of oral and cervicogenital HPV infection: Longitudinal analysis of the MHOC cohort study. *BMJ Open* **2022**, *12*, e056502. [CrossRef] [PubMed]
24. Melo, B.A.C.; Vilar, L.G.; Oliveira, N.R.; Lima, P.O.; Pinheiro, M.B.; Domingueti, C.P.; Pereira, M.C. Human papillomavirus infection and oral squamous cell carcinoma—A systematic review. *Braz. J. Otorhinolaryngol.* **2021**, *87*, 346–352. [CrossRef] [PubMed]
25. Antonsson, A.; de Souza, M.; Wood, Z.C.; Carroll, A.; Van, K.; Paterson, L.; Pandeya, N.; Whiteman, D.C. Natural history of oral HPV infection: Longitudinal analyses in prospective cohorts from Australia. *Int. J. Cancer* **2021**, *148*, 1964–1972. [CrossRef] [PubMed]
26. Eisenberg, M.C.; Campredon, L.P.; Brouwer, A.F.; Walline, H.M.; Marinelli, B.M.; Lau, Y.K.; Thomas, T.B.; Delinger, R.L.; Sullivan, T.S.; Yost, M.L.; et al. Dynamics and Determinants of HPV Infection: The Michigan HPV and Oropharyngeal Cancer (M-HOC) Study. *BMJ Open* **2018**, *8*, e021618. [CrossRef]
27. Cui, M.; Cheng, J.; Cheng, H.; Zhao, M.; Zhou, D.; Zhang, M.; Jia, J.; Luo, L. Characteristics of human papillomavirus infection among oropharyngeal cancer patients: A systematic review and meta-analysis. *Arch. Oral Biol.* **2024**, *157*, 105830. [CrossRef] [PubMed]
28. Blatt, S.; Pabst, A.; Zimmer, S.; Walter, C.; Al-Nawas, B.; Krüger, M. Clinical efficacy of an antibody-based detection system for human papilloma virus infection in oral squamous cell carcinoma. *Clin. Oral Investig.* **2021**, *25*, 2837–2843. [CrossRef] [PubMed]
29. Janecka-Widła, A.; Mucha-Małecka, A.; Majchrzyk, K.; Halaszka, K.; Przewoźnik, M.; Słonina, D.; Biesaga, B. Active HPV infection and its influence on survival in head and neck squamous-cell cancer. *J. Cancer Res. Clin. Oncol.* **2020**, *146*, 1677–1692. [CrossRef] [PubMed] [PubMed Central]
30. Ndiaye, C.; Alemany, L.; Diop, Y.; Ndiaye, N.; Diémé, M.J.; Tous, S.; Klaustermeier, J.E.; Alejo, M.; Castellsagué, X.; Bosch, F.X.; et al. The role of human papillomavirus in head and neck cancer in Senegal. *Infect. Agents Cancer* **2013**, *8*, 14. [CrossRef] [PubMed] [PubMed Central]
31. Kim, Y.; Joo, Y.H.; Kim, M.S.; Lee, Y.S. Prevalence of high-risk human papillomavirus and its genotype distribution in head and neck squamous cell carcinomas. *J. Pathol. Transl. Med.* **2020**, *54*, 411–418. [CrossRef] [PubMed]
32. Melchers, L.J.; Mastik, M.F.; Samaniego Cameron, B.; van Dijk, B.A.; de Bock, G.H.; van der Laan, B.F.; van der Vegt, B.; Speel, E.J.; Roodenburg, J.L.; Witjes, M.J.; et al. Detection of HPV-associated oropharyngeal tumours in a 16-year cohort: More than meets the eye. *Br. J. Cancer* **2015**, *112*, 1349–1357. [CrossRef] [PubMed]
33. Magaña-León, C.; Oros, C.; López-Revilla, R. Human papillomavirus types in non-cervical high-grade intraepithelial neoplasias and invasive carcinomas from San Luis Potosí, Mexico: A retrospective cross-sectional study. *Infect. Agents Cancer* **2015**, *10*, 33; Erratum in *Infect. Agents Cancer* **2016**, *11*, 11. [CrossRef] [PubMed]

34. Bettampadi, D.; Sirak, B.A.; Abrahamsen, M.E.; Reich, R.R.; Villa, L.L.; Ponce, E.L.; Giuliano, A.R. Factors Associated with Persistence and Clearance of High-Risk Oral Human Papillomavirus (HPV) Among Participants in the HPV Infection in Men (HIM) Study. *Clin. Infect. Dis.* **2021**, *73*, e3227–e3234. [CrossRef] [PubMed]
35. Nasioutziki, M.; Chatzistamatiou, K.; Loufopoulos, P.D.; Vavoulidis, E.; Tsampazis, N.; Pratilas, G.C.; Liberis, A.; Karpa, V.; Parcharidis, E.; Daniilidis, A.; et al. Cervical, anal and oral HPV detection and HPV type concordance among women referred for colposcopy. *Infect. Agents Cancer* **2020**, *15*, 22. [CrossRef] [PubMed]
36. Kornhaber, M.C.; Florence, T.; Davis, T.; Kingsley, K. Assessment of Oral Human Papillomavirus Prevalence in Pediatric and Adult Patients within a Multi-Ethnic Clinic Population. *Dent. J.* **2022**, *10*, 54. [CrossRef]
37. Garolla, A.; Graziani, A.; Grande, G.; Ortolani, C.; Ferlin, A. HPV-related diseases in male patients: An underestimated conundrum. *J. Endocrinol. Investig.* **2024**, *47*, 261–274. [CrossRef] [PubMed]
38. Wierzbicka, M.; Klussmann, J.P.; San Giorgi, M.R.; Wuerdemann, N.; Dikkers, F.G. Oral and laryngeal HPV infection: Incidence, prevalence and risk factors, with special regard to concurrent infection in head, neck and genitals. *Vaccine* **2021**, *39*, 2344–2350. [CrossRef]
39. Poljak, M.; Cuschieri, K.; Alemany, L.; Vorsters, A. Testing for Human Papillomaviruses in Urine, Blood, and Oral Specimens: An Update for the Laboratory. *J. Clin. Microbiol.* **2023**, *61*, e0140322. [CrossRef]
40. Barsouk, A.; Aluru, J.S.; Rawla, P.; Saginala, K.; Barsouk, A. Epidemiology, Risk Factors, and Prevention of Head and Neck Squamous Cell Carcinoma. *Med. Sci.* **2023**, *11*, 42. [CrossRef] [PubMed]
41. Vani, N.V.; Madhanagopal, R.; Swaminathan, R.; Ganesan, T.S. Dynamics of oral human papillomavirus infection in healthy populations and head and neck cancer. *Cancer Med.* **2023**, *12*, 11731–11745. [CrossRef] [PubMed]
42. Shen, F.; Du, Y.; Cao, X.; Chen, C.; Yang, M.; Yan, R.; Yang, S. Acceptance of the Human Papillomavirus Vaccine among General Men and Men with a Same-Sex Orientation and Its Influencing Factors: A Systematic Review and Meta-Analysis. *Vaccines* **2023**, *12*, 16. [CrossRef] [PubMed]
43. El Hussein, M.T.; Dhaliwal, S. HPV vaccination for prevention of head and neck cancer among men. *Nurse Pract.* **2023**, *48*, 25–32. [CrossRef] [PubMed]
44. Olusanya, O.A.; Tomar, A.; Thomas, J.; Alonge, K.; Wigfall, L.T. Application of the theoretical domains framework to identify factors influencing catch-up HPV vaccinations among male college students in the United States: A review of evidence and recommendations. *Vaccine* **2023**, *41*, 3564–3576. [CrossRef] [PubMed]
45. Amantea, C.; Foschi, N.; Gavi, F.; Borrelli, I.; Rossi, M.F.; Spontarelli, V.; Russo, P.; Gualano, M.R.; Santoro, P.E.; Moscato, U. HPV Vaccination Adherence in Working-Age Men: A Systematic Review and Meta-Analysis. *Vaccines* **2023**, *11*, 443. [CrossRef] [PubMed]
46. Magana, K.; Strand, L.; Love, M.; Moore, T.; Peña, A.; Ito Ford, A.; Vassar, M. Health inequities in human papillomavirus prevention, diagnostics and clinical care in the USA: A scoping review. *Sex. Transm. Infect.* **2023**, *99*, 128–136. [CrossRef] [PubMed]
47. Mehta, A.; Markman, B.; Rodriguez-Cintron, W. Don't jump down my throat: Gender gap in HPV vaccinations risk long term cancer threats. *Expert Rev. Vaccines* **2022**, *21*, 1045–1053. [CrossRef]
48. Vraga, E.K.; Brady, S.S.; Gansen, C.; Khan, E.M.; Bennis, S.L.; Nones, M.; Tang, R.; Srivastava, J.; Kulasingam, S. A review of HPV and HBV vaccine hesitancy, intention, and uptake in the era of social media and COVID-19. *Elife* **2023**, *12*, e85743. [CrossRef] [PubMed]
49. Deng, D.; Shen, Y.; Li, W.; Zeng, N.; Huang, Y.; Nie, X. Challenges of hesitancy in human papillomavirus vaccination: Bibliometric and visual analysis. *Int. J. Health Plan. Manag.* **2023**, *38*, 1161–1183. [CrossRef]
50. Morales-Campos, D.Y.; Zimet, G.D.; Kahn, J.A. Human Papillomavirus Vaccine Hesitancy in the United States. *Pediatr. Clin. N. Am.* **2023**, *70*, 211–226. [CrossRef] [PubMed]
51. Nowak, G.J.; Cacciatore, M.A. State of Vaccine Hesitancy in the United States. *Pediatr. Clin. N. Am.* **2023**, *70*, 197–210. [CrossRef] [PubMed]
52. Kopp, S.A.; Turk, D.E. Human Papillomavirus Vaccinations: Provider Education to Enhance Vaccine Uptake. *Clin. Pediatr.* **2023**, *62*, 840–848. [CrossRef] [PubMed]
53. Nogueira-Rodrigues, A.; Flores, M.G.; Macedo Neto, A.O.; Braga, L.A.C.; Vieira, C.M.; de Sousa-Lima, R.M.; de Andrade, D.A.P.; Machado, K.K.; Guimarães, A.P.G. HPV vaccination in Latin America: Coverage status, implementation challenges and strategies to overcome it. *Front. Oncol.* **2022**, *12*, 984449. [CrossRef] [PubMed]
54. Aguolu, O.G.; Malik, A.A.; Ahmed, N.; Omer, S.B. Overcoming Vaccine Hesitancy for Future COVID-19 and HIV Vaccines: Lessons from Measles and HPV Vaccines. *Curr. HIV/AIDS Rep.* **2022**, *19*, 328–343. [CrossRef] [PubMed]
55. Tankwanchi, A.S.; Jaca, A.; Ndlambe, A.M.; Zantsi, Z.P.; Bowman, B.; Garrison, M.M.; Larson, H.J.; Vermund, S.H.; Wiysonge, C.S. Non-COVID-19 vaccine hesitancy among migrant populations worldwide: A scoping review of the literature, 2000-2020. *Expert Rev. Vaccines* **2022**, *21*, 1269–1287. [CrossRef] [PubMed]
56. Harrington, N.; Chen, Y.; O'Reilly, A.M.; Fang, C.Y. The role of trust in HPV vaccine uptake among racial and ethnic minorities in the United States: A narrative review. *AIMS Public Health* **2021**, *8*, 352–368. [CrossRef] [PubMed]
57. Lott, B.E.; Okusanya, B.O.; Anderson, E.J.; Kram, N.A.; Rodriguez, M.; Thomson, C.A.; Rosales, C.; Ehiri, J.E. Interventions to increase uptake of Human Papillomavirus (HPV) vaccination in minority populations: A systematic review. *Prev. Med. Rep.* **2020**, *19*, 101163. [CrossRef] [PubMed]

58. Cho, D.; Ramondetta, L.; Garcini, L.; Lu, Q. HPVs Vaccination among Racial/Ethnic Minority College Students: Current Status and Future Direction. *J. Natl. Med. Assoc.* **2020**, *112*, 639–649. [CrossRef] [PubMed]
59. Mavi, J.; Kingsley, K. Analysis of a Pediatric Dental School Patient Population Revealed Increasing Trends of Limited English Proficiency (LEP) Patients: Implications for Pediatric Dental Public Health and Access to Care. *Pediatr. Rep.* **2022**, *14*, 276–287. [CrossRef]
60. Fisher, H.; Denford, S.; Audrey, S.; Finn, A.; Hajinur, H.; Hickman, M.; Mounier-Jack, S.; Mohamed, A.; Roderick, M.; Tucker, L.; et al. Information needs of ethnically diverse, vaccine-hesitant parents during decision-making about the HPV vaccine for their adolescent child: A qualitative study. *BMC Public Health* **2024**, *24*, 91. [CrossRef] [PubMed]
61. Frietze, G.; Padilla, M.; Cordero, J.; Gosselink, K.; Moya, E. Human Papillomavirus Vaccine Acceptance (HPV-VA) and Vaccine Uptake (HPV-VU): Assessing the impact of theory, culture, and trusted sources of information in a Hispanic community. *BMC Public Health* **2023**, *23*, 1781. [CrossRef] [PubMed]
62. Chan, D.N.S.; Li, C.; Law, B.M.H.; Choi, K.C.; Lee, P.P.K.; So, W.K.W. Factors affecting HPV vaccine uptake among ethnic minority adolescent girls: A systematic review and meta-analysis. *Asia Pac. J. Oncol. Nurs.* **2023**, *10*, 100279. [CrossRef] [PubMed]
63. Casey, S.M.; Paiva, T.; Perkins, R.B.; Villa, A.; Murray, E.J. Could oral health care professionals help increase human papillomavirus vaccination rates by engaging patients in discussions? *J. Am. Dent. Assoc.* **2023**, *154*, 10–23.e17. [CrossRef] [PubMed]
64. Chattopadhyay, A.; Weatherspoon, D.; Pinto, A. Human papillomavirus and oral cancer: A primer for dental public health professionals. *Community Dent. Health* **2015**, *32*, 117–128. [PubMed]
65. Maginot, R.; Esteves, C.; Kingsley, K. Changing Perspectives on Pediatric Human Papillomavirus (HPV) Vaccination among Dental Students and Residents Reveals Recent Increase in Vaccine Hesitancy. *Vaccines* **2022**, *10*, 570. [CrossRef] [PubMed]
66. Mann, S.K.; Kingsley, K. Human Papillomavirus (HPV) Vaccine Knowledge, Awareness and Acceptance among Dental Students and Post-Graduate Dental Residents. *Dent. J.* **2020**, *8*, 45. [CrossRef] [PubMed]
67. Xie, Y.J.; Liao, X.; Lin, M.; Yang, L.; Cheung, K.; Zhang, Q.; Li, Y.; Hao, C.; Wang, H.H.; Gao, Y.; et al. Community Engagement in Vaccination Promotion: Systematic Review and Meta-Analysis. *JMIR Public Health Surveill.* **2024**, *10*, e49695. [CrossRef] [PubMed]
68. Lu, Q.; Dawkins-Moultin, L.; Cho, D.; Tan, N.Q.P.; Hopfer, S.; Li, Y.; Ramondetta, L.; Xu, Y.; Lun, D.; Chen, M. A multilevel intervention to promote HPV vaccination among young adults in Texas: Protocol for a randomized controlled trial. *BMC Public Health* **2024**, *24*, 1506. [CrossRef]
69. Kreimer, A.R.; Bhatia, R.K.; Messeguer, A.L.; González, P.; Herrero, R.; Giuliano, A.R. Oral human papillomavirus in healthy individuals: A systematic review of the literature. *Sex. Transm. Dis.* **2010**, *37*, 386–391. [CrossRef]
70. Giuliano, A.R.; Felsher, M.; Waterboer, T.; Mirghani, H.; Mehanna, H.; Roberts, C.; Chen, Y.T.; Lynam, M.; Pedrós, M.; Sanchez, E.; et al. Oral Human Papillomavirus Prevalence and Genotyping Among a Healthy Adult Population in the US. *JAMA Otolaryngol. Head Neck Surg.* **2023**, *149*, 783–795; Erratum in *JAMA Otolaryngol. Head Neck Surg.* **2024**, *150*, 358. [CrossRef] [PubMed]
71. Du, J.; Ährlund-Richter, A.; Näsman, A.; Dalianis, T. Human papilloma virus (HPV) prevalence upon HPV vaccination in Swedish youth: A review based on our findings 2008-2018, and perspectives on cancer prevention. *Arch. Gynecol. Obstet.* **2021**, *303*, 329–335. [CrossRef] [PubMed]
72. Jacot-Guillarmod, M.; Pasquier, J.; Greub, G.; Bongiovanni, M.; Achtari, C.; Sahli, R. Impact of HPV vaccination with Gardasil® in Switzerland. *BMC Infect. Dis.* **2017**, *17*, 790. [CrossRef] [PubMed]

Disclaimer/Publisher's Note: The statements, opinions and data contained in all publications are solely those of the individual author(s) and contributor(s) and not of MDPI and/or the editor(s). MDPI and/or the editor(s) disclaim responsibility for any injury to people or property resulting from any ideas, methods, instructions or products referred to in the content.

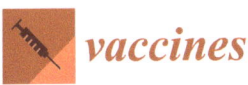

Article

Immunoinformatics Design and In Vivo Immunogenicity Evaluation of a Conserved CTL Multi-Epitope Vaccine Targeting HPV16 E5, E6, and E7 Proteins

Ni Guo [1,†], Zhixin Niu [1,†], Zhiling Yan [2], Weipeng Liu [1], Lei Shi [3], Chuanyin Li [1], Yuteng Yao [1,*] and Li Shi [3,*]

[1] Yunnan Key Laboratory of Vaccine Research & Development on Severe Infectious Disease, Institute of Medical Biology, Chinese Academy of Medical Sciences & Peking Union Medical College, Kunming 650118, China; guoni@student.pumc.edu.cn (N.G.); niuzhixinamber@163.com (Z.N.); liuweipeng@imbcams.com.cn (W.L.); chuanyinli@imbcams.com.cn (C.L.)

[2] Department of Gynaecologic Oncology, Peking University Cancer Hospital Yunnan & Yunnan Cancer Hospital & The Third Affiliated Hospital of Kunming Medical University, Kunming 650118, China; yanzhiling2021@126.com

[3] Department of Immunogenetics, Institute of Medical Biology, Chinese Academy of Medical Sciences & Peking Union Medical College, Kunming 650118, China; sansan33@imbcams.com.cn

* Correspondence: leoyyf@gmail.com (Y.Y.); shili.imb@gmail.com (L.S.)

† These authors contributed equally to this work.

Abstract: Human papillomavirus type 16 (HPV16) infection is responsible for more than 50% of global cervical cancer cases. The development of a vaccine based on cytotoxic T-lymphocyte (CTL) epitopes is a promising strategy for eliminating pre-existing HPV infections and treating patients with cervical cancer. In this study, an immunoinformatics approach was used to predict HLA-I-restricted CTL epitopes in HPV16 E5, E6, and E7 proteins, and a set of conserved CTL epitopes co-restricted by human/murine MHCs was screened and characterized, with the set containing three E5, four E6, and four E7 epitopes. Subsequently, the immunogenicity of the epitope combination was assessed in mice, and the anti-tumor effects of the multi-epitope peptide vaccine E5E6E7pep11 and the recombinant protein vaccine CTB-Epi11E567 were evaluated in the TC-1 mouse tumor model. The results demonstrated that mixed epitope peptides could induce antigen-specific IFN-γ secretion in mice. Prophylactic immunization with E5E6E7pep11 and CTB-Epi11E567 was found to provide 100% protection against tumor growth in mice. Moreover, both types of the multi-epitope vaccine significantly inhibited tumor growth and prolonged mouse survival. In conclusion, in this study, a multi-epitope vaccine targeting HPV16 E5, E6, and E7 proteins was successfully designed and evaluated, demonstrating potential immunogenicity and anti-tumor effects and providing a promising strategy for immunotherapy against HPV-associated tumors.

Keywords: human papilloma virus type 16 (HPV16); immunoinformatics; CTL epitope prediction; multi-epitope vaccine design; tumor immunotherapy

Citation: Guo, N.; Niu, Z.; Yan, Z.; Liu, W.; Shi, L.; Li, C.; Yao, Y.; Shi, L. Immunoinformatics Design and In Vivo Immunogenicity Evaluation of a Conserved CTL Multi-Epitope Vaccine Targeting HPV16 E5, E6, and E7 Proteins. *Vaccines* **2024**, *12*, 392. https://doi.org/10.3390/vaccines12040392

Academic Editor: Ralph A. Tripp

Received: 2 February 2024
Revised: 1 April 2024
Accepted: 7 April 2024
Published: 9 April 2024

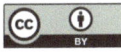

Copyright: © 2024 by the authors. Licensee MDPI, Basel, Switzerland. This article is an open access article distributed under the terms and conditions of the Creative Commons Attribution (CC BY) license (https://creativecommons.org/licenses/by/4.0/).

1. Introduction

Persistent infection with human papillomaviruses (HPVs) contributes to the global cervical cancer burden [1,2]. More than 200 HPV types have been identified and further classified into high-risk (HR) and low-risk (LR) HPV based on their association with cervical cancer. HPV16 represents the most significant high-risk human papillomavirus (HR-HPV), accounting for more than half of cervical cancer cases worldwide [2,3]. Although current vaccines have demonstrated significant efficacy in preventing cervical cancer, they are unable to clear pre-existing HPV infections. Developing therapeutic HPV vaccines presents numerous challenges, including the rapid identification of viable target antigens, issues regarding cross-protection due to antigenic diversity and antigenic variation, immune evasion within the tumor microenvironment, as well as the assessment of vaccine immunogenicity and long-term safety [4,5].

Cytotoxic T lymphocytes (CTLs) play an essential role in the host's defense against viral infections. When a cell is infected by viruses, fragments of viral proteins are presented on the host cell surface via major histocompatibility complex (MHC) class I molecules. Cytotoxic T cells recognize these protein fragments—also known as epitopes—in conjunction with MHC class I molecules, activating specific $CD8^+$ T cytotoxic T cell or $CD4^+$ helper T cell responses, thereby facilitating virus and infected cell clearance [6,7]. Epitope-based vaccines leverage the functionality of CTLs in clearing viruses and offer several advantages compared to traditional vaccines. Firstly, they can elicit a broader CTL response by being engineered to carry multiple epitopes from various parts of the pathogen. Secondly, they can be more rapidly produced, thus enabling rapid adaptation in response to viral mutations and epidemics. Furthermore, this type of vaccine contains only critical immunogenic regions of the pathogen to stimulate effective immunity, excluding other components that might cause adverse effects [8].

In studies on HPV16-associated cervical cancer vaccines, researchers are endeavoring to develop multi-epitope vaccines that target viral oncoproteins co-expressed by tumor cells. The E6 and E7 proteins, the principal oncogenic proteins of HR-HPVs, are persistently expressed in tumors, making them constant immunological targets and prime candidates for vaccine development [9]. The results of some studies have indicated that although the E5 protein has reduced oncogenic potential, it can enhance cellular receptor activity and play a role in certain HPV-related cancers [10–12].

Vaccine developers have long been devoted to designing vaccines with precise, efficient, and extensive immune responses more quickly and accurately. Due to co-evolution with humans, HPV16 has evolved into four variant lineages (A, B, C, and D) and sixteen sublineages: A1–A3 (EUR), A4 (As), B1–B4 (AFR-1), C1–C4 (AFR-2), D1 (NA), D2 (AA2), D3 (AA1), and D4 (AA1) [13]. The results of several large-scale case–control studies have shown that HPV variant lineages are associated with the disease risk, persistence, and resulting histological types of lesions in different populations [14–16]. In our previous study, we found significant differences in the distribution of mutations in the LCR, E1, and E7 genes of HPV16, and these mutations showed different amounts and frequencies in different HPV16 lineages [17–19]. These findings suggest that the variation in and mutation of HPV16 may contribute to the immune evasion of the virus and the establishment of persistent infection, leading to cervical cancer. Therefore, selecting highly conserved CTL epitopes can aid the vaccine in providing protection against diverse HPV16 lineages.

In recent years, immunoinformatics tools have become increasingly important in vaccine design. Such tools enable researchers to efficiently predict potential CTL epitopes. Using immunoinformatics tools for the prediction and analysis of CTL epitopes in antigens can guide vaccine development toward greater precision [20]. Accordingly, in the current study, we initially obtained the conserved CTL epitopes of HPV16 E5, E6, and E7 proteins capable of binding to high-frequency distributed HLA-class I molecules using immunoinformatics predictions, constructed a combined mixed-peptide vaccine and a recombinant protein vaccine incorporating these epitopes, and assessed their immunogenicity and protective efficacy against tumors in mice.

2. Materials and Methods

2.1. Sequence Retrieval of the HPV16 Genome and E5, E6, and E7 Proteins

Sixty-eight distinct HPV16 whole-genome sequences classified into sixteen sublineage variants were obtained from the PaVE database (https://pave.niaid.nih.gov/explore/variants/variant_genomes, accessed on 10 September 2022) and the data included in a previous study [13,21]. With reference to the accession numbers of these isolates, the corresponding E5, E6, and E7 protein IDs were retrieved from the NCBI (https://ncbi.nlm.nih.gov/, accessed on 10 September 2022), and the protein sequences were downloaded in FASTA format. The lineage (traditionally by geographical region) and sublineage (by numeric-alphabetic nomenclature), strain name, genome ID number, and protein ID number are summarized in Table S1.

2.2. Immunoinformatics Prediction

The T-Cell Epitope Prediction Tools from the Immune Epitope Database (IEDB, version 2.26) analysis resource (http://tools.iedb.org/mhci/, accessed on 17 September 2022) were used for protein epitope prediction analysis. NetMHCPan 4.1 EL was chosen as the default optimal prediction method, which can be used to comprehensively evaluate the ability of a peptide to bind MHC molecules and the likelihood that the peptide will be naturally processed and presented to derive a score for each epitope. The E5, E6, or E7 protein sequence of the HPV16 Ref isolate (NC_001526) was used for prediction. Based on the recommendations of the IEDB, only frequently occurring HLA class I alleles, which occur in at least 1% of the global population, were selected for analysis. The respective genotypic frequency in the global population was calculated using data from studies conducted around the globe provided by the Allele Frequency Net Database (AFND, http://allelefrequencies.net/, accessed on 20 September 2022). The peptide lengths were limited to 8–11 amino acids for the selected HLA class I. Mouse MHC-I-(H-2b-)-restricted CTL epitope prediction was performed using the same tools and parameters described above.

2.3. Conserved CTL Epitope Identification and Population Coverage Analysis

The conservancy analysis tool (http://tools.iedb.org/conservancy/, accessed on 25 September 2022) provided by the IEDB (version 2.26) was used to assess the conservancy of the epitopes. FASTA protein sequences of E5, E6, and E7 derived from 68 HPV16 reference isolates were entered after the removal of duplicate protein sequences to calculate the degree of conservancy of selected epitopes across all HPV16 sublineages. Population coverage for each candidate epitope was analyzed using the IEDB population coverage calculation tool (http://tools.iedb.org/population/, accessed on 26 September 2022), which is based on the allele frequencies of individuals from 115 countries and 21 different ethnic groups (divided into 16 different geographical regions) provided by the HLA Allele Frequency Database (2020 update). The calculation of coverage was carried out based on the world population, and we selected the MHC I separate calculation option for CTL responses.

2.4. Immunogenicity, Antigenicity and Toxicity Evaluation of Candidate Epitopes

The immunogenicity of each candidate's conserved CTL epitope was predicted using the class I immunogenicity analysis tool provided by the IEDB (http://tools.iedb.org/immunogenicity, accessed on 28 September 2022). The properties of the amino acids and their position in the peptide segment were used as the main parameters to evaluate the immunogenicity of the peptide MHC (pMHC) complex. Protective antigenic or non-antigenic predictions were performed for each epitope peptide using the VaxiJen v2.0 server. The AllerTOP v.2 server (https://www.ddg-pharmfac.net/AllerTOP/, accessed on 28 September 2022) was used to predict and identify potential allergens in candidate epitope peptides. The ToxinPred2 server (https://webs.iiitd.edu.in/raghava/toxinpred2/batch.html, accessed on 28 September 2022) was used to predict the toxicity of each candidate peptide.

2.5. Preparation of the Mixed-Peptide Vaccine

The candidate epitope peptides were chemically synthesized by GeneScript (Nanjing, China) with $\geq$95% purity. Each peptide was dissolved to its highest attainable concentration and subsequently diluted to a uniform 1 mg/mL using phosphate-buffered saline (PBS, 0.01 M, pH = 7.4). These preparations were then mixed with the CpG ODN 1826 adjuvant to generate a composite peptide vaccine designated as E5E6E7pep11. The final formulation of E5E6E7pep11 consisted of a concentration of 5 µg of each peptide and 20 µg of the adjuvant per 100 µL volume.

2.6. Construction of Recombinant Protein Vaccines

The conserved CTL epitope was linearly linked through the use of an "AAY" spacer sequence, and a cholera toxin B subunit (CTB) was conjugated at the N-terminus to function as an intramolecular adjuvant, thereby enhancing the immunogenicity of the multi-epitope vaccine construct.

The gene sequence for recombinant protein CTB-Epi11E567 was codon optimized using GeneOptimizer™ (Thermo Fisher Scientific, Waltham, MA, USA) and then synthesized by Sangon Biotech (Shanghai, China). To construct the expression vector, the gene was amplified by polymerase chain reaction (PCR) with the following primer pairs: forward primer 5′-accctcgagggatccgaattcATGATCAAACTGAAATTCGGC-3′ and reverse primer 5′-caggtcgacaagcttgaattcCAGGGTGCCCATCAGCAG-3′. Afterward, the amplified fragments with the homology arm of the linearized vector were cloned into a linearized pCold-TF vector digested by EcoR I using 2× Hieff Clone® Universal Enzyme Premix (Yeasen, Shanghai, China), and the expression vector pCold-TF-CTB-Epi11E567 was constructed.

The pCold-TF-CTB-Epi11E567 was transformed into competent *E. coli* (BL21). These cells were then cultured in LB medium containing 100 µg/mL of ampicillin at 37 °C with shaking until an OD600 of approximately 0.6 was reached, at which point IPTG was added to a final concentration of 0.5 mM to induce expression. The culture was then incubated at 15 °C to promote protein expression. After 24 h of expression, cells were harvested via centrifugation and resuspended in an ultrasonic buffer for lysis via sonication in an ice bath. The cell lysates were centrifuged at $12,000 \times g$ for 20 min at 4 °C to separate the supernatant containing the soluble target protein. The target protein, featuring a 6 × His-TF tag, was then purified via affinity chromatography using BeyoGold™ His-tag Purification Resin (Beyotime Biotechnology, Shanghai, China). Subsequently, the 6 × His-TF tag protein was removed via cutting with HRV 3C Protease (Takara Bio, Shiga, Japan) and passage through BeyoGold™ His-tag Purification Resin. The protein was further validated through 10% SDS-PAGE and Coomassie Blue staining, and its concentration was quantified using the BCA method (Thermo Fisher Scientific, Waltham, MA, USA). The recombinant protein was then filter sterilized through a 0.22 µm membrane and stored at -80 °C.

2.7. Physiochemical Property Evaluation

The ProtParam tool provided by Expasy 3.0 (http://web.expasy.org/protparam, accessed on 1 March 2023) was used to predict the physicochemical properties of the recombinant protein CTB-Epi11E567 and Epi11E567. Parameters including molecular weight (MW), theoretical isoelectric point, aliphatic index, instability index, and grand average of hydropathicity (GRAVY) were computed.

2.8. Cell Line and Mice

The TC-1 cell line was used to construct a mouse cervical cancer model, which comprises primary lung epithelial cells from C57BL/6 mice, immortalized with HPV16 E6 and E7 oncoproteins and transformed with the c-Ha-ras oncogene, donated by Prof. Yanbing Ma (Chinese Academy of Medical Sciences and Peking Union Medical College). TC-1 cells were cultured with RPMI 1640 (CORING, Corning, NY, USA) medium containing 10% fetal bovine serum (Thermo Fisher Scientific, MA, USA) in an incubator at 37 °C with 5% CO_2. The C57BL/6 mice (female, 6–8 weeks of age) were obtained from the Central Animal Service Center, Institute of Medical Biology, Chinese Academy of Medical Sciences (IMBCAMS), and housed in specific pathogen-free (SPF) animal experimental barrier systems. All animal-related experiments were approved by the Laboratory Animal Ethics Committee of the IMBCAMS (approval number: DWSP2023060084).

2.9. IFN-γ ELISpot Assay

The C57BL/6 mice were randomly assigned to three groups, each containing four animals ($n = 4$). The groups were inoculated intramuscularly (i.m.) with 100 µL of either PBS, 20 µg of CpG ODN 1826, or E5E6E7pep11 (5 µg/peptide and 20 µg of ODN 1826 per mouse) as vaccine formulations. The mice were administered an immunization dose on days 0, 7, and 14. One week following the final immunization dose, the mice were euthanized, and their spleens were aseptically harvested. The spleens were then processed through a 70 μm cell strainer and subjected to Ficoll density gradient centrifugation to isolate single splenocytes. These cells were resuspended in a serum-free medium for subsequent cell counting.

The ELISpot assay was performed using the ELISpot Plus Kit: Mouse IFN-γ (Mabtech, Kista, Sweden) in accordance with the manufacturer's instructions. In brief, 4×10^5 cells were seeded into each well of a 96-well plate that had been pre-coated with an antibody to capture IFN-γ. The cells were incubated at 37 °C with 5% CO_2 in the presence of stimulants for 24 h. Following incubation, the plate was washed, and the cells were sequentially incubated with R4-6A2-biotin antibody and streptavidin-ALP. The addition of BCIP/NBT-plus substrate facilitated the development of spots, which were subsequently enumerated using an ImmunoSpot® Analyzer (Cellular Technology Limited, Shaker Heights, Cleveland, OH, USA). A total of 11 epitope peptides were combined to create a peptide pool (11p-pool) as a specific stimulant for cellular immune response with a final concentration of 2 μg/mL per peptide. Similarly, peptide pools containing E5 protein epitopes (E5-pool), E6 protein epitopes (E6-pool), and E7 protein epitopes (E7-pool) were formulated at equivalent single-peptide working concentrations. Serum-free medium was used as a negative stimulus control and PHA was used as a positive stimulus control. Three replicates were set up for each well.

2.10. In Vivo Tumor Prevention Studies

The C57BL/6 mice were randomly divided into 4 groups of 6 mice each ($n = 6$) and received intramuscular injections of 100 μL of E5E6E7pep11 (5 μg/peptide and 20 μg of CpG ODN 1826) or CTB-Epi11E567 (100 μg) at 7, 14, and 21 days prior to tumor challenge. Control groups were also established and administered with PBS and CpG ODN 1826 (20 μg) for comparison. The mice received a subcutaneous injection (s.c.) of 1×10^5 TC-1 cells in the lower right dorsal area 7 days after the final vaccination. Tumor size was measured and recorded at three-day intervals post-inoculation. The endpoint of survival was determined when tumors reached the ethical limit (diameter = 15 mm), at which point the mice were euthanized.

2.11. In Vivo Tumor Treatment Study

The mice were grouped for treatment experiments in the same manner as in the prophylactic study. In contrast, the mice were pre-challenged with 1×10^5 TC-1 cells on day 0 and given one dose of vaccine intramuscularly on days 3, 10, and 17 following tumor challenge. The dosage administered was consistent with that described in the tumor prevention study. Tumor measurements and survival endpoint determination were performed as previously described.

2.12. Statistical Analysis

Two-way ANOVA was used to statistically analyze the data from the ELISpot assay, and the log-rank (Mantel–Cox) test was used to compare and plot the survival curves, with a p-value of less than 0.05 considered statistically significant. All statistical analyses and graphing were carried out in GraphPad Prism 8.

3. Results

3.1. Epitope Prediction and Selection

Below, an integrated flowchart is used to illustrate the step-by-step process utilized for epitope prediction and selection. The brief results of our computational analyses are summarized in Figure 1.

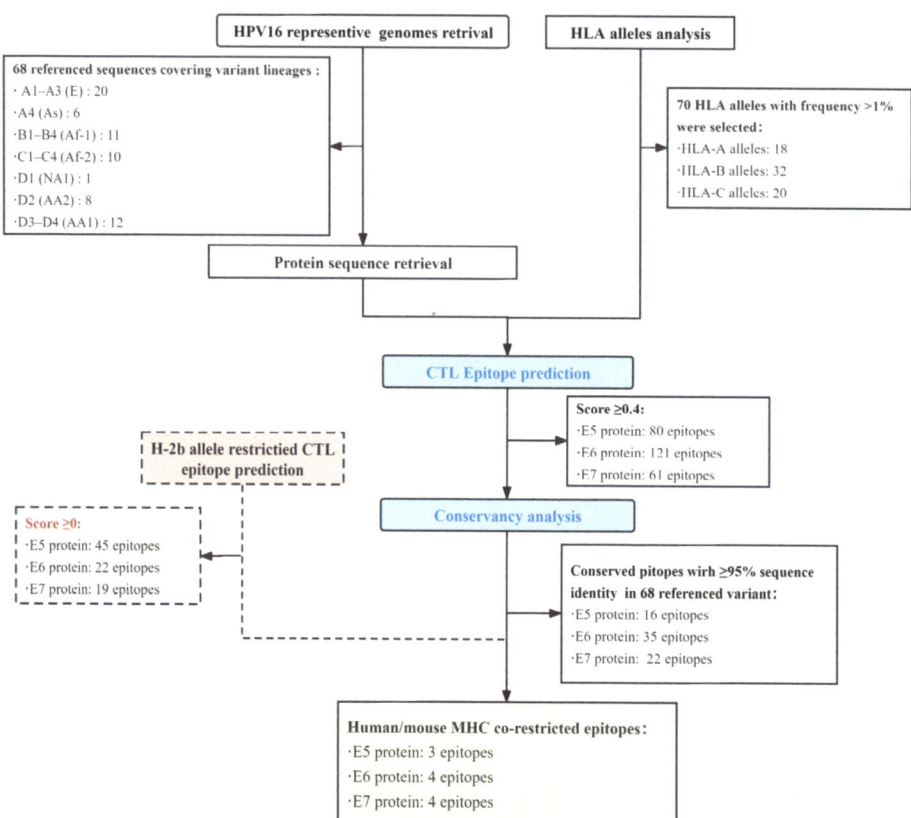

Figure 1. Flowchart and brief results of epitope prediction and screening in the present study.

In the immunoinformatics analysis, the binding affinities of HPV16 E5, E6, and E7 protein epitopes to the 70 global high-frequency HLA class I alleles, enumerated in Table S2, were, respectively, predicted using the NetMHCPan 4.1 EL model. Epitopes with score values > 0.4 were retained, yielding a total of 80 E5 (Table S3), 121 E6 (Table S4), and 61 E7 epitopes (Table S5).

To enhance the cross-reactivity of epitopes among different HPV16 variants, we performed a conservation analysis of epitopes that scored higher than the cut-off value and removed epitopes that were more than 95% conserved among the 68 reference variants, including 16 E5 (Table S6), 35 E6 (Table S7), and 22 E7 epitopes (Table S8). To facilitate subsequent functional validation of epitopes in a mouse model, we conducted CTL epitope prediction based on the H-2b alleles. Upon setting a threshold with a total score > 0, we identified 45 E5, 22 E6, and 19 E7 H-2b-restricted CTL epitopes, as shown in Table S9. In the final selection process, conserved CTL epitopes restricted by both human and murine MHC molecules were retained as candidates for vaccine construct development, including 3 E5, 4 E6, and 4 E7 epitopes. The locations of the predicted CTL/CD8[+] T cell epitopes in the E5, E6, and E7 proteins were mapped and are presented in Figure 2. In addition, the HLA-I alleles presenting these epitopes are also annotated.

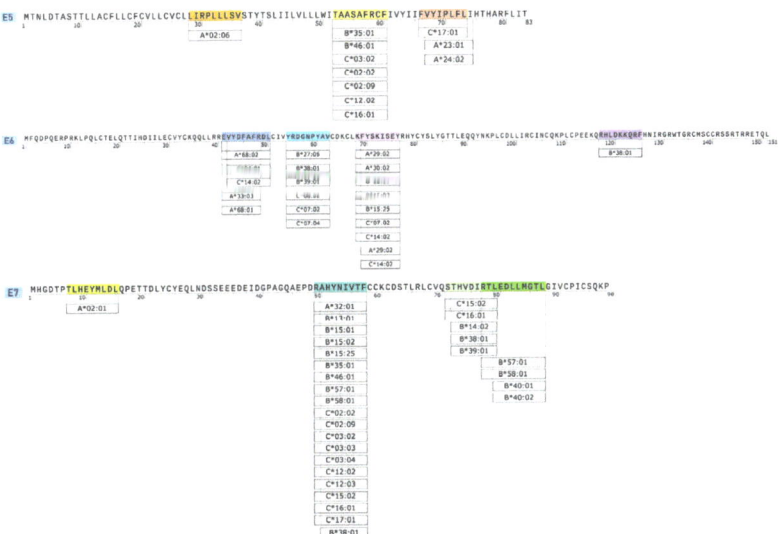

Figure 2. CTL/CD8$^+$ candidate epitope location maps plotted for the E5, E6, and E7 proteins.

3.2. Characterization of CTL Epitopes for Vaccine Development

The results of the population coverage analysis, as shown in Tables 1 and S10, indicate that the combination of the 11 candidate epitopes can cover 98.42% of the global population. Notably, epitope E7p9 demonstrates the highest coverage rate, reaching 70.50%, thus suggesting that it possesses extensive potential applicability. We predicted the immunogenicity and antigenicity of 14 candidate epitopes, and the results, as presented in Table 1, indicate that epitopes E5p2, E5p3, E6p4, E6p5, E7p9, and E7p10 exhibit favorable immunogenicity (scores > 0). Moreover, E6p4, E7p9, E7p10, and E7p11 demonstrate pronounced antigenicity (scores > 0.4). In the allergenicity evaluation, the AllerTOP v.2 analysis classified only E6p5, E7p10, and E7p11 as potential allergens. With regard to toxicity, the prediction results of the ToxinPred sever revealed that all 11 candidate epitopes were non-toxic.

Table 1. Characterization of conserved CTL candidate epitopes for vaccine construction.

Protein	Epitope	Sequence	Position	Length	Coverage	Immunogenicity	Antigency	Allergenicity	Toxicity
E5	E5p1	LIRPLLLSV	28–36	9	1.95%	−0.12	0.33	Non-Allergen	Non-Toxin
	E5p2	TAASAFRCF	52–60	9	30.81%	0.01	0.26	Non-Allergen	Non-Toxin
	E5p3	FVYIPLFLI	66–73	9	28.62%	0.2	0.39	Non-Allergen	Non-Toxin
E6	E6p4	EVYDFAFRDL	41–50	10	32.66%	0.34	1.46	Non-Allergen	Non-Toxin
	E6p5	YRDGNPYAV	54–62	9	44.37%	0.04	0.39	Allergen	Non-Toxin
	E6p6	KFYSKISEY	68–76	9	37.65%	−0.33	0.23	Non-Allergen	Non-Toxin
	E6p7	RHLDKKQRF	117–125	9	3.23%	−0.46	0.35	Non-Allergen	Non-Toxin
E7	E7p8	TLHEYMLDL	7–15	9	39.08%	−0.05	0.33	Non-Allergen	Non-Toxin
	E7p9	RAHYNIVTF	49–57	9	70.50%	0.18	0.59	Non-Allergen	Non-Toxin
	E7p10	STHVDIRTL	71–79	9	16.98%	0.27	0.58	Allergen	Non-Toxin
	E7p11	RTLEDLLMGTL	77–87	11	17.96%	−0.02	0.64	Allergen	Non-Toxin

3.3. Evaluation of Antigen-Specific IFN-γ Response

To evaluate the ability of the candidate epitopes to induce specific cellular immune responses in vivo, immunogenicity studies were conducted in C57BL/6 mice. Following three doses of immunization at one-week intervals with a mixture of epitope peptides formulated with the CpG ODN 1826 adjuvant, E5E6E7pep11, the ability of splenocytes from the mice to secrete antigen-specific IFN-γ upon stimulation with peptide pools was assessed using the ELISpot assay. As shown in Figure 3, E5E6E7pep11-immunized mice induced higher levels of antigen-specific IFN-γ secretion compared to the other two groups; CpG injection alone did not induce IFN-γ secretion from CD8+ T cells. In addition, the E5 epitope was identified as the probable dominant epitope for triggering specific immune responses.

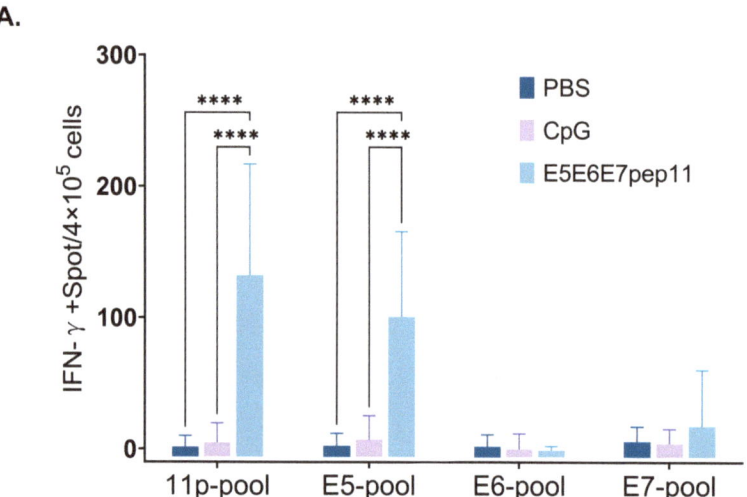

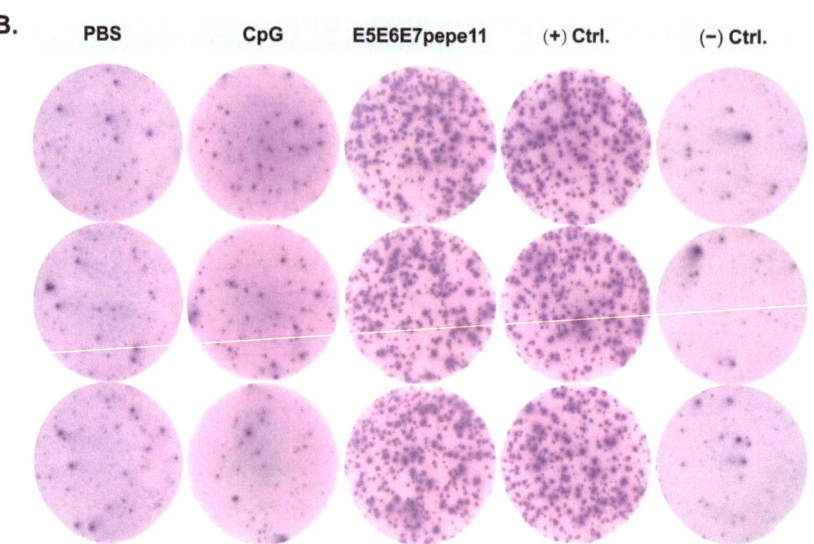

Figure 3. Induction of antigen-specific IFN-γ response in C57BL/6 mice vaccinated with E5E6E7pep11. C57BL/6 mice (n = 4) were inoculated intramuscularly (i.m.) with 100 µL of either PBS, CpG ODN 1826, or E5E6E7pep11 on days 0, 7, and 14. Splenic lymphocytes were collected 1 week after the second immunization process and then stimulated in vitro with the 11p-pool, E5-pool, E6-pool, and E7-pool. (**A**) The number of IFN-γ spot-forming cells (SFCs) detected using ELISpot was subtracted from the SFCs stimulated by serum-free medium as a negative control. (**B**) Representative ELISpot images, using 11p-pool as a specific stimulus, PMA as a non-specific stimulus (positive control), and serum-free medium as a negative stimulus (negative control). **** $p < 0.0001$.

3.4. Construction and Expression of Recombinant Multi-Epitope Protein

Following the confirmation of the immunogenic efficacy of the mixed peptide vaccine, we proceeded to develop a recombinant protein vaccine comprising 11 epitopes for subsequent in vivo anti-tumor efficacy studies. Based on the amino acid sequence, we predicted the physicochemical properties of the vaccine expression product CTB-Epi11E567, which contains a total of 302 amino acids and possesses a molecular weight (MW) of 34.05 kDa, a theoretical isoelectric point (pI) of 8.27, an aliphatic index of 91.59, an instability index of 34.80, and a grand average of hydropathicity (GRAVY) of −0.007. These results indicate that the long peptide expressed by our therapeutic vaccine was hydrophilic and stable.

3.5. Prophylactic Efficacy of the Multi-Epitope Vaccine

The prophylactic anti-tumor effects of E5E6E7pep11 and CTB-Epi11E567 were further evaluated using a syngeneic model grafted with TC-1. As in the immunization program shown in Figure 4A, the C57BL/6 mice were immunized with three separate doses at one-week intervals prior to subcutaneous challenge with TC-1 cells. The survival status of the mice was continuously recorded for a period of two months following tumor challenge, and the survival curves for each group were plotted. Mice in the PBS placebo control group and the CpG adjuvant-only control group exhibited continuous tumor growth, and all reached ethical endpoint criteria within 40 days post-tumorigenesis. In contrast, vaccination with the E5E6E7pep11 and CTB-Epi11E567 vaccines demonstrated a complete prophylactic anti-tumor effect. The survival rate in mice was 100%, and the state of being tumor-free was maintained until the end of the observation period, which was day 80 post-challenge (Figure 4B).

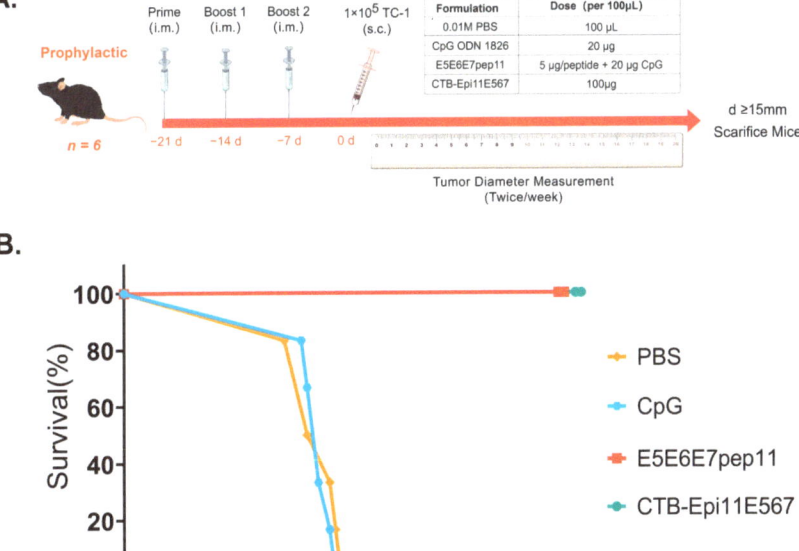

Figure 4. Prophylactic anti-tumor immunity induced by multi-epitope vaccines. (**A**) The C57BL/6 mice (n = 6) were intramuscularly vaccinated (i.m.) with 100 μL of PBS, CpG ODN 1826 (20 μg), E5E6E7pep11 (5 μg/peptide and 20 μg CpG ODN 1826), or CTB-Epi11E567 (100 μg) at 7, 14, and 21 days prior to the 1×10^5 TC-1 cell challenge. (**B**) Percentage survival of each group of mice within 80 days of tumor challenge. The mice were euthanized when their tumor diameter reached ≥ 15 mm.

3.6. Therapeutic Efficacy of the Multi-Epitope Vaccine

The therapeutic potential of E5E6E7pep11 and CTB-Epi11E567 in treating established tumors was also assessed. The mice were subjected to a subcutaneous challenge of

1×10^5 TC-1 cells on day 0, followed by 1 dose of vaccination on days 3, 10, and 17. The tumor volume and survival status of the mice were continuously monitored and recorded. Mice whose tumor volumes met the ethical endpoint criteria were euthanized. In cases where no tumor development occurred or tumor progression was slow, the mice were uniformly euthanized upon the conclusion of the observation period, which was day 80 post-tumor challenge (Figure 5A). In the above experiments, the CpG adjuvant control group displayed complete non-immunogenicity and no antitumor efficacy as expected; therefore, this group was omitted from the current assay. Instead, a mixture of peptide pep11 group without adjuvants was included to investigate the contribution of adjuvants to the therapeutic efficacy of the mixed epitope peptide. In comparison with the PBS control group, mice treated with E5E6E7pep11 and CTB-Epi11E567 vaccines exhibited significantly slower tumor growth, with approximately 67% (4/6) and 50% (3/6) of the mice remaining tumor free up to 80 days post tumor challenge, respectively. Furthermore, despite the favorable anti-tumor therapeutic efficacy evinced by E5E6E7pep11, vaccination with the adjuvant-free mixed peptides (pep11) failed to achieve the desired therapeutic effect, with no significant survival benefit observed in this group as compared to the PBS control group (Figure 5B,C).

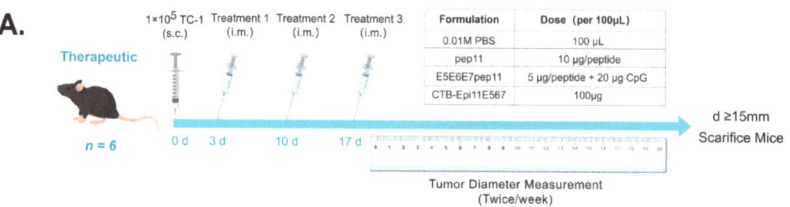

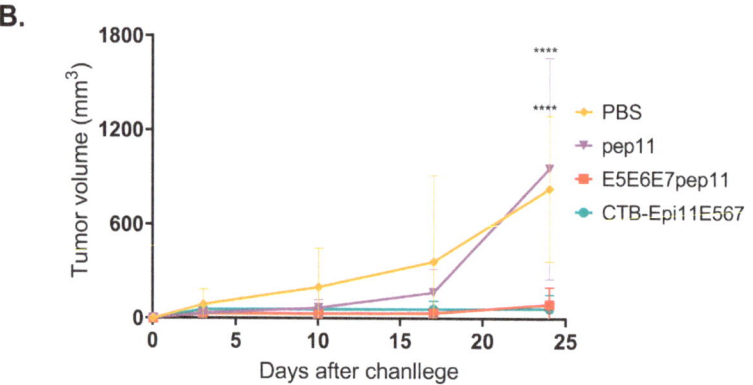

Figure 5. *Cont.*

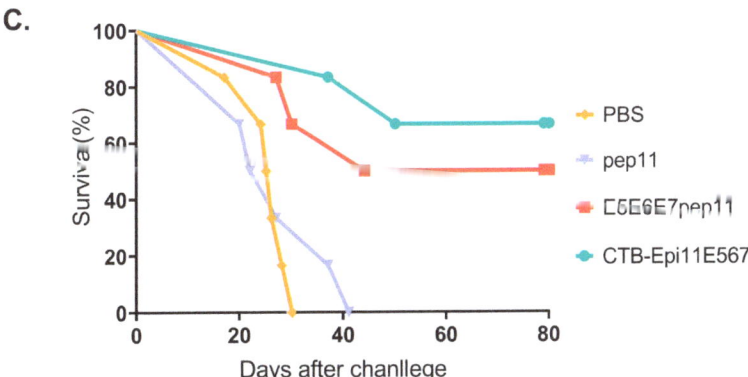

Figure 5. Therapeutic anti-tumor immune effects induced by multi-epitope vaccines. (**A**) The C57BL/6 mice (n = 6) were intramuscularly vaccinated (i.m.) with 100 µL of PBS, pep11 (5 µg/peptide), E5E6E7pep11 (5 µg/peptide and 20 µg CpG ODN 1826), or CTB-Epi11E567 (100 µg) at 3, 10, and 17 days post-challenge of 1×10^5 TC-1 cells. (**B**) Tumor volume was measured biweekly, and the average tumor sizes for each group of mice were computed to graph the kinetics of tumor growth. (**C**) Percentage survival of each group of mice within 80 days of tumor challenge. **** $p < 0.0001$.

4. Discussion

Although a variety of therapeutic HPV vaccines are already under active development, such as VGX3100, a DNA vaccine targeting the HPV16 E6/E7 fusion protein, there is currently no successful vaccine on the market to eliminate established HPV infections [5]. Relying on traditional laboratory strategies, vaccine development is generally a time-consuming and costly endeavor [22]. Rapid advances in biotechnology and immunoinformatic technology have made it possible to rapidly identify potential antigenic epitopes by means of huge amounts of immune library data and machine learning-based information tools [23]. In the current study, we harnessed the predictive capacity of the NetMHCPan 4.1 EL method for in silico prediction to expedite the identification and screening of antigenic epitopes [24,25]. Fortified by a substantial corpus of experimental data, the algorithm was proven to be capable of pinpointing peptide fragments that are potential candidates for binding to specific MHC class molecules, thus potentially triggering T-cell responses. We ascertained a total of 16 E5 epitopes, 35 E6 epitopes, and 22 E7 epitopes, and have corroborated the immunogenic potential of 11 CTL epitopes in B6 mice.

The epitope recognition of CTLs is restricted by specific human leukocyte antigen (HLA) molecules, which are highly polymorphic in the general population. Therefore, screening for antigenic peptides that bind to HLA in the broader population is critical for the development of therapeutic vaccines to enable mass population vaccination [26–28]. The overall population coverage of the candidate epitope combinations that we ultimately obtained reached 98.42%, indicating that vaccines constructed based on these epitopes are suitable for populations with diverse genetic backgrounds. Specifically, individual epitopes such as E5p2, E6p4, E6p5, E6p6, E7p8, and E7p9 can cover over 30% of the general population; notably, the E7p9 epitope was able to sufficiently bind with 20 HLA-I class molecules, implying a broader applicability of these epitope vaccines across different ethnic groups.

Current therapeutic strategies for HPV16 are focused on E6 and E7, two proteins closely associated with cervical carcinogenesis [9–11,29]. In this study, we included the E5 oncogenic protein as one of the target antigens and used three CTL candidate epitopes located in the conserved region of the E5 protein to construct a multi-epitope vaccine. Some studies have suggested that the E5 protein could be a potential target for cervical cancer therapy [30,31]. Although frequently deleted in the advanced stages of cervical cancer, the E5 protein indeed participates in multiple signaling pathways regulating malignant transformation [12,32–35]. E5 is widely expressed on the surface of cervical epithelial cells in the early stages of cervical lesions; therefore, the targeting of immune epitopes of the E5 protein could represent a promising therapeutic strategy [36]. Yi-Fang Chen et al. identified VCLLIRPLL$_{25-33}$ as a restricted CTL epitope in Db-C57BL/6 mice and verified in a mouse model that inoculation of this epitope peptide in combination with CpG ODN 1826 induced HPV16-associated tumor elimination [30]. The design of the multi-epitope vaccine reflects a comprehensive strategy aimed at enhancing the immune response by concurrently targeting multiple oncogenic proteins of HPV16. Compared to vaccines that target a limited number of antigens, multi-epitope vaccines theoretically offer more comprehensive protection by targeting a broader spectrum of antigens. For example, in a previous study, Liao S et al. demonstrated that the incorporation of the E5 peptide alongside E6 and E7 peptides significantly enhanced tumor protection, surpassing the protective effects observed with either E5 alone or E6 + E7 alone [37]. In the validation assay of epitope immunogenicity, we stimulated splenocytes using different peptide pools in vitro with the aim of carrying out a dominant epitope analysis, and the results showed that the E5 epitope peptide combination appeared to be the main reason for the cells being induced to secrete antigen-specific IFN-γ, which suggested that the E5 antigenic epitope may play a role in anti-tumor immunity. However, since the mouse tumor model used in this study was constructed based on the TC-1 cell line, which does not express the E5 oncoprotein on its surface, the demonstrated anti-tumor efficacy might be derived to a greater degree from the E6 and E7 epitopes. Several previous studies have demonstrated the good immunogenicity and antitumor protective effects of some of our candidate E6 and E7 epitope peptides, similar to our results on the TC-1 tumor model [38–41]. For instance, Jemon et al. developed a heterologous virus-like particle vaccine containing the EVYDFAFRDL$_{48-57}$ epitope peptide from the HPV16 E6 protein and the helper T-cell epitope PADRE, resulting in a significant delay in tumor growth and improved survival rates in a TC-1 mouse tumor model [40]. In another study, He X et al. combined the E7HHH$_{49-57}$ epitope peptide with CoPoP liposomes to create a peptide-liposome vaccine. This formulation successfully triggered an effective CD8+ T-cell response in mice and demonstrated efficacy in eradicating or reversing TC-1 tumor growth [41]. This evidence presented indicated that while the E6 and E7 epitopes did not substantially stimulate antigen-specific IFN-γ secretion in immunogenicity assessment assays, this does not rule out the immunogenic potential of these epitopes. This observation could be due to the immune system's preferential recognition of one or more E5 epitope peptides, leading to competitive inhibition in recognizing the other epitopes. Assessment of vaccine protective efficacy on a TC-1 tumor model expressing E5 protein is very valuable for gaining deeper insights into the contribution of E5, E6, and E7 epitopes in antitumor immunity, which is worth further exploring in future studies.

Although the results of some studies have substantiated the therapeutic anti-tumor efficacy of minimal epitope peptides, there is also evidence suggesting that synthetic long peptide vaccines may elicit more robust antigen-specific CD8$^+$ T cell responses and potentiate greater tumor treatment effects compared to short peptide vaccines. This could be attributed to the additional steps of antigen uptake, processing, and presentation by antigen-presenting cells (APCs) that long peptides undergo in the body [42–44]. The immune efficacy of the recombinant protein vaccine in the form of a synthetic long peptide and a mixed minimal epitope peptide vaccine was assessed simultaneously in our study, and we observed that the long peptide vaccine, CTB-Epi11E567, appeared to possess an advantage in terms of therapeutic anti-tumor efficacy. However, this result could be ascribed to disparities in the vaccine dosage. The authors of future studies may further explore the immunogenicity of the vaccine across a broader range of doses. Overall, both vaccine modalities demonstrated significant prophylactic and therapeutic anti-tumor effects in mice. Additionally, the significance of adjuvants in peptide-based vaccine formulations has been underscored in previous studies [43,45–47]. In this study, to augment the immunogenicity of the vaccine, we incorporated the adjuvant CpG ODN 1826, an agonist of pattern-recognition receptor nine (TLR9) widely used as a vaccine adjuvant, into the peptide vaccine. We discerned that the CpG adjuvant played a crucial role when combined with the short peptide form of the vaccine owing to the fact that the inoculation with epitope peptides alone did not engender effective anti-tumor protection, aligning with the results of previous studies [48]. The cholera toxin B subunit (CTB) has long been recognized as a potent mucosal adjuvant, and evidence from a recent study indicates its promise as a systemic adjuvant [49]. In this study, CTB was used as an intramolecular adjuvant to prepare recombinant protein vaccines to facilitate broader in vivo immune stimulation. In addition, we found that N-terminal fusion CTB conferred better stability and solubility of the multi-epitope peptide as evidenced by the difference in the physicochemical properties of CTB-Epi11E567 and Epi11E567, which was more conducive to protein expression, purification, and preservation.

In this study, we present the available epitope combinations and validate the immune effects of these epitopes in mice. However, the differences between mouse and human MHCs led to some limitations in the epitope screening process, as some conserved CTL epitopes with high scores were not selected for further experimental validation in mice. The construction of H-2 humanized mouse models may facilitate further in vivo evaluations of more epitopes in the future. Additionally, both forms of the multi-epitope vaccines achieved a 100% anti-tumor protective effect in prophylactic anti-tumor trials; however, there was a lack of evaluation of long-term immune protection and protective efficacy following re-challenge with the tumor. The detection of immune memory cells will contribute to a more comprehensive evaluation of the vaccines. As helper CD4 T cells play a crucial role in enhancing the proliferation of CTL clones and guiding their transformation into effector and memory cells, incorporating Th epitopes may direct the vaccine-induced anti-tumor response towards sustainable and comprehensive regulation [50–52].

5. Conclusions

In this study, we employed immunoinformatics approaches to identify 11 conserved cytotoxic T lymphocyte (CTL) epitopes targeting the HPV16 oncoproteins. Subsequently, we developed peptide vaccines and recombinant protein vaccines incorporating these epitopes. Initial assessment of the immunogenicity of these epitopes and the anti-tumor efficacy of the vaccines was conducted using a murine tumor model. Our findings present a promising selection of candidate epitopes and introduce a viable approach for the rapid development of therapeutic multi-epitope vaccines against HPV16, with the potential for widespread population coverage.

Supplementary Materials: The following supporting information can be downloaded at https://www.mdpi.com/article/10.3390/vaccines12040392/s1, Table S1. Protein ID of E5, E6, and E7 proteins of 68 referenced HPV16 isolates; Table S2. 70 selected HLA alleles (>1%) in worldwide population; Table S3. Selected epitopes of HPV16 E5 predicted against the HLA class I loci; Table S4. Selected epitopes of HPV16 E6 predicted against the HLA class I loci; Table S5. Selected epitopes of HPV16 E7 predicted against the HLA class I loci; Table S6. Conserved CTL epitopes of E5 protein with ≥95% conservation amongst 68 reference variant strains; Table S7. Conserved CTL epitopes of E6 protein with ≥95% conservation amongst 68 reference variant strains; Table S8. Conserved CTL epitopes of E7 protein with ≥95% conservation amongst 68 reference variant strains; Table S9. Selected H-2b restricted CTL epitope of HPV16 E5, E6 and E7 protein; Table S10. Population Coverage of individual candidate epitope in word.

Author Contributions: Conceptualization, Y.Y. and L.S. (Li Shi); methodology, N.G., Z.N., L.S. (Lei Shi), and C.L.; formal analysis, N.G., Z.N., Z.Y., and W.L.; investigation, Z.Y. and L.S. (Lei Shi); resources, Z.Y. and L.S. (Lei Shi); data curation, C.L.; writing—original draft, N.G.; writing—review and editing, Z.N., W.L., Y.Y., and L.S. (Li Shi); funding acquisition, Z.Y., W.L., Y.Y., and L.S. (Li Shi). All authors have read and agreed to the published version of the manuscript.

Funding: This work was supported by a grant from the CAMS Innovation Fund for Medical Sciences (CIFMS 2021-I2M-1-004); the Yunnan Provincial Science and Technology Department (202002AA100009); NMPA Key Laboratory for Quality Control and Evaluation of Vaccines and Biological Products; Yunnan Province Xingdian Talent Support Program (2024); and the Yunnan Provincial Innovation Team of Therapeutic Neutralizing Antibody (202405AS350026).

Institutional Review Board Statement: The animal study protocol was approved by the Laboratory Animal Ethics Committee of the IMBCAMS, and the ethics approval number is DWSP2023060084 (Approval date: 8 June 2023). Any procedures involving the care and use of animals were conducted in compliance with national and international laws and policies.

Informed Consent Statement: Not applicable.

Data Availability Statement: The original contributions presented in this study are included in the article and Supplementary Materials, further inquiries can be directed to the first authors and corresponding authors.

Conflicts of Interest: The authors declare no conflicts of interest. The funders had no role in the design of the study, data collection, analyses and interpretation, writing of the manuscript, or decision to publish the results.

References

1. Deshmukh, A.A.; Damgacioglu, H.; Georges, D.; Sonawane, K.; Ferlay, J.; Bray, F.; Clifford, G.M. Global burden of HPV-attributable squamous cell carcinoma of the anus in 2020, according to sex and HIV status: A worldwide analysis. *Int. J. Cancer* **2022**, *152*, 417–428. [CrossRef] [PubMed]
2. Sung, H.; Ferlay, J.; Siegel, R.L.; Laversanne, M.; Soerjomataram, I.; Jemal, A.; Bray, F. Global Cancer Statistics 2020: GLOBOCAN Estimates of Incidence and Mortality Worldwide for 36 Cancers in 185 Countries. *CA Cancer J. Clin.* **2021**, *71*, 209–249. [CrossRef] [PubMed]
3. de Sanjose, S.; Quint, W.G.; Alemany, L.; Geraets, D.T.; Klaustermeier, J.E.; Lloveras, B.; Tous, S.; Felix, A.; Bravo, L.E.; Shin, H.R.; et al. Human papillomavirus genotype attribution in invasive cervical cancer: A retrospective cross-sectional worldwide study. *Lancet Oncol.* **2010**, *11*, 1048–1056. [CrossRef]
4. Fan, T.; Zhang, M.; Yang, J.; Zhu, Z.; Cao, W.; Dong, C. Therapeutic cancer vaccines: Advancements, challenges, and prospects. *Signal Transduct. Target Ther.* **2023**, *8*, 450. [CrossRef] [PubMed]
5. Mo, Y.; Ma, J.; Zhang, H.; Shen, J.; Chen, J.; Hong, J.; Xu, Y.; Qian, C. Prophylactic and Therapeutic HPV Vaccines: Current Scenario and Perspectives. *Front. Cell Infect. Microbiol.* **2022**, *12*, 909223. [CrossRef] [PubMed]
6. Coleman, N.; Birley, H.D.; Renton, A.M.; Hanna, N.F.; Ryait, B.K.; Byrne, M.; Taylor-Robinson, D.; Stanley, M.A. Immunological events in regressing genital warts. *Am. J. Clin. Pathol.* **1994**, *102*, 768–774. [CrossRef]
7. Stanley, M. Immune responses to human papillomavirus. *Vaccine* **2006**, *24* (Suppl. 1), S16–S22. [CrossRef] [PubMed]
8. Ma, B.; Maraj, B.; Tran, N.P.; Knoff, J.; Chen, A.; Alvarez, R.D.; Hung, C.F.; Wu, T.C. Emerging human papillomavirus vaccines. *Expert. Opin. Emerg. Drugs* **2012**, *17*, 469–492. [CrossRef]
9. Pal, A.; Kundu, R. Human Papillomavirus E6 and E7: The Cervical Cancer Hallmarks and Targets for Therapy. *Front. Microbiol.* **2019**, *10*, 3116. [CrossRef]
10. Gutierrez-Xicotencatl, L.; Pedroza-Saavedra, A.; Chihu-Amparan, L.; Salazar-Piña, A.; Maldonado-Gama, M.; Esquivel-Guadarrama, F. Cellular Functions of HPV16 E5 Oncoprotein during Oncogenic Transformation. *Mol. Cancer Res.* **2021**, *19*, 167–179. [CrossRef]
11. Kim, M.K.; Kim, H.S.; Kim, S.H.; Oh, J.M.; Han, J.Y.; Lim, J.M.; Juhnn, Y.S.; Song, Y.S. Human papillomavirus type 16 E5 oncoprotein as a new target for cervical cancer treatment. *Biochem. Pharmacol.* **2010**, *80*, 1930–1935. [CrossRef] [PubMed]
12. Ilahi, N.E.; Bhatti, A. Impact of HPV E5 on viral life cycle via EGFR signaling. *Microb. Pathog.* **2020**, *139*, 103923. [CrossRef] [PubMed]
13. Burk, R.D.; Harari, A.; Chen, Z. Human papillomavirus genome variants. *Virology* **2013**, *445*, 232–243. [CrossRef] [PubMed]
14. Mirabello, L.; Yeager, M.; Cullen, M.; Boland, J.F.; Chen, Z.; Wentzensen, N.; Zhang, X.; Yu, K.; Yang, Q.; Mitchell, J.; et al. HPV16 Sublineage Associations With Histology-Specific Cancer Risk Using HPV Whole-Genome Sequences in 3200 Women. *J. Natl. Cancer Inst.* **2016**, *108*, djw100. [CrossRef] [PubMed]
15. Clifford, G.M.; Tenet, V.; Georges, D.; Alemany, L.; Pavón, M.A.; Chen, Z.; Yeager, M.; Cullen, M.; Boland, J.F.; Bass, S.; et al. Human papillomavirus 16 sub-lineage dispersal and cervical cancer risk worldwide: Whole viral genome sequences from 7116 HPV16-positive women. *Papillomavirus Res.* **2019**, *7*, 67–74. [CrossRef] [PubMed]
16. Londesborough, P.; Ho, L.; Terry, G.; Cuzick, J.; Wheeler, C.; Singer, A. Human papillomavirus genotype as a predictor of persistence and development of high-grade lesions in women with minor cervical abnormalities. *Int. J. Cancer* **1996**, *69*, 364–368. [CrossRef]

17. Dai, S.; Li, C.; Yan, Z.; Zhou, Z.; Wang, X.; Wang, J.; Sun, L.; Shi, L.; Yao, Y. Association of Human Papillomavirus Type 16 Long Control Region Variations with Cervical Cancer in a Han Chinese Population. *Int. J. Med. Sci.* **2020**, *17*, 931–938. [CrossRef] [PubMed]
18. Yao, Y.; Yan, Z.; Dai, S.; Li, C.; Yang, L.; Liu, S.; Zhang, X.; Shi, L.; Yao, Y. Human Papillomavirus Type 16 E1 Mutations Associated with Cervical Cancer in a Han Chinese Population. *Int. J. Med. Sci.* **2019**, *16*, 1042–1049. [CrossRef] [PubMed]
19. Zhou, Z.; Yang, H.; Yang, L.; Yao, Y.; Dai, S.; Shi, L.; Li, C.; Yang, L.; Yan, Z.; Yao, Y. Human papillomavirus type 16 E6 and E7 gene variations associated with cervical cancer in a Han Chinese population. *Infect. Genet. Evol.* **2019**, *73*, 13–20. [CrossRef]
20. De Groot, A.S.; Moise, L.; Terry, F.; Gutierrez, A.H.; Hindocha, P.; Richard, G.; Hoft, D.F.; Ross, T.M.; Noe, A.R.; Takahashi, Y.; et al. Better Epitope Discovery, Precision Immune Engineering, and Accelerated Vaccine Design Using Immunoinformatics Tools. *Front. Immunol.* **2020**, *11*, 442. [CrossRef]
21. Smith, B.; Chen, Z.; Reimers, L.; van Doorslaer, K.; Schiffman, M.; Desalle, R.; Herrero, R.; Yu, K.; Wacholder, S.; Wang, T.; et al. Sequence imputation of HPV16 genomes for genetic association studies. *PLoS ONE* **2011**, *6*, e21375. [CrossRef] [PubMed]
22. Karch, C.P.; Burkhard, P. Vaccine technologies: From whole organisms to rationally designed protein assemblies. *Biochem. Pharmacol.* **2016**, *120*, 1–14. [CrossRef] [PubMed]
23. Soria-Guerra, R.E.; Nieto-Gomez, R.; Govea-Alonso, D.O.; Rosales-Mendoza, S. An overview of bioinformatics tools for epitope prediction: Implications on vaccine development. *J. Biomed. Inform.* **2015**, *53*, 405–414. [CrossRef] [PubMed]
24. Hoof, I.; Peters, B.; Sidney, J.; Pedersen, L.E.; Sette, A.; Lund, O.; Buus, S.; Nielsen, M. NetMHCpan, a method for MHC class I binding prediction beyond humans. *Immunogenetics* **2009**, *61*, 1–13. [CrossRef] [PubMed]
25. Mei, S.; Li, F.; Leier, A.; Marquez-Lago, T.T.; Giam, K.; Croft, N.P.; Akutsu, T.; Smith, A.I.; Li, J.; Rossjohn, J.; et al. A comprehensive review and performance evaluation of bioinformatics tools for HLA class I peptide-binding prediction. *Brief. Bioinform.* **2020**, *21*, 1119–1135. [CrossRef] [PubMed]
26. Terasaki, P.I. A brief history of HLA. *Immunol. Res.* **2007**, *38*, 139–148. [CrossRef] [PubMed]
27. Rothbard, J.B. Antigen presentation. One size fits all. *Curr. Biol.* **1994**, *4*, 653–655. [CrossRef] [PubMed]
28. Stern, L.J.; Wiley, D.C. Antigenic peptide binding by class I and class II histocompatibility proteins. *Structure* **1994**, *2*, 245–251. [CrossRef] [PubMed]
29. Kumar, A.; Yadav, I.S.; Hussain, S.; Das, B.C.; Bharadwaj, M. Identification of immunotherapeutic epitope of E5 protein of human papillomavirus-16: An in silico approach. *Biologicals* **2015**, *43*, 344–348. [CrossRef] [PubMed]
30. Chen, Y.F.; Lin, C.W.; Tsao, Y.P.; Chen, S.L. Cytotoxic-T-lymphocyte human papillomavirus type 16 E5 peptide with CpG-oligodeoxynucleotide can eliminate tumor growth in C57BL/6 mice. *J. Virol.* **2004**, *78*, 1333–1343. [CrossRef]
31. Liu, D.W.; Tsao, Y.P.; Hsieh, C.H.; Hsieh, J.T.; Kung, J.T.; Chiang, C.L.; Huang, S.J.; Chen, S.L. Induction of CD8 T cells by vaccination with recombinant adenovirus expressing human papillomavirus type 16 E5 gene reduces tumor growth. *J. Virol.* **2000**, *74*, 9083–9089. [CrossRef] [PubMed]
32. DiMaio, D.; Petti, L.M. The E5 proteins. *Virology* **2013**, *445*, 99–114. [CrossRef] [PubMed]
33. Suprynowicz, F.A.; Disbrow, G.L.; Krawczyk, E.; Simic, V.; Lantzky, K.; Schlegel, R. HPV-16 E5 oncoprotein upregulates lipid raft components caveolin-1 and ganglioside GM1 at the plasma membrane of cervical cells. *Oncogene* **2008**, *27*, 1071–1078. [CrossRef] [PubMed]
34. Maufort, J.P.; Shai, A.; Pitot, H.C.; Lambert, P.F. A role for HPV16 E5 in cervical carcinogenesis. *Cancer Res.* **2010**, *70*, 2924–2931. [CrossRef]
35. Campo, M.S.; Graham, S.V.; Cortese, M.S.; Ashrafi, G.H.; Araibi, E.H.; Dornan, E.S.; Miners, K.; Nunes, C.; Man, S. HPV-16 E5 down-regulates expression of surface HLA class I and reduces recognition by CD8 T cells. *Virology* **2010**, *407*, 137–142. [CrossRef] [PubMed]
36. Chang, J.L.; Tsao, Y.P.; Liu, D.W.; Huang, S.J.; Lee, W.H.; Chen, S.L. The expression of HPV-16 E5 protein in squamous neoplastic changes in the uterine cervix. *J. Biomed. Sci.* **2001**, *8*, 206–213. [CrossRef] [PubMed]
37. Liao, S.; Zhang, W.; Hu, X.; Wang, W.; Deng, D.; Wang, H.; Wang, C.; Zhou, J.; Wang, S.; Zhang, H.; et al. A novel "priming-boosting" strategy for immune interventions in cervical cancer. *Mol. Immunol.* **2015**, *64*, 295–305. [CrossRef] [PubMed]
38. Blatnik, R.; Mohan, N.; Bonsack, M.; Falkenby, L.G.; Hoppe, S.; Josef, K.; Steinbach, A.; Becker, S.; Nadler, W.M.; Rucevic, M.; et al. A Targeted LC-MS Strategy for Low-Abundant HLA Class-I-Presented Peptide Detection Identifies Novel Human Papillomavirus T-Cell Epitopes. *Proteomics* **2018**, *18*, e1700390. [CrossRef] [PubMed]
39. Riemer, A.B.; Keskin, D.B.; Zhang, G.; Handley, M.; Anderson, K.S.; Brusic, V.; Reinhold, B.; Reinherz, E.L. A conserved E7-derived cytotoxic T lymphocyte epitope expressed on human papillomavirus 16-transformed HLA-A2+ epithelial cancers. *J. Biol. Chem.* **2010**, *285*, 29608–29622. [CrossRef]
40. Jemon, K.; Young, V.; Wilson, M.; McKee, S.; Ward, V.; Baird, M.; Young, S.; Hibma, M. An enhanced heterologous virus-like particle for human papillomavirus type 16 tumour immunotherapy. *PLoS ONE* **2013**, *8*, e66866. [CrossRef]
41. He, X.; Zhou, S.; Quinn, B.; Jahagirdar, D.; Ortega, J.; Abrams, S.I.; Lovell, J.F. HPV-Associated Tumor Eradication by Vaccination with Synthetic Short Peptides and Particle-Forming Liposomes. *Small* **2021**, *17*, e2007165. [CrossRef] [PubMed]
42. Li, W.; Joshi, M.D.; Singhania, S.; Ramsey, K.H.; Murthy, A.K. Peptide Vaccine: Progress and Challenges. *Vaccines* **2014**, *2*, 515–536. [CrossRef] [PubMed]

43. Zwaveling, S.; Ferreira Mota, S.C.; Nouta, J.; Johnson, M.; Lipford, G.B.; Offringa, R.; van der Burg, S.H.; Melief, C.J. Established human papillomavirus type 16-expressing tumors are effectively eradicated following vaccination with long peptides. *J. Immunol.* **2002**, *169*, 350–358. [CrossRef] [PubMed]
44. Rosalia, R.A.; Quakkelaar, E.D.; Redeker, A.; Khan, S.; Camps, M.; Drijfhout, J.W.; Silva, A.L.; Jiskoot, W.; van Hall, T.; van Veelen, P.A.; et al. Dendritic cells process synthetic long peptides better than whole protein, improving antigen presentation and T-cell activation. *Eur. J. Immunol.* **2013**, *43*, 2554–2565. [CrossRef] [PubMed]
45. Wu, C.Y.; Monie, A.; Pang, X.; Hung, C.F.; Wu, T.C. Improving therapeutic HPV peptide-based vaccine potency by enhancing CD4+ T help and dendritic cell activation. *J. Biomed. Sci.* **2010**, *17*, 88. [CrossRef] [PubMed]
46. Zom, G.G.; Willems, M.; Khan, S.; van der Sluis, T.C.; Kleinovink, J.W.; Camps, M.G.M.; van der Marel, G.A.; Filippov, D.V.; Melief, C.J.M.; Ossendorp, F. Novel TLR2-binding adjuvant induces enhanced T cell responses and tumor eradication. *J. Immunother. Cancer* **2018**, *6*, 146. [CrossRef] [PubMed]
47. Sabbatini, P.; Tsuji, T.; Ferran, L.; Ritter, E.; Sedrak, C.; Tuballes, K.; Jungbluth, A.A.; Ritter, G.; Aghajanian, C.; Bell-McGuinn, K.; et al. Phase I trial of overlapping long peptides from a tumor self-antigen and poly-ICLC shows rapid induction of integrated immune response in ovarian cancer patients. *Clin. Cancer Res.* **2012**, *18*, 6497–6508. [CrossRef]
48. Maynard, S.K.; Marshall, J.D.; MacGill, R.S.; Yu, L.; Cann, J.A.; Cheng, L.I.; McCarthy, M.P.; Cayatte, C.; Robbins, S.H. Vaccination with synthetic long peptide formulated with CpG in an oil-in-water emulsion induces robust E7-specific CD8 T cell responses and TC-1 tumor eradication. *BMC Cancer* **2019**, *19*, 540. [CrossRef] [PubMed]
49. Hou, J.; Liu, Y.; Hsi, J.; Wang, H.; Tao, R.; Shao, Y. Cholera toxin B subunit acts as a potent systemic adjuvant for HIV-1 DNA vaccination intramuscularly in mice. *Hum. Vaccin. Immunother.* **2014**, *10*, 1274–1283. [CrossRef]
50. Borst, J.; Ahrends, T.; Bąbała, N.; Melief, C.J.M.; Kastenmüller, W. CD4(+) T cell help in cancer immunology and immunotherapy. *Nat. Rev. Immunol.* **2018**, *18*, 635–647. [CrossRef]
51. Sanami, S.; Rafieian-Kopaei, M.; Dehkordi, K.A.; Pazoki-Toroudi, H.; Azadegan-Dehkordi, F.; Mobini, G.R.; Alizadeh, M.; Nezhad, M.S.; Ghasemi-Dehnoo, M.; Bagheri, N. In silico design of a multi-epitope vaccine against HPV16/18. *BMC Bioinform.* **2022**, *23*, 311. [CrossRef] [PubMed]
52. Grabowska, A.K.; Kaufmann, A.M.; Riemer, A.B. Identification of promiscuous HPV16-derived T helper cell epitopes for therapeutic HPV vaccine design. *Int. J. Cancer* **2015**, *136*, 212–224. [CrossRef] [PubMed]

Disclaimer/Publisher's Note: The statements, opinions and data contained in all publications are solely those of the individual author(s) and contributor(s) and not of MDPI and/or the editor(s). MDPI and/or the editor(s) disclaim responsibility for any injury to people or property resulting from any ideas, methods, instructions or products referred to in the content.

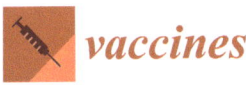

Article

Elimination of Human Papillomavirus 16-Positive Tumors by a Mucosal rAd5 Therapeutic Vaccination in a Pre-Clinical Murine Study

Molly R. Braun [1,*], Anne C. Moore [1,2,3], Jonathan D. Lindbloom [1], Katherine A. Hodgson [1], Emery G. Dora [1] and Sean N. Tucker [1]

[1] Vaxart Inc., 170 Harbor Way Suite 300, South San Francisco, CA 94080, USA; anne.moore@ucc.ie (A.C.M.); edora@vaxart.com (E.G.D.); stucker@vaxart.com (S.N.T.)
[2] School of Biochemistry and Cell Biology, University College Cork, T12 XF62 Cork, Ireland
[3] National Institute of Bioprocessing Research and Training, A94 X099 Dublin, Ireland
* Correspondence: mbraun@vaxart.com

Abstract: Therapeutic vaccination can harness the body's cellular immune system to target and destroy cancerous cells. Several treatment options are available to eliminate pre-cancerous and cancerous lesions caused by human papillomaviruses (HPV), but may not result in a long-term cure. Therapeutic vaccination may offer an effective, durable, and minimally intrusive alternative. We developed mucosally delivered, recombinant, non-replicating human adenovirus type 5 (rAd5)-vectored vaccines that encode HPV16's oncogenic proteins E6 and E7 alongside a molecular dsRNA adjuvant. The induction of antigen-specific T cells and the therapeutic efficacy of rAd5 were evaluated in a mouse model of HPV tumorigenesis where E6E7-transformed cells, TC-1, were implanted subcutaneously in C57BL/6 mice. After tumor growth, mice were treated intranasally with rAd5 vaccines expressing the wildtype form of E6E7 (rAd5-16/E6E7$_{Wt}$) in combination with an anti-PD-1 antibody or isotype control. Animals treated with rAd5-16/E6E7$_{Wt}$ with and without anti-PD-1 had significant reductions in tumor volume and increased survival compared to controls. Further, animals treated with rAd5-16/E6E7$_{Wt}$ had increased CD4+ and CD8+ tumor-infiltrating lymphocytes (TILs) and produced a cytotoxic tumor microenvironment. In a second study, the immunogenicity of a non-transformative form of E6E7 (rAd5-16/E6E7$_{Mu}$) and a vaccine encoding predicted T cell epitopes of E6E7 (rAd5-16/E6E7$_{epi}$) were evaluated. These vaccines elicited significant reductions in TC-1 tumor volume and increased survival of animals. Antigen-specific CD8+ T effector memory cells were observed in the animals treated with E6E7-encoding rAd5, but not in the rAd5-empty group. The work described here demonstrates that this mucosal vaccination can be used therapeutically to elicit specific cellular immunity and further identifies a clinical candidate with great potential for the treatment and prevention of human cervical cancer.

Keywords: human papillomavirus; therapeutic vaccination; mucosal immunity; CD8+ T cell responses

1. Introduction

Most cervical cancers, as well as oropharyngeal and anogenital cancers, are caused by persistent infection with human papillomavirus (HPV) [1]. There are over 200 types of HPV, with HPV16 and HPV18 being responsible for 71% of cervical cancers [2]. Prophylactic vaccines against the viral L1 capsid protein are currently in use and are highly protective against the most common and high-risk HPVs (hrHPVs), including HPV16. However, these vaccines are only effective if administered prior to infection and have no therapeutic effects [3]. Most infections are spread through sexual contact and are cleared by the body without intervention, with persistent infection occurring in approximately 10% of patients [4]. The development of cervical intraepithelial neoplasia (CIN), abnormal changes in the cells lining the cervix, is caused by these persistent infections. Severity is graded by a

Citation: Braun, M.R.; Moore, A.C.; Lindbloom, J.D.; Hodgson, K.A.; Dora, E.G.; Tucker, S.N. Elimination of Human Papillomavirus 16-Positive Tumors by a Mucosal rAd5 Therapeutic Vaccination in a Pre-Clinical Murine Study. *Vaccines* 2024, 12, 955. https://doi.org/10.3390/vaccines12090955

Academic Editors: Yufeng Yao and Li Shi

Received: 2 July 2024
Revised: 7 August 2024
Accepted: 13 August 2024
Published: 23 August 2024

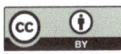

Copyright: © 2024 by the authors. Licensee MDPI, Basel, Switzerland. This article is an open access article distributed under the terms and conditions of the Creative Commons Attribution (CC BY) license (https://creativecommons.org/licenses/by/4.0/).

scale from CIN1 to CIN3, with CIN3 being the most severe form. When left untreated, these abnormal cell pathologies can lead to cervical cancer [5]. Currently, the standard of care to treat CIN2-3 involves invasive surgical methods such as ablation or excision of a large section of the cervix [6]. While these methods have worked well when employed properly and in a timely manner, treatment may not result in durable protection. Immunotherapy treatments via a therapeutic vaccine can specifically target precancerous and malignant cells that express HPV oncoproteins, generating a more targeted approach to treatment. Further, by training the immune system to target HPV+ cells, therapeutic vaccination may provide more durable protection from re-occurrence than traditional methods of treating CIN2-3 [7]. Excitingly, there have been many recent advances in the field of immunotherapy, particularly in therapeutic vaccination, which aims to provide non-invasive, more durable treatments to prevent progression to cervical cancer. Previous work using therapeutic vaccination to treat cervical cancer has shown efficacy correlated with a robust HPV-specific T cell response [8]. Therefore, a successfully implemented therapeutic vaccine must be able to stimulate these immune responses.

HPV is a double-stranded circular DNA virus. During infection, viral proteins E6 and E7 modify the cell cycle to promote viral genome amplification using the host cell's machinery. In some cases, the viral genome may integrate with the host genome, allowing the continual presence of these proteins [9,10]. Unchecked expression of E6 and E7 causes unregulated cell entry into S-phase, leading to oncogenesis. As E6 and E7 are the causative agents of pre-cancerous and cancerous pathologies, stimulation of cytotoxic cellular immunity specific to these proteins has often been the objective of therapeutic vaccination [11]. Many studies have demonstrated that targeting these two antigens can lead to tumor and/or lesion regression and viral clearance [12–21]. We have developed a mucosal vaccine platform known as Vector-Adjuvant-Antigen Standardized Technology (VAAST®), which utilizes non-replicating recombinant human adenovirus type 5 (rAd5) to express an antigen of interest as well as a molecular dsRNA adjuvant within the same target cell [22–26]. The dsRNA forms a short hairpin RNA structure that is expressed independently from the same rAd5 vector as the antigen of interest. This hairpin structure can stimulate cellular innate immune sensors when expressed within a cell, directing an immune response to the very cell where the antigen is expressed, and increase overall immunogenicity. When used in clinical trials, these vaccines are formulated into enterically coated tablets that can be administered orally to humans to stimulate mucosal and systemic immune responses [22–27]. After delivery to the ileum [25], rAd5 is believed to be taken up by epithelial and resident immune cells where the transgene is expressed in the context of MHC I or cross-presented on dendritic cells via MHC I and MHC II. Effector T cells recognize the presented vaccine antigens and elicit cell-mediated immunity in the mucosa [28]. Despite delivery to the ileum, evidence of mucosal activation and transit throughout the body has been observed in humans using this platform. In a phase II influenza challenge study, oral rAd5 encoding the influenza haemagglutinin gene was administered prior to pandemic H1 influenza challenge. The vaccine elicited HA-specific antibodies, mucosal homing B cells, and protected subjects from intranasal challenge with influenza [23]. Additionally, phase I and phase II clinical trials have shown antigen-specific antibodies in saliva and nasal secretions [29,30] as well as upregulation of the mucosal homing marker $\alpha 4\beta 7+$ on B and T cells [22,23]. Therefore, although this oral tablet vaccine is administered in humans via the intestinal mucosa, there is direct evidence of mucosal cross-talk beyond the intestinal site of delivery.

In recent years, the use of checkpoint inhibitors (CPIs), antibodies that block inhibitory signals between antigen-presenting cells and cytotoxic T cells, have been widely used to treat a variety of cancers including lung cancer, bladder cancer, and head and neck cancers [31], in addition to malignant cervical cancer [32]. One main target of these CPI therapies is programmed cell death protein 1 (PD-1), which is expressed on CTLs and, when activated via engagement of PD-L1, dampens the cytotoxic capacity of T cells. This pathway is often exploited by tumor cells to suppress the local immune response [33]. Expression of PD-1 and its receptor PD-L1 has been found in cells from patients with cervical cancer [34].

Previous studies have demonstrated that there are advantages in combining CPIs with therapeutic vaccination [19,35–37]. Therefore, the addition of antibodies targeting PD-1 to immunotherapies may improve disease outcomes.

In this study, we examined the antitumor effects of mucosal therapeutic vaccination with rAd5 encoding the HPV16 genes E6 and E7. rAd5 was tested with anti-PD-1 antibodies to examine if the combination of vaccination with a CPI could enhance the therapeutic efficacy of treatment. HPV16 does not infect animals nor lead to the mucosal tumorigenesis seen in humans, limiting methods to study therapeutic vaccination pre-clinically [38]. In a proof-of-concept experiment, we employed a commonly available HPV tumorigenesis model that uses the TC-1 cell line, murine C57BL/6 lung cells generated by transduction with HPV16 E6, E7, and the variant H-ras activated by the G12V mutation [39,40]. These cells can be cultured in vitro and implanted subcutaneously into C57BL/6 mice, providing a surrogate model to test therapeutic vaccinations [19,39]. Intranasal vaccination was used as a mucosal proxy for oral delivery as oral gavage methods deliver the vaccine to the stomach, rather than the intestines, leaving rAd5 susceptible to the stomach's low-pH environment [41]. However, previous studies with rAd5 vaccines show that immunological readouts in mice aligned with positive immunogenicity readouts in human clinical trials [27,42].

We found that the HPV16-specific rAd5, when administered to TC-1 tumor-bearing mice, led to a significant reduction in tumor volume and increased survival. This was true when the vaccinating antigen was the wildtype form of E6 and E7, encoded selected mutations, or was co-administered with anti-PD-1. Tumor-infiltrating lymphocytes (TILs) were increased in E6E7-specific vaccination and generated a ratio of Treg/CD8+ T cells that has been previously associated with improved clinical outcomes [43]. Relative percentages of CD4+ and CD8+ T cells remained consistent between the groups treated with E6/E7-containing rAd5 compared to controls; however, there was a significant increase in E7-specific CD8+ T cells in these groups, which was largely made up by T effector memory cells. Our results indicate that these mucosal E6/E7-expressing rAd5 vectors are efficacious and immunogenic in a mouse model of HPV-derived tumorigenesis and may represent an effective, non-invasive, and potent therapeutic for the treatment of HPV-related cancers.

2. Materials and Methods

2.1. rAd5 Generation

The transgene expressed by the rAd5-16/E6E7$_{Wt}$ vaccine was generated based on the published sequence of HPV16 E6 (GenBank Accession Number ANY26540.1) and E7 (GenBank Accession Number AIQ82815.1). A tPA signal sequence is upstream of the E6E7 gene and a furin cleavage site separates E6 and E7. For rAd5-16/E6E7$_{Mu}$, E6 mutations L57G, E154A, T156A, Q157A, and L158A and E7 mutations H2P, C24G, E46A, and L67R were introduced. rAd5-16/E6E7$_{Mu.1}$ shares the same mutations are rAd5-16/E6E7$_{Mu}$, except for E7 L67R. For rAd5-16/E6E7$_{epi}$, MHC class I binding predictions were made in May 2019 using the IEDB analysis resource ANN tool [44,45]. Amino acids 18–26, 42–56, and 126–143 of E6 and 4–23, 62–77, and 81–90 of E7 were included without spacers, furin cleavage sites, or tPA sequences. The transgene sequences described above were inserted into the E1 region of a recombinant plasmid containing the rAd5 genome lacking the E1 and E3 genes. A third rAd5 construct was used that did not contain a transgene sequence (rAd5-empty). A sequence encoding the molecular dsRNA adjuvant was included downstream of the transgene region in all constructs. Both E6/E7 and the dsRNA are under the control of CMV promoters. The rAd5 vaccines were generated and propagated as previously described [46].

2.2. ELISpot

C57BL/6 mice (n = 2–8/group, female, 6–8 weeks old, Jackson Labs, Bar Harbor, ME, USA) or J:DO mice (n = 3–8/group, female, 6–8 weeks old, Jackson Labs), were vaccinated three times one week apart with 1×10^8 infectious units (IUs)/animal. On day 21, one week after final vaccination, 5×10^5 splenocytes were cultured in duplicate wells with a pool of overlapping peptides spanning the coding sequence of E6 or of E7. These peptides, which were synthesized as 15-mers overlapping by 11 amino acids (JPT GmbH, Berlin, Germany), were reconstituted in DMSO and subsequently diluted in RPMI-based cell culture medium at 0.2 µg/well. After overnight incubation, the numbers of spot forming units (SFUs) of IFNγ per million splenocytes was determined. Spots were counted using an AID ELISPOT reader or by Zellnet Consulting (Fort Lee, NJ, USA). Animal work was performed at Vaxart, Inc. (South San Francisco, CA, USA). The animal procedures used in the current study were submitted to the Institutional Animal Care and Use Committee (IACUC).

2.3. TC-1 Challenge Model

TC-1 cells (ATCC, Manassas, VA, USA) were grown as a monolayer at 37 °C with 5% CO_2 in RPMI 1640 supplemented with 2 mM L-glutamine (31870-025, Thermofisher, Waltham, MA, USA), 1 mM sodium pyruvate (11360-039, Thermofisher), 0.1 mM non-essential amino acids (11140-035, Thermofisher), 50 µM β-mercaptoethanol (31350-010, Thermofisher), 1% penicillin/streptomycin (15140-122, Thermofisher), and 10% fetal bovine serum (P30-3306, Pan Biotech, Aidenbach, Germany). For tumor implantation, cells were detached from the plate with trypsin-0.05% EDTA (25300054, Thermofisher) and 1×10^6 TC-1 cells in 200 µL of RPMI 1640 without phenol red were injected into the right flank of 50 C57BL/6JRj mice (female, 7 weeks old, Janiver Labs, Le Genest-Saint-Isle, France). Animals were randomized into groups of 10 by mean tumor volume when tumors reached 20–60 mm^3 or 100–200 mm^3 for the small and large tumor models, respectively (Vivo Manager software 1.11E-02, Biosystems, Couternon, France). All work described was performed by Oncodesign Services (Dijon, France). The animal procedures used in the current study were submitted to the Institutional Animal Care and Use Committee of Oncodesign (Oncomet), approved by French authorities (CNREEA agreement No. 91 (Oncodesign)).

2.4. Therapeutic Immunization and Immunotherapy

Therapeutic vaccinations were given by intranasal administration of rAd5 (1×10^8 infectious units (IUs)/animal) on the day of randomization and repeated twice more, seven days apart. The anti-murine PD-1 monoclonal antibody (RMP1-14, BioXcell, Lebanon, NH, USA) or rat IgG2a as an isotype control (2A3, BioXcell) was administered twice weekly during vaccination by intraperitoneal injection at a dose of 10 mg/kg. In experiments with rAd5-16/E6E7$_{Wt}$, animals were treated as follows: (i) PBS; (ii) rAd5-empty + iso; (iii) rAd5-empty + anti-PD-1; (iv) rAd5-16/E6E7$_{Wt}$ + iso; or (v) rAd5-16/E6E7$_{Wt}$ + anti-PD-1. For experiments with modified E6E7, animals were treated as follows: (i) PBS; (ii) rAd5-empty; (iii) rAd5-16/E6E7$_{Mu}$; (iv) rAd5-16/E6E7$_{epi}$. Animals were monitored for clinical signs (viability and behavior) every day. Body weights were measured twice a week. The length and width of the tumor were measured twice a week with calipers and the volume of the tumor was estimated by the following formula: tumor volume = (width2 × length)/2 [47]. Animals were euthanized if the tumor exceeded 10% of the normal body weight or reached 1500 mm^3. All work described was performed by Oncodesign Services (Dijon, France).

2.5. Analysis of Tumor Infiltrating Cells (TILs) by Flow Cytometry

TC-1 tumors were established in the flank as described above and allowed to grow to a mean volume of 111.5 mm^3 on day 13 post-tumor induction. Five mice per group were randomized into each group and were treated on days 13 and 20 with one of the following regimes: (i) rAd-empty + iso; (ii) rAd-16/E6E7$_{Wt}$ + iso; or (iii) rAd-16/E6E7$_{Wt}$ + anti-PD-1. All doses and routes were the same as previously described. Animals were monitored daily and tumors volumes were determined twice a week. On day 24, all animals were euthanized and tumors were removed, weighed, mechanically disrupted with a scalpel, and then crushed with a 1 mL syringe plunger on a 70 µm sieve. One million cells were resuspended in staining buffer (PBS, 0.2% BSA, 0.02% NaN3). Cells were stained for T cell subsets with FoxP3 PE, CD8a PerCP, CD3 V450, CD4 VioGreen, and CD45 APC-Cy7. The stained cells were analyzed with a flow cytometer (LSR II, BD Biosciences, Durham, NC, USA). Flow cytometry data were acquired until either 50,000 CD45+ events were recorded for each sample or a maximum duration of 2 min elapsed. All work described was performed by Oncodesign Services (Dijon, France).

2.6. Flow Cytometry on Blood Cells from Small Tumor Model Animals

Blood was collected by jugular vein puncture of TC-1 mice on days 14 and 21, one day after vaccine treatments. Prior to staining, red blood cells (RBCs) were lysed with Versalyse lysing buffer (A09777, Beckman coulter, Brea, CA, USA) for 10–15 min. Cells were stained with the viability dye Viakrom 808 (Beckman Coulter), followed by staining with Dextramer E749-57 APC (Immudex, Copenhagen, Denmark, Allele H-2Db). Cells were then stained with CD45 BV605 (103155, Biolegend, San Diego, CA, USA), CD3 PE (130-120-160, Miltenyi, Bergisch Gladbach, Germany), CD4 PE-Vio770 (130-123-894, Miltenyi), CD8 BV785 (100750, Biolegend), CD62L (BV421 104436, Biolegend), and CD44 VioBright FITC (130-120-213, Miltenyi). Cells were fixed with Cytofix buffer (554655, BD Biosciences) and then run on a flow cytometer (Cytoflex LX, Beckman Coulter). All work described was performed by Oncodesign Services (Dijon, France).

2.7. Statistics

Mean and standard error of the mean (SEM) are shown for all data points except when $n \leq 3$, in which only mean and individual datapoints are shown. For ELISpot analysis and analysis of blood cells at various timepoints, an ordinary two-way ANOVA with Tukey's multiple comparison test was used. For TIL analysis, a Mann–Whitney t-test was used. Statistics were performed using GraphPad Prism (Version 10.0.3).

3. Results

3.1. Immunogenicity of Wildtype and Modified E6E7 Therapeutic Vaccines for HPV16

The E6 and E7 proteins of HPV16, when unchecked, may cause dysregulation of the cell cycle and tumorigenesis. Several studies have previously mutated HPV16 E6 and/or E7 proteins to reduce the risk associated with the oncogenic potential of these proteins [20,21,48]. Eliminating the oncogenic potential of E6 and E7 in a vaccine could further increase safety and therapeutic acceptance. Therefore, in addition to testing the immunogenicity of wildtype (Wt) E6 and E7 as therapeutic antigens (rAd5-16/E6E7$_{Wt}$), an rAd5 vaccine was generated with mutations that disrupt E6's ability to bind p53 and PTPN13 and E7's ability to bind Rb and mi2β (rAd5-16/E6E7$_{Mu}$) (Figure 1A) [21]. In a second approach, a construct was generated to express the minimal epitopes required for immunogenicity and efficacy (rAd5-16/E6E7$_{epi}$), utilizing the Immune Epitope Database & Tools, a resource that uses MHC class I binding, peptide processing, and immunogenicity predictions to identify consequential epitopes [49]. As a comparator, a vaccine was tested which only contains the molecular dsRNA adjuvant (rAd5-empty) (Figure 1A).

Immunogenicity of rAd5 vectors encoding either the wildtype or mutated HPV16 E6E7 were first examined by ELISpot assay to measure specific T cell responses; C57BL/6 mice were intranasally vaccinated on day 0 and day 28. T cells from splenocytes were assessed for antigen-specific IFNγ production one week after the final vaccination. A non-significant decrease in E6 immunogenicity and a significant increase in E7 immunogenicity was observed when comparing rAd5-16/E6E7$_{Mu}$ with rAd5-16/E6E7$_{Wt}$ (Figure 1B). Additionally, no significant differences in T cell responses to E6 or E7 were detected when the mutated E6E7 (rAd5-16/E6E7$_{Mu}$) and minimal epitope vaccine (rAd5-16/E6E7$_{epi}$) were compared in C57BL/6 mice (Figure 1C). E7 has a strong H-2Db-restricted CD8+ T cell epitope (RAHYNIVTF, known as R9F) in C57BL/6 mice that can dominate the immune response. Therefore, we wanted to test if the rAd5 vaccines were immunogenic in outbred mice with more heterologous MHC class I variation. Thus, the outbred mouse strain J:DO was used to provide a better sense of the T cell response with a diverse background of

MHC alleles. Mice were vaccinated with rAd5-16/E6E7$_{Wt}$ and a vaccine nearly identical to rAd5-16/E6E7$_{Mu}$ (which differs by one amino acid in E7 L67R, termed rAd5-16/E6E7$_{Mu.1}$) and IFNγ-producing T cells were assessed by ELISpot. Similar trends were observed in J:DO mice as in C57BL/6 mice with no significant differences between E6 responses and significant increases in E7 responses (Figure S1).

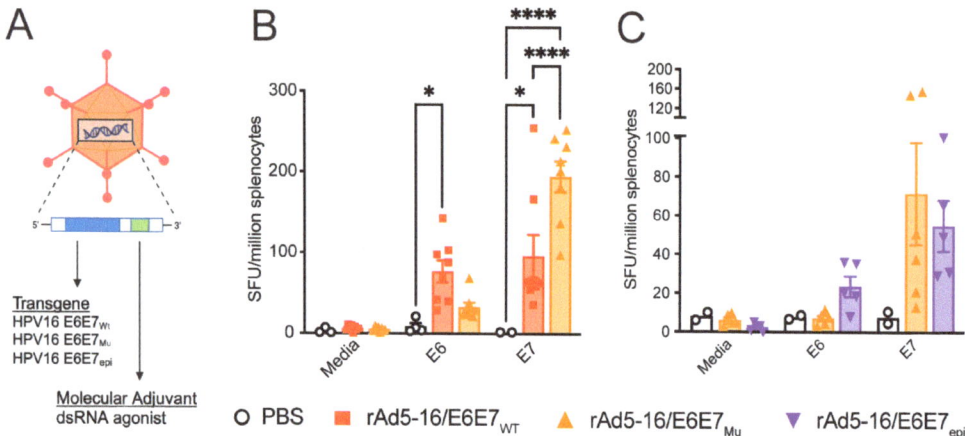

Figure 1. rAd5 vaccines from VAAST platform induce antigen-specific T cells. (**A**) Illustration of the rAd5 vector used during vaccination. The transgene region (blue) represents the antigen included in the construct upstream of the molecular dsRNA adjuvant (green). (**B**,**C**) Antigen-specific T cells expressing IFNγ in C57BL/6 mice intranasally vaccinated with rAd after stimulation with media, E6, or E7 peptide pools. Spot forming units (SFUs) per million spleen cells are shown. Mean and SEM, two-way ANOVA. n = 2–8 mice/group. Error bars not shown when $n \leq 3$. p = 0.01 to 0.05 (*), $p < 0.0001$ (****).

3.2. Mucosal Application of Antigen-Specific rAd5 Reduces Tumor Size

To test the efficacy of rAd5-16/E6E7$_{Wt}$, we utilized the TC-1 solid tumor growth model. HPV-E6/E7-expressing TC-1 cells were injected subcutaneously into the hind flank of C57BL/6 mice on day 0 and allowed to grow for several days before mice were treated with an intranasal administration of the rAd5-16/E6E7$_{Wt}$ vaccine, rAd5-empty vaccine, or PBS (untreated). In addition to vaccination, mice were administered the CPI monoclonal antibody against PD-1 (anti-PD-1) or an isotype control (Figure 2A,D). These combinations were tested in a small tumor model study, where mice were immunized on day 7 after the tumors had reached a mean volume of 28.3 mm^3, and then again on days 14 and 21 (Figure 2A). Administration of rAd5-16/E6E7$_{Wt}$ with isotype administration reduced tumor growth and induced tumor shrinkage in all animals up to day 39, at which point 2/10 tumors re-grew and one animal reached the humane endpoint before the study end (Figures 2B,C and S2A). The use of the anti-PD-1 with rAd5-16/E6E7$_{Wt}$ vaccine trended slightly better for survival (10/10 survived), but this result was not significantly different (Figures 2B,C and S2A). Animals treated with rAd5-empty with or without anti-PD-1 or treated with PBS did not control tumor growth and met the ethical criteria for euthanasia before the study end (Figures 2B,C and S2A). Overall, mice immunized with rAd5-16/E6E7$_{Wt}$ overwhelmingly survived the tumor challenge, compared to 0% in the control groups.

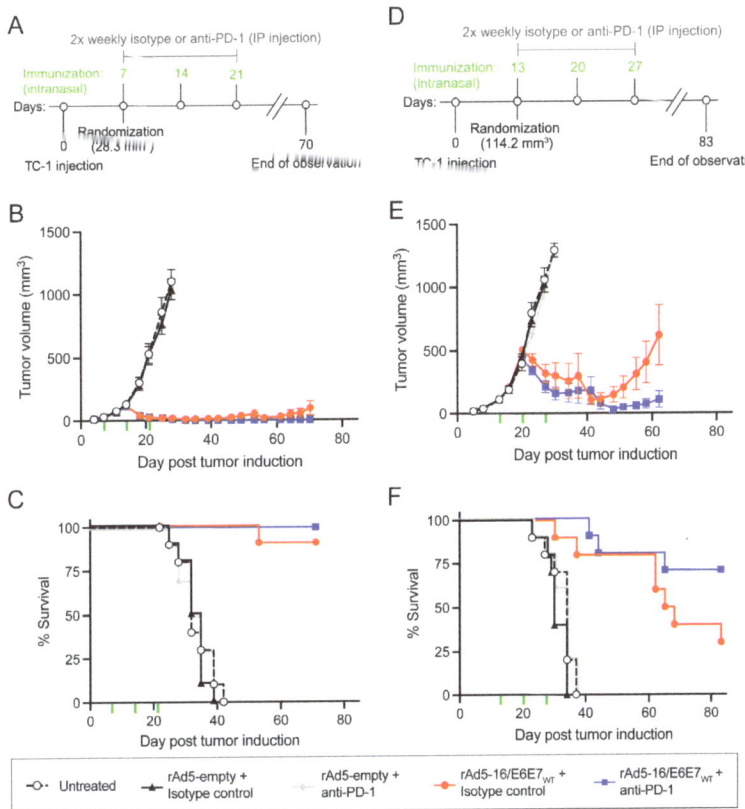

Figure 2. Intranasal administration of rAd5 vaccine expressing wildtype E6-E7 can eliminate and prevent tumor growth in mice. (**A**) Overview of small tumor model timeline. Vaccinations started on day 7 once tumors reached an average of 28.3 mm^3. (**B**) Tumor volumes were measured in treatment groups through to the study end. Curves are shown for data points where at least 80% of animals were present. Vaccination is indicated by green hash-marks. (**C**) Survival curve of small tumor model indicating time until ethical criteria for euthanasia were met. (**D**) Overview of large tumor model timeline. Vaccinations started on day 13 once tumors reached an average of 114.2 mm^3. (**E**) Tumor volume in treatment groups through to the study end. Curves are shown for data points where at least 80% of animals were present. Vaccination is indicated by green hash-marks. (**F**) Survival curve of large tumor model indicating time until ethical criteria for euthanasia were met. Mean and SEM. $n = 10$ mice/group.

To investigate if rAd5 vaccines could have therapeutic efficacy later in tumor progression, TC-1 tumor cells were injected as before but randomization and treatment occurred when tumors reached a mean volume of 114.2 mm^3 on day 13 (large tumor model). Animals were vaccinated as above, followed by subsequent vaccinations on days 20 and 27 with twice-weekly injections of anti-PD-1 or the isotype control (Figure 2D). The group administered rAd5-16/E6E7$_{Wt}$ with anti-PD-1 was able to control tumor growth, up to day 40, at which point 2/10 mice reached a humane endpoint (Figures 2E,F and S2B). Within this group, 70% (7/10) of animals survived to the end of the experiment on day 83. rAd5-16/E6E7$_{Wt}$ with the isotype control was also able to substantially control tumor growth effects and improve survival with 80% of mice surviving (8/10) to day 60 (33 days after the last immunization), before four additional animals reached a humane endpoint by day 80, resulting in a day 83 survival rate of 30% (Figures 2E,F and S2B). Mice left untreated or treated with rAd5-empty with anti-PD-1 or the isotype control were not able to control

3.3. Immunization with Ad-HPV-16 Generates a Cytotoxic Tumor Microenvironment

Tumors can elicit Treg cells to dampen the local immune response and promote further tumor growth [50]. It was previously observed that the TILs of individuals who had a higher ratio of Tregs to CD8+ T cells had unfavorable clinical outcomes [43]. To understand how E6E7-specific rAd5 vaccines were able to control tumor growth, TILs were analyzed by flow cytometry using the large tumor model. TC-1 tumor cells were injected and allowed to grow to a mean volume of 111.5 mm^3 before intranasal immunization with rAd5-16/E6E7$_{Wt}$ with or without anti-PD-1 and compared to immunization with rAd5-empty on day 13 post TC-1 injection (Figure 3A). Mice were vaccinated again seven days later and tumors were harvested on day 24, when initial tumor regression was observed but tumors were still of sufficient mass to permit cell isolation and analysis (Figure 3A,B). Lymphocytes were normalized per unit volume of tumor isolated to allow comparisons across groups. rAd5-16/E6E7$_{Wt}$ with or without the anti-PD-1 checkpoint inhibitor induced a significant increase in the number of CD4+ and CD8+ T cells in the tumor mass along with an increase in Treg cells (defined as CD45 + CD3 + CD4 + FoxP3+) (Figure 3C–E). Although there was in increase in Treg cells in addition to CD8+ T cells in vaccinated animals, the increase in the latter was much greater. Therefore, a lower Treg/CD8+ T cell ratio was observed in rAd5-16/E6E7$_{Wt}$, in the presence or absence of anti-PD-1, compared to rAd5-empty and the isotype antibody (Figure 3F). This demonstrates that immunization with rAd5-16/E6E7$_{Wt}$ alone or in combination with anti-PD1 modulates the inter-tumoral immune response towards an overall cytotoxic tumor microenvironment.

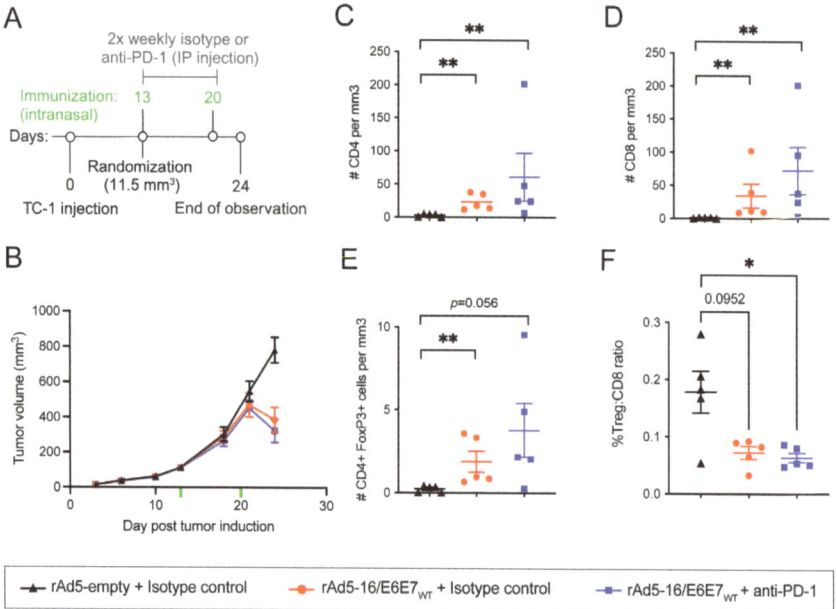

Figure 3. E6E7-specific rAd5 vaccines induce tumor infiltrating lymphocytes. (**A**) Overview of large tumor model timeline for TIL analysis. (**B**) Mean tumor volume per group until tumor collection. Treatment began when mean tumor volumes reached 111.5 mm^3 on day 13. Vaccination is indicated by green hash marks. (**C**) number of CD4 T cells per mm^3 of tumor. (**D**) number of CD8 T cells per mm^3 of tumor. (**E**) number of Treg cells per mm^3 of tumor. (**F**) Ratio of Treg T cells to CD8 T cells. $n = 5$ mice/group. Mean and SEM. B-D Mann–Whitney t-test. $n = 5$ mice/group. $p = 0.01$ to 0.05 (*), $p = 0.001$ to 0.01 (**).

3.4. Vaccination with rAd5 Vectors Expressing Non-Oncogenic E6E7 Led to Tumor Reduction

Although rAd5-16/E6E7$_{Mu}$ and rAd5-16/E6E7$_{epi}$ were immunogenic in ELISpot assays (Figures 1C and S1), we sought to understand if mutating the key oncogenic sites of E6 and E7 in the vaccine affected the ability of the vaccine to elicit an efficacious immune response. Thus, the small tumor model utilized in Figure 2A,B was employed with these constructs. On study day 0, TC-1 tumors were induced by subcutaneous injection of 1×10^6 TC-1 cells into the right flank of C57BL/6 mice. Animals were randomized into treatment groups when tumors reached 49.0 mm^3 on day 6. Groups were then treated with PBS (untreated), rAd5-empty, rAd5-16/E6E7$_{Mu}$, or rAd5-16/E6E7$_{epi}$ by intranasal application three times, seven days apart (Figure 4A). Blood samples were taken on days 14 and 21 for flow cytometry analysis. After randomization and initial treatment on day 6, tumors continued to grow until day 13, at which point there was no significant difference in tumor size between treatment groups (Figures 4B,C and S2D). Animals received additional treatments on day 13 and day 20. After day 13, tumors in the untreated group and the group treated with rAd5-empty continued to increase in volume until humane endpoints were reached, whereas tumor volume in the groups treated with rAd5-16/E6E7$_{Mu}$ or rAd5-16/E6E7$_{epi}$ began to decrease in size through to the end of the study at day 49 (Figures 4B and S2D). The effect of rAd5-16/E6E7$_{Mu}$ was particularly pronounced as tumor volume completely regressed in all animals with lasting regression in 5/10 animals (Figure S2D).

3.5. Mucosal Application of Antigen-Specific rAd5 Generates Antigen-Specific T$_{EM}$ Cells in a Small Tumor Model

As oncogenesis is driven by E6 and E7, which are intracellular targets, cellular immunity after rAd5-16/E6E7$_{Mu}$ and rAd5-16/E6E7$_{epi}$ treatment was characterized by flow cytometry one day after the second and third treatment (days 14 and 21) to look for changes in T cell distributions as well as the generation of antigen-specific T cells (Figure 4A,D,E). Blood was sampled from animals from the group treated with rAd5, but not the untreated group. The percentage of CD3+ cells within the CD45+ population was consistent between groups, except for a statistically significant increase in overall percentage of T cells in the group treated with rAd5-16/E6E7$_{Mu}$ compared to rAd5-empty at day 14. This difference was not present at day 21, one day after the second treatment (Figure S3A). Among CD3+ T cells, there were no differences in overall distribution of either CD8+ T cells or CD4+ T cells at either sampling day between the various groups (Figure S3B,C).

To further characterize the cellular immune response, we next examined the cellular markers CD44 and CD62L in the T cell population to distinguish between naïve, central memory (T$_{CM}$), and effector memory (T$_{EM}$) T cells. There were no significant differences or consistent trends in the distribution between CD8+ T cell subsets (Figure S3D–F). As T$_{EM}$ cells are the main drivers of cellular cytotoxicity towards cancerous cells, we sought to understand if E7-specific T cells were being produced by rAd5 treatments using a dextramer with the known R9F (E749-57) H-2 Db allele (DexE7) bound to MHC class I. On day 14, after two treatments, the rAd5-16/E6E7$_{Mu}$ group had a significant increase in E7-specific T cells compared to the rAd5-empty group. At day 21, after three treatments, both the rAd5-16/E6E7$_{Mu}$ group and the rAd5-16/E6E7$_{epi}$ group had significantly increased percentages of DexE7-specific CD8+ T cells with rAd5-16/E6E7$_{Mu}$ having a significantly higher response to both rAd5-empty and rAd5-16/E6E7$_{epi}$ (Figure 4D). Of the DexE7+ CD8+ T cells, most cells were T$_{EM}$ cells, representing a critical cell population for cell-mediated control of HPV tumorigenesis (Figure 4E).

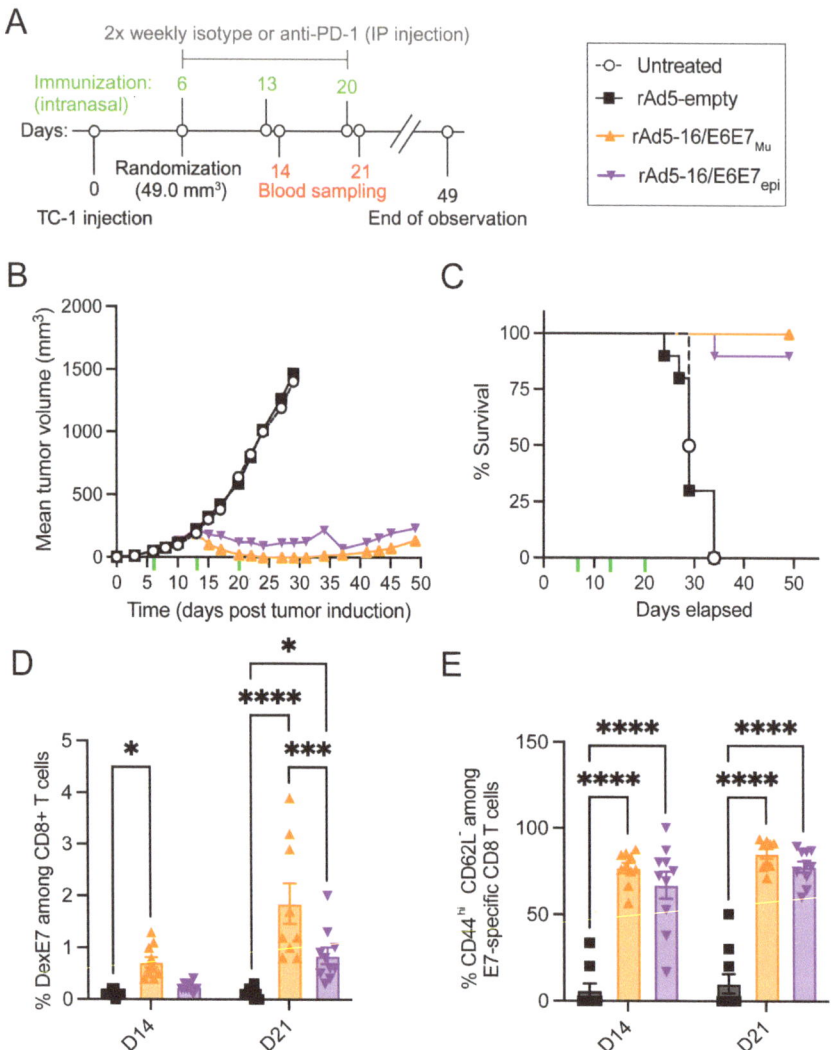

Figure 4. E6-E7-specific rAd5 vaccines with oncogenic mutations prevent tumor growth in mice bearing subcutaneous TC-1 tumors and generate antigen-specific T_{EM} cells. (**A**) Overview of small tumor model timeline. Vaccinations, indicated by green hash marks, started on day 6 once tumors reached an average of 49.0 mm^3. (**B**) Tumor volume in treatment groups through to the study end. Curves are shown for data points where at least 80% of animals were present. (**C**) Survival curve of small tumor model indicating time until ethical criteria for euthanasia were met. (**D**) Percentage of CD8+ T cells specific to HPV16 E7. (**E**) Percentage of E7-specfic T cells among E7-specific cells. n = 10 mice/group, mean and SEM, two-way ANOVA. p = 0.01 to 0.05 (*), p = 0.001 to 0.0001 (***), p < 0.0001 (****).

4. Discussion

Therapeutic vaccination, designed to stimulate cell-mediated immunity, may provide revolutionary new options for the treatment of many cancers by stimulating life-long memory anti-tumor responses. HPV-specific therapeutic vaccination may also provide a less invasive, more easily administered, and more widely available treatment for CIN2/3. Here, we demonstrate that mucosally administered adenovirus-based vaccines expressing HPV16 antigens are highly efficacious at killing HPV16-immortalized epithelial cells in a mouse model. These vaccines induced high levels of antigen-specific T cells in inbred and outbred mice and induced a favorable ratio of cytotoxic to regulatory T cells in tumors, overall leading to efficacy and animal survival in the TC-1 tumorigenesis murine model.

The first objective of this study was to determine the immunogenicity of candidate HPV 16 E6 and E7 antigens expressed by the adenovirus type 5 vector. We show that E6E7-specific rAd5 vaccination leads to the generation of specific T cell responses in C57BL/6 and J:DO mice. Mutations in the wildtype antigen led to some changes in the measured T cell responses in C57BL/6 mice. Specifically, when comparing rAd5-16/E6E7$_{Wt}$ and rAd5-16/E6E7$_{Mu}$, the latter yielded a decreased SPU count after E6 stimulation, whereas an increase in SPU was observed after E7 stimulation in splenocytes from vaccinated C57BL/6 mice. It is possible that the specific mutations in rAd5-16/E6E7$_{Mu}$ change the peptide processing for MHC class I presentation. For example, an E6 intermediate affinity epitope, identified by the IEDB analysis resource ANN tool, is present between amino acid residues 52–60 in wildtype HPV16 E6 (FAFRDLCIV). The L57G substitution of rAd5-16/E6E7$_{Mu}$ may disrupt this H-2Db epitope, leading to a reduced T cell response. This was not, however, observed when tested in J:DO mice. It could additionally be speculated that the E7 E46A mutation in rAd5-16/E6E7$_{Mu}$, which is three positions upstream of the dominant H-2Db RAHYNIVTF epitope, further enhances processing and presentation. Future studies are required to determine the relative contribution of predicted H-2Db and H-2Kb epitopes to the overall T cell responses to these antigens.

Importantly, we show that rAd-16E6E7 vaccines drive tumor regression at both early and late stages of tumor growth and generate a cytotoxic tumor microenvironment. The addition of the anti-PD-1 antibody increased the durability of the vaccine-induced anti-tumor response by at least 20 days in the large tumor model. Further, we showed that HPV16 E6/E7 vaccines which contain previously described mutations that inhibit E6 and E7 oncogenic properties, or contain only predicted immunodominant epitopes, maintained the ability to control HPV16+ tumorigenesis through to the study end on day 49. This effect was especially pronounced in the rAd5-16/E6E7$_{Mt}$ group, with complete regression of tumors in all mice and lasting regression in half of the mice. These findings support the further development of mucosally administered therapeutic adenovirus vaccines against HPV.

Antigen-specific cytotoxic CD8+ T cells play critical roles in immunotherapies [51] and thus it is important that any therapeutic vaccine be able to generate this type of response. We sought to understand how T cell dynamics changed in response to antigen-specific vaccination. When examining the TILs generated by rAd5-16/E6E7$_{Wt}$, we observed an increase in CD4+, CD8+, and Treg cells. Treg cells are typically associated with suppression of the effector T cell response [50]. We found that although there was an increase in Tregs infiltrating the tumor compared to tumors from control animals, the ratio of Treg/CD8+ T cells suggested a more cytotoxic tumor microenvironment and aligned with that observed in human subjects with better clinical outcomes [43]. Further, in the small tumor model, administration of the rAd5 encoding E6 and E7 with mutations did not appear to alter the overall distribution of CD4+ and CD8+ T cells, but rAd5 encoding E6E7 genes were able to generate antigen-specific CD8+ T$_{EM}$ cells in the periphery, with rAd5-16/E6E7$_{Mt}$ generating a more pronounced response than rAd5-16/E6E7$_{epi}$.

A few limitations of this study can be considered. First, in humans this vaccine platform is typically delivered to the ileum via enterically coated tablets; it is possible that oral delivery in mice would expose rAd5 to the low pH of the stomach, interfering with the vaccine's potency [41]. However, previous studies with rAd5 vaccines show agreement in immunological readouts when comparing intranasal and oral delivery in hamsters [27,42,52]. Another limitation of this study is the use of a subcutaneous tumor model when, in humans, HPV induces mucosal tumors. While this proof-of-concept experiment shows promise for biological relevance, future studies may include modeling these vaccines in orthotopic tumor models to better predict clinical efficacy [53].

The generation of antigen-specific T cells in humans is important in the control of HPV tumorigenesis. It has been suggested that the exclusion of antigen-specific CD8+ T cells from the epithelium may play a key role in the progression of intraepithelial neoplasia [54]. Further, α4β7+ CD8+ T cells are better able to enter the cervical mucosa and are associated with cervical lesion clearance compared to those excluded from the epithelium [54]. Studies with an electroporated DNA vaccine candidate suggested that the ability to elicit potent antigen-specific T cell responses correlated with histopathological regression and a reduction in HPV viral DNA detection [20]. The mucosal rAd5 VAAST platform employed here has been used to generate mucosal homing T cells in human clinical trials investigating the platform's prophylactic effects. In a phase II influenza clinical trial comparing the immunogenicity and efficacy of this mucosal rAd5 compared to a licensed injected vaccine, rAd5 was able to generate significantly more T cells expressing the mucosal homing marker α4β7+ [22]. The generation of antigen-specific T cells has also been demonstrated with the VAAST platform in a phase I COVID-19 clinical trial where rAd5 generated more cytotoxic T cell responses compared to the responses generated by an injected mRNA vaccination [55]. Although the therapeutic, rather than prophylactic, efficacy of the VAAST platform has not yet been tested in humans, the ability to generate mucosal homing cytotoxic CD8+ T cells combined with the preclinical results described here suggest that this platform may be able to generate a potent and effective T cell response that targets the provenance of HPV tumorigenesis.

Overall, we show the generation of antigen-specific CD8+ T cells induced by therapeutic vaccination via a mucosal route while also demonstrating a reduction in tumor volume and increased survival in a murine model.

5. Conclusions

These proof-of-concept results suggest that the rAd5 platform provides a promising technology in humans to treat HPV-derived cervical dysplasia. Currently, several therapeutic vaccines for HPV have completed placebo-controlled clinical trials and have largely been administered via injection or electroporation. A systematic review of different HPV16 and HPV18 E6 and E7 vaccines demonstrated a total overall proportion of regression from CIN2/3 to CIN1 at 0.54 compared a placebo group at 0.27 [56]. These numbers represent a meaningful reduction in the advancement of cervical cancer; yet, there remains room for improvement. Future research into the clinical use of mucosal rAd5 as a therapeutic could include investigation of optimal dose regimes, including investigations into the spacing between doses to allow for optimal contraction and expansion of antigen-specific T cells. Further, it is tantalizing to imagine that a non-invasive treatment, like the one described here, could be administered early in cervical cancer diagnosis, even at the point of infection identification, before CIN2-3 is reached.

While treatment options exist for CIN2-3, these treatments can be invasive or require frequent interventions. In low- and middle-income countries (LMICs), the introduction of preventative HPV vaccination campaigns began later with only 41% of LMICs introducing these vaccines by 2019 [57], leaving the burden of infection falling more heavily in regions where access to healthcare services and cold chain logistics is limited. A vaccine strategy, like the one described here, which can be therapeutically administered to activate necessary mucosal immune responses, using an easy-to-administer thermostable tablet, could have an even greater global impact on the treatment of pre-cancerous lesions, thereby preventing the development of malignant cervical cancer, particularly in regions where healthcare access is limited.

Supplementary Materials: The following supporting information can be downloaded at: https://www.mdpi.com/article/10.3390/vaccines12090955/s1. Supplementary Figure S1: rAd5 vaccines expressing WT and non-oncogenic E6E7 induce specific T cells in J:DO mice. Spot forming units (SFU) measuring IFNγ in rAd5-vaccinated J:DO mice after stimulation with media, E6, or E7 peptide pools. Mean and SEM, two-way ANOVA. n = 3–8 mice/group. p = 0.01 to 0.05 (*), p = 0.001 to 0.01 (**). Supplementary Figure S2: Individual tumor volumes of C57BL/6 mice bearing subcutaneous TC-1 tumors. Individual tumor volumes, measured in mm3, of the individual mice from the (A) small tumor model with rAd5-E6E7WT, (B) large tumor model with rAd5-16/E6E7WT, (C) large tumor model with rAd5-16/E6E7WT for TIL analysis and (D) small tumor model with rAd5-16/E6E7Mu and rAd5-16/E6E7epi. Supplementary Figure S3: rAd5 expressing non-oncogenic E6E7 does not change overall distribution of CD4+ and CD8+ T cells. (A) CD3+, (B) CD8+, (C) CD4+, (D) effector memory CD8+, (E) central memory CD8+, or (F) naïve CD8+ T cells did not alter in relative percentage between vaccination groups. Small differences were not statically significant unless specified n = 10 mice/group, mean and SEM, two-way ANOVA. $p = 0.001$ to 0.01 (**).

Author Contributions: Conceptualization, A.C.M., K.A.H. and S.N.T.; data curation, M.R.B.; formal analysis, M.R.B., A.C.M. and J.D.L.; investigation, M.R.B., A.C.M., K.A.H. and S.N.T.; methodology, A.C.M., J.D.L., K.A.H. and E.G.D.; supervision, S.N.T.; writing—original draft, M.R.B.; writing—review and editing, M.R.B., A.C.M. and S.N.T. All authors have read and agreed to the published version of the manuscript.

Funding: This research was funded by Vaxart, Inc. (South San Francisco, CA, USA).

Institutional Review Board Statement: The animal study protocol was approved by the Institutional CNREEA agreement No. 91 approved on 7 April 2024.

Informed Consent Statement: Not applicable.

Data Availability Statement: Raw data are available upon request for the purposes of reproducing or adding to the analysis except in cases where data or information encroaches on the intellectual property of Vaxart, Inc. All data discussed in this article are available in the main or Supplementary Materials.

Acknowledgments: We wish to thank Oncodesign Services for their careful work and prompt communication and Kayan Tam for her assistance in generating figures for this publication.

Conflicts of Interest: Authors M.R.B, J.D.L, E.G.D. and S.N.T. are employed by Vaxart Inc. and receive stock. Authors A.C.M. and K.A.H. were employed by Vaxart, Inc. The authors declare that this study received funding from Vaxart, Inc. The experiments were designed and analyzed by Vaxart Inc. using material developed by Vaxart Inc.

References

1. De Sanjose, S.; Serrano, B.; Tous, S.; Alejo, M.; Lloveras, B.; Quiros, B.; Clavero, O.; Vidal, A.; Ferrandiz-Pulido, C.; Pavon, M.A.; et al. Burden of Human Papillomavirus (HPV)-Related Cancers Attributable to HPVs 6/11/16/18/31/33/45/52 and 58. *JNCI Cancer Spectr.* **2018**, *2*, pky045. [CrossRef]
2. Muhr, L.S.A.; Eklund, C.; Dillner, J. Towards quality and order in human papillomavirus research. *Virology* **2018**, *519*, 74–76. [CrossRef]
3. Hildesheim, A.; Gonzalez, P.; Kreimer, A.R.; Wacholder, S.; Schussler, J.; Rodriguez, A.C.; Porras, C.; Schiffman, M.; Sidawy, M.; Schiller, J.T.; et al. Impact of human papillomavirus (HPV) 16 and 18 vaccination on prevalent infections and rates of cervical lesions after excisional treatment. *Am. J. Obstet. Gynecol.* **2016**, *215*, 212.e1–212.e15. [CrossRef] [PubMed]
4. Ho, G.Y.; Bierman, R.; Beardsley, L.; Chang, C.J.; Burk, R.D. Natural history of cervicovaginal papillomavirus infection in young women. *N. Engl. J. Med.* **1998**, *338*, 423–428. [CrossRef] [PubMed]
5. Ljubojevic, S.; Skerlev, M. HPV-associated diseases. *Clin. Dermatol.* **2014**, *32*, 227–234. [CrossRef]
6. Khallouf, H.; Grabowska, A.K.; Riemer, A.B. Therapeutic Vaccine Strategies against Human Papillomavirus. *Vaccines* **2014**, *2*, 422–462. [CrossRef]
7. Hoffman, S.R.; Le, T.; Lockhart, A.; Sanusi, A.; dal Santo, L.; Davis, M.; McKinney, D.A.; Brown, M.; Poole, C.; Willame, C.; et al. Patterns of persistent HPV infection after treatment for cervical intraepithelial neoplasia (CIN): A systematic review. *Int. J. Cancer* **2017**, *141*, 8–23. [CrossRef] [PubMed]
8. Stern, P.L.; van der Burg, S.H.; Hampson, I.N.; Broker, T.R.; Fiander, A.; Lacey, C.J.; Kitchener, H.C.; Einstein, M.H. Therapy of human papillomavirus-related disease. *Vaccine* **2012**, *30* (Suppl. S5), F71–F82. [CrossRef]
9. Cheng, S.; Schmidt-Grimminger, D.C.; Murant, T.; Broker, T.R.; Chow, L.T. Differentiation-dependent up-regulation of the human papillomavirus E7 gene reactivates cellular DNA replication in suprabasal differentiated keratinocytes. *Genes Dev.* **1995**, *9*, 2335–2349. [CrossRef]
10. Moody, C.A.; Laimins, L.A. Human papillomavirus oncoproteins: Pathways to transformation. *Nat. Rev. Cancer* **2010**, *10*, 550–560. [CrossRef]
11. Chabeda, A.; Yanez, R.J.R.; Lamprecht, R.; Meyers, A.E.; Rybicki, E.P.; Hitzeroth, I.I. Therapeutic vaccines for high-risk HPV-associated diseases. *Papillomavirus Res.* **2018**, *5*, 46–58. [CrossRef] [PubMed]
12. Borysiewicz, L.K.; Fiander, A.; Nimako, M.; Man, S.; Wilkinson, G.W.; Westmoreland, D.; Evans, A.S.; Adams, M.; Stacey, S.N.; Boursnell, M.E. A recombinant vaccinia virus encoding human papillomavirus types 16 and 18, E6 and E7 proteins as immunotherapy for cervical cancer. *Lancet* **1996**, *347*, 1523–1527. [CrossRef] [PubMed]

13. Ding, Z.; Ou, R.; Ni, B.; Tang, J.; Xu, Y. Cytolytic activity of the human papillomavirus type 16 E711-20 epitope-specific cytotoxic T lymphocyte is enhanced by heat shock protein 110 in HLA-A*0201 transgenic mice. *Clin. Vaccine Immunol.* **2013**, *20*, 1027–1033. [CrossRef]
14. Juarez, V.; Pasolli, H.A.; Hellwig, A.; Garbi, N.; Arregui, A.C. Virus-Like Particles Harboring CCL19, IL-2 and HPV16 E7 Elicit Protective T Cell Responses in HLA-A2 Transgenic Mice. *Open Virol. J.* **2012**, *6*, 270–276. [CrossRef] [PubMed]
15. Khan, S.; Oosterhuis, K.; Wunderlich, K.; Bunnik, E.M.; Bhaggoe, M.; Boedhoe, S.; Karia, S.; Steenbergen, R.D.M.; Bosch, L.; Serroyen, J. Development of a replication-deficient adenoviral vector-based vaccine candidate for the interception of HPV16- and HPV18-induced infections and disease. *Int. J. Cancer* **2017**, *141*, 393–404. [CrossRef] [PubMed]
16. Lee, S.J.; Yang, A.; Wu, T.C.; Hung, C.F. Immunotherapy for human papillomavirus-associated disease and cervical cancer: Review of clinical and translational research. *J. Gynecol. Oncol.* **2016**, *27*, e51. [CrossRef]
17. McCarthy, C.; Youde, S.J.; Man, S. Definition of an HPV18/45 cross-reactive human T-cell epitope after DNA immunisation of HLA-A2/KB transgenic mice. *Int. J. Cancer* **2006**, *118*, 2514–2521. [CrossRef]
18. Perez, S.; Zimet, G.D.; Tatar, O.; Stupiansky, N.W.; Fisher, W.A.; Rosberger, Z. Human Papillomavirus Vaccines: Successes and Future Challenges. *Drugs* **2018**, *78*, 1385–1396. [CrossRef]
19. Rice, A.E.; Latchman, Y.E.; Balint, J.P.; Lee, J.H.; Gabitzsch, E.S.; Jones, F.R. An HPV-E6/E7 immunotherapy plus PD-1 checkpoint inhibition results in tumor regression and reduction in PD-L1 expression. *Cancer Gene Ther.* **2015**, *22*, 454–462. [CrossRef]
20. Trimble, C.L.; Trimble, C.L.; Morrow, M.P.; Kraynyak, K.A.; Shen, X.; Dallas, M.; Yan, J.; Edwards, L.; Parker, R.L.; Denny, L.; et al. Safety, efficacy, and immunogenicity of VGX-3100, a therapeutic synthetic DNA vaccine targeting human papillomavirus 16 and 18 E6 and E7 proteins for cervical intraepithelial neoplasia 2/3: A randomised, double-blind, placebo-controlled phase 2b trial. *Lancet* **2015**, *386*, 2078–2088. [CrossRef]
21. Wieking, B.G.; Vermeer, D.W.; Spanos, W.C.; Lee, K.M.; Vermeer, P.; Lee, W.T.; Xu, Y.; Gabitzsch, E.S.; Balcaitis, S.; Balint, J.P., Jr.; et al. A non-oncogenic HPV 16 E6/E7 vaccine enhances treatment of HPV expressing tumors. *Cancer Gene Ther.* **2012**, *19*, 667–674. [CrossRef] [PubMed]
22. McIlwain, D.R.; Chen, H.; Rahil, Z.; Bidoki, N.H.; Jiang, S.; Bjornson, Z.; Kolhatkar, N.S.; Martinez, C.J.; Gaudilliere, B.; Hedou, J. Human influenza virus challenge identifies cellular correlates of protection for oral vaccination. *Cell Host Microbe* **2021**, *29*, 1828–1837.e5. [CrossRef] [PubMed]
23. Liebowitz, D.; Gottlieb, K.; Kolhatkar, N.S.; Garg, S.J.; Asher, J.M.; Nazareno, J.; Kim, K.; McIlwain, D.R.; Tucker, S.N. Efficacy, immunogenicity, and safety of an oral influenza vaccine: A placebo-controlled and active-controlled phase 2 human challenge study. *Lancet Infect. Dis.* **2020**, *20*, 435–444. [CrossRef]
24. Kim, L.; Liebowitz, D.; Lin, K.; Kasparek, K.; Pasetti, M.F.; Garg, S.J.; Gottlieb, K.; Trager, G.; Tucker, S.N. Safety and immunogenicity of an oral tablet norovirus vaccine, a phase I randomized, placebo-controlled trial. *JCI Insight* **2018**, *3*, e121077. [CrossRef] [PubMed]
25. Kim, L.; Martinez, C.J.; Hodgson, K.A.; Trager, G.R.; Brandl, J.R.; Sandefer, E.P.; Doll, W.J.; Liebowitz, D.; Tucker, S.N. Systemic and mucosal immune responses following oral adenoviral delivery of influenza vaccine to the human intestine by radio controlled capsule. *Sci. Rep.* **2016**, *6*, 37295. [CrossRef]
26. Liebowitz, D.; Lindbloom, J.D.; Brandl, J.R.; Garg, S.J.; Tucker, S.N. High titre neutralising antibodies to influenza after oral tablet immunisation: A phase 1, randomised, placebo-controlled trial. *Lancet Infect. Dis.* **2015**, *15*, 1041–1048. [CrossRef]
27. Johnson, S.; Martinez, C.I.; Tedjakusuma, S.N.; Peinovich, N.; Dora, E.G.; Birch, S.M.; Kajon, A.E.; Werts, A.D.; Tucker, S.N. Oral Vaccination Protects Against Severe Acute Respiratory Syndrome Coronavirus 2 in a Syrian Hamster Challenge Model. *J. Infect. Dis.* **2022**, *225*, 34–41. [CrossRef]
28. Flitter, B.A.; Braun, M.R.; Tucker, S.N. Drop the Needle; A Temperature Stable Oral Tablet Vaccine Is Protective against Respiratory Viral Pathogens. *Vaccines* **2022**, *10*, 593. [CrossRef]
29. Cummings, J.F.; Tucker, S. Potent Immune Responses to Norovirus G1.1 Evaluated in Elderly Subjects following Oral Tablet Delivery in a Phase 1 Placebo-Controlled Study. In Proceedings of the World Vaccine Congress 2022, Barcelona, Spain, 11–14 October 2022.
30. Johnson, S.; Martinez, C.I.; Jegede, C.B.; Gutierrez, S.; Cortese, M.C.; Martinez, J.; Garg, S.J.; Peinovich, N.; Dora, E.G.; Tucker, S.N. SARS-CoV-2 oral tablet vaccination induces neutralizing mucosal IgA in a phase 1 open label trial. *medRxiv* **2022**. [CrossRef]
31. Ribas, A.; Wolchok, J.D. Cancer immunotherapy using checkpoint blockade. *Science* **2018**, *359*, 1350–1355. [CrossRef]
32. Li, C.; Cang, W.; Gu, Y.; Chen, L.; Xiang, Y. The anti-PD-1 era of cervical cancer: Achievement, opportunity, and challenge. *Front. Immunol.* **2023**, *14*, 1195476. [CrossRef] [PubMed]
33. Callahan, M.K.; Postow, M.A.; Wolchok, J.D. CTLA-4 and PD-1 Pathway Blockade: Combinations in the Clinic. *Front. Oncol.* **2014**, *4*, 385. [CrossRef] [PubMed]
34. Chen, Z.; Pang, N.; Du, R.; Zhu, Y.; Fan, L.; Cai, D.; Ding, Y.; Ding, J. Elevated Expression of Programmed Death-1 and Programmed Death Ligand-1 Negatively Regulates Immune Response against Cervical Cancer Cells. *Mediat. Inflamm.* **2016**, *2016*, 6891482. [CrossRef] [PubMed]
35. Fu, J.; Malm, I.J.; Kadayakkara, D.K.; Levitsky, H.; Pardoll, D.; Kim, Y.J. Preclinical evidence that PD1 blockade cooperates with cancer vaccine TEGVAX to elicit regression of established tumors. *Cancer Res.* **2014**, *74*, 4042–4052. [CrossRef]

36. Peng, S.; Tan, M.; Li, Y.D.; Cheng, M.A.; Farmer, E.; Ferrall, L.; Gaillard, S.; Roden, R.B.S.; Hung, C.F.; Wu, T.C. PD-1 blockade synergizes with intratumoral vaccination of a therapeutic HPV protein vaccine and elicits regression of tumor in a preclinical model. *Cancer Immunol. Immunother.* **2021**, *70*, 1049–1062. [CrossRef]
37. Mkrtichyan, M.; Chong, N.; Abu Eid, R.; Wallecha, A.; Singh, R.; Rothman, J.; Khleif, S.N. Anti-PD-1 antibody significantly increases therapeutic efficacy of Listeria monocytogenes (Lm)-LLO immunotherapy. *J. Immunother. Cancer* **2013**, *1*, 15. [CrossRef]
38. Roberts, J.N.; Buck, C.B.; Thompson, C.D.; Kines, R.; Bernardo, M.; Choyke, P.L.; Lowy, D.R.; Schiller, J.T. Genital transmission of HPV in a mouse model is potentiated by nonoxynol-9 and inhibited by carrageenan. *Nat. Med.* **2007**, *13*, 857–861. [CrossRef]
39. Berraondo, P.; Nouze, C.; Preville, X.; Ladant, D.; Leclerc, C. Eradication of large tumors in mice by a tritherapy targeting the innate, adaptive, and regulatory components of the immune system. *Cancer Res.* **2007**, *67*, 8847–8855. [CrossRef]
40. Lin, K.Y.; Guarnieri, F.G.; Staveley-O'Carroll, K.F.; Levitsky, H.I.; August, J.T.; Pardoll, D.M.; Wu, T.C. Treatment of established tumors with a novel vaccine that enhances major histocompatibility class II presentation of tumor antigen. *Cancer Res.* **1996**, *56*, 21–26.
41. McConnell, E.L.; Basit, A.W.; Murdan, S. Measurements of rat and mouse gastrointestinal pH, fluid and lymphoid tissue, and implications for in-vivo experiments. *J. Pharm. Pharmacol.* **2008**, *60*, 63–70. [CrossRef]
42. Braun, M.R.; Martinez, C.I.; Dora, E.G.; Showalter, L.J.; Mercedes, A.R.; Tucker, S.N. Mucosal immunization with Ad5-based vaccines protects Syrian hamsters from challenge with omicron and delta variants of SARS-CoV-2. *Front. Immunol.* **2023**, *14*, 1086035. [CrossRef]
43. Jordanova, E.S.; Gorter, A.; Ayachi, O.; Prins, F.; Durrant, L.G.; Kenter, G.G.; van der Burg, S.H.; Fleuren, G.J. Human leukocyte antigen class I, MHC class I chain-related molecule A, and CD8+/regulatory T-cell ratio: Which variable determines survival of cervical cancer patients? *Clin. Cancer Res.* **2008**, *14*, 2028–2035. [CrossRef] [PubMed]
44. Nielsen, M.; Lundegaard, C.; Worning, P.; Lauemoller, S.L.; Lamberth, K.; Buus, S.; Brunak, S.; Lund, O. Reliable prediction of T-cell epitopes using neural networks with novel sequence representations. *Protein Sci.* **2003**, *12*, 1007–1017. [CrossRef]
45. Lundegaard, C.; Lamberth, K.; Harndahl, M.; Buus, S.; Lund, O.; Nielsen, M. NetMHC-3.0: Accurate web accessible predictions of human, mouse and monkey MHC class I affinities for peptides of length 8-11. *Nucleic Acids Res.* **2008**, *36*, W509–W512. [CrossRef]
46. Scallan, C.D.; Tingley, D.W.; Lindbloom, J.D.; Toomey, J.S.; Tucker, S.N. An adenovirus-based vaccine with a double-stranded RNA adjuvant protects mice and ferrets against H5N1 avian influenza in oral delivery models. *Clin. Vaccine Immunol.* **2013**, *20*, 85–94. [CrossRef] [PubMed]
47. Simpson-Herren, L.; Lloyd, H.H. Kinetic parameters and growth curves for experimental tumor systems. *Cancer Chemother. Rep.* **1970**, *54*, 143–174. [PubMed]
48. Boursnell, M.E.; Rutherford, E.; Hickling, J.K.; Rollinson, E.A.; Munro, A.J.; Rolley, N.; McLean, C.S.; Borysiewicz, L.K.; Vousden, K.; Inglis, S.C. Construction and characterisation of a recombinant vaccinia virus expressing human papillomavirus proteins for immunotherapy of cervical cancer. *Vaccine* **1996**, *14*, 1485–1494. [CrossRef] [PubMed]
49. IEDB Analysis Resource. Available online: http://tools.iedb.org/main/tcell/ (accessed on 2 February 2019).
50. Scott, E.N.; Gocher, A.M.; Workman, C.J.; Vignali, D.A.A. Regulatory T Cells: Barriers of Immune Infiltration into the Tumor Microenvironment. *Front. Immunol.* **2021**, *12*, 702726. [CrossRef]
51. Raskov, H.; Orhan, A.; Christensen, J.P.; Gogenur, I. Cytotoxic CD8(+) T cells in cancer and cancer immunotherapy. *Br. J. Cancer* **2021**, *124*, 359–367. [CrossRef]
52. Langel, S.N.; Johnson, S.; Martinez, C.I.; Tedjakusuma, S.N.; Peinovich, N.; Dora, E.G.; Kuehl, P.J.; Irshad, H.; Barrett, E.G.; Werts, A.D.; et al. Adenovirus type 5 SARS-CoV-2 vaccines delivered orally or intranasally reduced disease severity and transmission in a hamster model. *Sci. Transl. Med.* **2022**, *14*, eabn6868. [CrossRef]
53. Zottnick, S.; Voss, A.L.; Riemer, A.B. Inducing Immunity Where It Matters: Orthotopic HPV Tumor Models and Therapeutic Vaccinations. *Front. Immunol.* **2020**, *11*, 1750. [CrossRef] [PubMed]
54. Trimble, C.L.; Clark, R.A.; Thoburn, C.; Hanson, N.C.; Tassello, J.; Frosina, D.; Kos, F.; Teague, J.; Jiang, Y.; Barat, N.C. Human papillomavirus 16-associated cervical intraepithelial neoplasia in humans excludes CD8 T cells from dysplastic epithelium. *J. Immunol.* **2010**, *185*, 7107–7114. [CrossRef] [PubMed]
55. Tucker, S.N. Oral Tablet Vaccination to SARS-CoV-2 Induces Long Lasting Cross-reactive Mucosal Antibody Responses in Humans. In Proceedings of the World Vaccine Congress 2022, Barcelona, Spain, 11–14 October 2022.
56. Ibrahim Khalil, A.; Zhang, L.; Muwonge, R.; Sauvaget, C.; Basu, P. Efficacy and safety of therapeutic HPV vaccines to treat CIN 2/CIN 3 lesions: A systematic review and meta-analysis of phase II/III clinical trials. *BMJ Open* **2023**, *13*, e069616. [CrossRef] [PubMed]
57. Bruni, L.; Saura-Lazaro, A.; Montoliu, A.; Brotons, M.; Alemany, L.; Diallo, M.S.; Afsar, O.Z.; LaMontagne, D.S.; Mosina, L.; Contreras, M. HPV vaccination introduction worldwide and WHO and UNICEF estimates of national HPV immunization coverage 2010–2019. *Prev. Med.* **2021**, *144*, 106399. [CrossRef]

Disclaimer/Publisher's Note: The statements, opinions and data contained in all publications are solely those of the individual author(s) and contributor(s) and not of MDPI and/or the editor(s). MDPI and/or the editor(s) disclaim responsibility for any injury to people or property resulting from any ideas, methods, instructions or products referred to in the content.

MDPI AG
Grosspeteranlage 5
4052 Basel
Switzerland
Tel.: +41 61 683 77 34

Vaccines Editorial Office
E-mail: vaccines@mdpi.com
www.mdpi.com/journal/vaccines

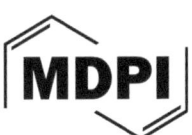

Disclaimer/Publisher's Note: The title and front matter of this reprint are at the discretion of the Guest Editors. The publisher is not responsible for their content or any associated concerns. The statements, opinions and data contained in all individual articles are solely those of the individual Editors and contributors and not of MDPI. MDPI disclaims responsibility for any injury to people or property resulting from any ideas, methods, instructions or products referred to in the content.